BOTTOM LINE YEAR BOOK 2004

BY THE EDITORS OF
Bottom Line
PERSONAL
www.BottomLineSecrets.com

Copyright © 2004 by Boardroom® Inc.

10 9 8 7 6 5 4 3 2

All rights reserved. No part of this book may be reproduced in any form or by any means without written permission from the publisher.

ISBN 0-88723-300-7

Bottom Line® Books publishes the opinions of expert authorities in many fields. The use of a book is not a substitute for legal, accounting, health or other professional services. Consult competent professionals for answers to your specific questions.

Offers, prices, addresses, telephone numbers and Web sites listed in this book are accurate at the time of publication, but they are subject to frequent change.

Bottom Line® Books is a registered trademark of
Boardroom® Inc.
281 Tresser Boulevard, Stamford, CT 06901

Printed in the United States of America

Contents

PART ONE: YOUR HEALTH

1 • HEALTH NEWS AND BREAKTHROUGHS

Hidden Health Trap: The Impact of Your Gender 1
New Miracle Drug: Your Morning Coffee 3
Best Home Medical Tests 5
Reliable Health Web Sites 6
Full-Body CT Scan Hype 7
The Miracle Heart Drugs 13 Million Americans Take 7
Best Time to Take Heart Pills 8
Ibuprofen Linked to High Blood Pressure? 9
When to Take Your Daily Aspirin 9
Aspirin and Heart Attack Risk 9
Trans Fatty Acids Are Worse Than Butter 9
The Right Waist Measurement 10
Hypertension and Rosacea May Be Linked 10
New Test to Predict Heart Attack Risk 10
Faster Test for Heart Attack Now in the ER 10
Bypass Surgery Danger for Women 10
Heart-Bypass Surgery Side Effect 11
Falling Blood Pressure Alert 11
Hot Tub Health Risk 11
Don't Stand Up Quickly After a Meal 11
Better Stroke Prevention 12
Flu Vaccine Cuts Stroke Risk 12
Warning for Women Smokers 12
Another Secondhand Smoke Warning 12
Quit Smoking Without Gaining Weight 13
Diabetes Drug Danger 13
Knee Surgery May Not Help Arthritis 13
New Alzheimer's Test 13
Don't Believe the HGH Hype 14
No More Snoring 14
Aspirin for a Healthier Colon 14
Thyroid Disease Could Be the Cause of Your Symptoms 14
Better Lyme Disease Test 16
Most Common Sites for Melanoma 16
New Medications for Psoriasis 16
Ultrasound Speeds Healing of Broken Bones 16
Screening for Osteoporosis 17
Vitamin A Warning 17
Painkiller Trap for Broken Bones 17
Should You Have Your Fillings Removed? 17
Better Than Novocaine 18
Let Your Dentist Know If You Have Heart Problems 18
Booster Shots for Adults 18
Adieu to the Flu 18
When to Treat a Fever 18
Vitamin E Makes Colds and Flu Worse 19
Sinus Relief 19
Best Time to Give Antihistamines to Children 20
Migraine/Bacteria Connection 20
Some Migraine Drugs Worsen the Pain 21
Acetaminophen/Alcohol Alert 21
Pill Dosage Danger 21
Don't Mix Bananas and These Antidepressants 21
How Long to Keep Foods 21
Does Bottled Water Spoil? 22
Superbugs in Poultry 22
Deli Meat Danger 22
Organic Food Trap 22

2 • GETTING THE VERY BEST MEDICAL CARE

How to Survive a Trip to the ER 23
Great ER Service–Guaranteed 24
Don't Be Afraid to Visit a Hospital Patient 24
Older Drugs May Be Better Than Newer Versions 24
How to Get Drugs Not Yet FDA Approved 25
How Dangerous Medication Mistakes Can Be Avoided 25
Self-Defense Against Prescription Mistakes 26
Drug Overdosing Danger 26
New-Drug Dangers 27
All About Generics 27
Has Your Medication Been Switched? 27
Check Your Medication Dosage 28
Are Drug Companies Calling the Shots? 28
Why You Really Need to Have an Annual Physical 29
Why You Must Know the Medical History of
   Your Family 29
Do Your Own Medical Research 31
Beware of "Normal" Test Results 32
Female Doctors Have Better Bedside Manners ... 33
Doctors Making House Calls Again? 33
How to Relax at the Dentist 33
Important Presurgery Test 33
Stop Herbs Before Surgery 34
No Need for Lengthy Presurgery Fasting 34
Safer Surgery 34
Do You Need to See a Dietitian? 34

3 • QUICK FIXES FOR COMMON PROBLEMS

How to Get to Sleep and Stay Asleep 35
How to Prevent Nighttime Visits to the Bathroom 37
Nighttime Leg Cramp Relief 37
A Simple Way to Avoid Infectious Diseases 37
Exercise to Reduce Colds 38
Feed a Cold, Starve a Fever 38
Natural Decongestant 38
Drug-Free Relief for Hay Fever 38
Natural Way to Treat Constipation 38
Better Treatment for Carpal Tunnel Syndrome ... 39
Acupressure Cure for Hiccups 39
What to Do If You Feel Faint 39
No Stitches Necessary 39
Should You Ice an Injury or Use Heat? 40
Folk Remedies for Summer Ills 40
Quick Action Helps Stop Outbreaks of Poison Ivy 41
Stress-Busters to Go 41
Quick Stress Reduction 42
Easy Way to Swallow Pills 42
Simple Ways to Stay Healthy 42

4 • FITNESS MADE SIMPLE

Outsmart These Fat Triggers to Lose Weight 43
Can That Weight Really Be Right? 45
Turn Off Hunger 45
Most People Don't Realize When They're Full 45
Stop Food Cravings and Lose Weight 45
Reduced-Fat Foods Could Cause Weight Gain 46
Healthier Peanut Butter 47
Weight-Loss Secrets That Really Work 47
A Harvard MD Weighs in on the Eating Debate 48
Always Have Breakfast 50
Beware of Unintended Weight Loss 50

Easy Way to Increase Fat Burning 50
Two Big Benefits of Magnesium 50
How to Avoid Injury When Working Out 51
Short Bursts of Exercise for Bigger Benefits 52
Take the Stairs 52
Best Time to Exercise 53
The No-Exercise Workout 53
Heartburn from Exercise 53
Exercise in a Pill? 54
New Exercise Guidelines 54
Better Fitness Walking 54
Exercising with Asthma 54
Painless Ways to Build Exercise into Your Routine 54
Can Fat Be Fit? 56
Enjoy a Better Body Image at Any Age 56
Choosing a Gym Doesn't Have to Be a Workout 58

5 • THE BEST IN NATURAL HEALING

Should You Forgo Surgery? 59
How to Survive a Medical Emergency Without a Doctor 61
The Ultimate Disease-Fighting Diet 62
Simple Way to Boost Health 64
How to Strengthen Your Immune System Easily 64
How to Stay Healthy 65
Cranberries Protect Against Disease 67
The Simple Drink That Fights Cancer, Heart Disease,
   Colds and Cavities 67
Tea Drinking Builds Strong Bones 68
Better Tea Drinking 68
When Herbs Are Safer Than Drugs 69
Oregano Oil May Replace Antibiotics 70
Are You Aging Too Fast? 70
Think Positively and Live Longer 71
The Wrinkle-Cure Diet 71
Add a Decade to Your Life 72
Natural Treatment for Alzheimer's 73
Olive Oil Helps Prevent Cognitive Decline 73
Tired? Forgetful? You May Need More B Vitamins 73
Smart Food Choices Boost Brainpower 75
Little-Known Benefit of Watermelon 76
Cancer-Fighting Condiment 76
New Benefits of Broccoli 76
Another Natural Cancer Fighter 76
Stop Pain Fast with Self-Hypnosis 76
Lower Your Cholesterol Without Drugs 78
Drinking Water Protects the Heart 79
Eggs Can Be Part of a Heart-Healthy Diet 79
Chocolate Is Good for the Heart 80
Exercise Lowers Cholesterol 80
Honey May Protect Against Heart Disease 80
Vitamins After Heart Surgery 80
Cut Stroke Risk Easily 80
Folate Lowers Risk of Stroke 81
Use Ginger to Ease Arthritic Knee Pain 81
Secrets of Avoiding Digestive Problems 81
Kidney Stones and Soy Foods Don't Mix 83
If You Have a Food Allergy… 83
Traffic Trap 83
Moderate Wine Drinking May Prevent the
   Common Cold 83
How to Reverse Hearing Loss 83
Canned or Fresh Produce? 84
Cook Tomatoes for More Lycopene 84

Potassium Warning 84
Get More Vitamin C from Orange Juice 84
Sweet Sleep Aid 84

6 • STRICTLY PERSONAL

Best Ways to Boost Your Sexual Fitness 85
Natural Aphrodisiacs 87
Sex Makes You Look Younger...............................89
Working Out Can Improve Your Sex Life.............89
Biking Can Cause Sexual Dysfunction in Women 89
Daily Exercise Protects Against Impotency.........89
Better Than Viagra 89
Impotence/Cardiovascular Disease Link 90
Carrots Combat Ovarian Cancer...........................90
Grape Juice as a Breast Cancer Preventive 90
Better Breast Cancer Detection 90
More Accurate Mammograms...............................90
Mammograms Can Help Predict Stroke Risk 91
HRT and Breast Cancer Risk.................................91
Alternatives to Hormone Replacement 92
Postmenopausal Breathing Remedy 93
Menstrual Cycle Red Flag 93
Bone Loss Warning 93
Beware of Diagnosing Your Own Yeast Infections 93
Best Therapies for Prostate Cancer 93
Prostate Cancer Fighter..95
Garlic and Chives Reduce Prostate Cancer Risk 95
Reverse Prostate Cancer 96
Better Prostate Cancer Detection 96
The Best Prostate Cancer Surgery 96
Getting Help for Drug or Alcohol Addiction 96

PART TWO: YOUR MONEY

7 • MONEY MATTERS

Secrets of Shrewd Money Management in a
   Volatile Economy 97
Hidden Threats to Your Financial Security 99
Where to Get Money for an Emergency............100
To Avoid Big Money Mistakes…Ignore Your Intuition 101
How to Choose an Internet Bank........................103
On-Line Banking Dangers 103
Check-Writing Alert...103
When You Prefer to Be Billed by Mail… 103
Before You Cosign… 104
Credit Card Alert 104
Easy Way to Get a Better Credit Card Deal 104
Improve Your Credit Report 104
How to Ease Your Debt Burden 104
When Choosing a Debt Consolidator… 105
It Pays to Use a Mortgage Broker 105
Double-Check Your Mortgage Escrow Account 106
How to Handle a Mortgage Buyout 106
Save 50% When Refinancing 107
Extra Deduction for Refinancing........................107
The Right Money Strategies for Different Ages 107
How Safe Is Your Money?....................................109
For a Simpler Divorce… 110
Postnuptial Agreement Basics 110
Couples Can Stop Fighting Over Money..........110
Teaching Grandkids About Money 112
What Not to Say to Children About Money.....112
Protect Elderly Relatives from Financial Abuse 112

8 • INSURANCE SAVVY

Life Insurance Checkup: Save Big Money Now..............113
New Sales Gimmick for Whole Life Insurance 115
Are You Missing a Life Insurance Policy?........115
Umbrella Policies Protect Against Lawsuits 115
Better Home Insurance...116
Insurance Trap 116
Lower Insurance Costs by Paying Bills on Time..............116
Insurance Premiums Headed Up 116
Report All Car Accidents 117
Save 25% or More on Car Insurance 117
How to Get All the Medical Insurance You Are Due......118
When You Can't Resolve a Health
   Insurance Problem…..119
Second Opinions and Your HMO 119
Higher Co-Pays at Certain Hospitals 119
How to Minimize Health Insurance Costs........119
Cheaper Long-Term-Care Insurance 120
Check Your Long-Term-Care Coverage 120
Nursing Home and Home-Health-Care Cost Danger 120

9 • TAX GUIDE

How to Profit from the New Tax Law 121
Tax-Friendly States..123
Learn About Taxes Before You Move 123
Tax-Deductible Moving Expenses......................123
24 Sources of Tax-Free Income 124
How to Get Maximum Tax Benefit from Your Home......126
It's Now Easier to Use the Home-Sale Exclusion............127
Tax-Free Home-Sale Loophole............................129
File Even If You Can't Afford to Pay Your Tax Bill 129
Uncle Sam Will Help Pay Your Medical Bills ..130
Checking for the AMT..131
Vacation Tax Breaks 131
Keep More Gambling Winnings 133
Some Divorce Costs Are Deductible 134
How Unmarried Couples Can Save Big on Taxes 134
Big Loopholes in Preparing Your Tax Return ..136
IRS Warns of "Dirty Dozen" Tax Scams 137
Don't Make Mistakes with Your
   Social Security Number 138
Simple Ways to Avoid Underpayment Penalties.............138
Tax Cost of Settling a Debt 140
Avoid Underreporting Penalties 140
Should You Pay Taxes with a Credit Card? 140
How to Give a Collectible to Charity 140
When You Can't Pay on Time 140
Electronic Refund Trap 141
Has Your Refund Check Been Intercepted? 141
Even Honest People Get in Trouble with the IRS—
   What to Do If You're Accused 141
Audit Targets Now 142
Tax Breaks Can Help You Buy
   Long-Term-Care Insurance 143
What the IRS Doesn't Want You to Know
   About Its Audit Process...................................143
Is Your Tax Professional Doing a Good Job?...144
Smart Reasons to File an Amended Tax Return 146
Inside the IRS 147

v

10 • BETTER INVESTING

10 Principles for a Tricky Market 149
Manage Investments Monthly 150
Read All Investment Statements 150
When to Hire an Investment Adviser 151
Find Investment Analysts with the Best Records 151
How to Profit from Today's Headlines 151
Stick with What You Have 153
Wall Street Research You Can Trust 153
How to Protect Yourself from Bad Broker Advice 154
Self-Defense Against Increasing Brokerage Fees 154
High-Net-Worth Services Now Available to
   More People 154
Easy Way to Find High-Dividend Stocks 155
Brokerage Statement Reminder 155
Smarter Investing with Dollar Cost Averaging 155
How to Profit from Insider Trading Legally 156
Don't Miss These Signs 156
What Mutual Funds Won't Tell You 157
Use Expense Erosion 158
Corporate Bond Warning 158
Better Way to Buy Bonds 158
Don't Hang on to These Savings Bonds 159
Smart CD Buying 159
Second Homes Are Seldom Good Investments 159
Investment Real Estate Can Supercharge
   Your Portfolio 159
10 Top Tax Strategies for a Shrunken Portfolio 161
How to Get a Deduction for Big Losses 163
Wealth Preservation Loopholes 164
How to Avoid Taxes When Buying and
   Selling Mutual Funds 165
Silver Lining to the Bear Market 166
Rebalance Your Portfolio Without Having to Pay
   Huge Capital Gains Taxes 166
Tax-Deductible Investment Expenses 168
Don't Make Costly Tax Return Mistakes 169

11 • CONSUMER CONFIDENTIAL

How to Bargain for the Absolutely Best Price 171
Beware of "Gotcha" Fees 173
Cheaper Diamonds 173
Penny-Pincher's Guide to Saving Money 173
Cost-Cutting Secrets 175
Best Coupon Savings 176
Painless Ways to Save from *Bottom Line* Readers 176
Keep Up with Safety Recalls 177
If You Break an Item in a Store… 177
On-Line Auctions: The Latest Strategies 178
Swap Good Deeds 179
How to Get the Best Prices On-Line 179
Keep Your Old Monitor and Save 179
Easier Merchandise Returns 179
How to Shrink Your Medical Bills by 25% or More ... 180
Check Hospital Bills Carefully 182
Work with Your Doctor to Reduce Costs 182
Cheaper Contact Lenses 182
How to Save on Prescription Drugs 182
Cutting Medication Costs 183
More Savings on Drugs 183
If You're Overcharged for a Funeral… 184
How to Buy a Diamond Ring 184
When to Buy a New Mattress 184
How to Buy Better Sunglasses 184
Electronics at a Discount 185
Save on Detergent 185
Low-Cost Alternatives to Cleaning Products 185
How to Avoid Carpet-Cleaner Scams 185
A Home Energy Audit Can Cut Energy Bills in Half .. 186
More Energy Savers 186
For Much Lower Heating Costs… 186
Cut Air-Conditioning Costs 187
Save $100 Just by Changing Lightbulbs 187
Appliances That Pay for Themselves 188
Finding a Good Contractor 189
Contractor Self-Defense 189
Home Appliance Smarts 190
No More Repair Rip-Offs 190
Repair Appliances Yourself 190
How to Hire a Moving Company 190

PART THREE: YOUR FINANCIAL FUTURE

12 • RETIREMENT WISDOM

Retire on Less…and Live Well 191
Will You Have Enough to Retire? 193
Learning to Enjoy Your Nest Egg 194
Don't Let These Financial Mistakes
   Destroy Your Retirement Dreams 195
How to Guarantee Income for Life 196
Lump Sum vs. Pension for Life 197
Dangerous Pension Errors to Avoid 197
Beware of the Social Security Integration Trap 198
If You Plan to Retire and Marry at the Same Time… .. 198
Retirees Beware 198
Roth IRA Conversion Trap 198
If You Inherit an IRA… 199
Early Retirement Withdrawals Without Penalty 199
Better Ways to Roll Over a 401(k) to an IRA 199
401(k) vs. IRA Withdrawals 199
What 401(k) Reports Don't Tell You 199
Is Your Keogh Plan Creditor-Proof? 200
Secrets of Paying Less Tax on Social Security Benefits .. 200
Keep Your W-2s 202
Rehearse Your Retirement 202
Better Retirement Locations 202

13 • PROTECTING YOUR ESTATE

Estate Planning for Terribly Tricky Times 203
Secure Your Family's Future 205
State Death Tax Alert 206
Estate Planning After Divorce 207
Wealth Planning for Blended Families 207
How to Help Charity and Your Family—and
   Disinherit the IRS 208
Self-Defense for Executor/Heirs 210
Make Your Estate Easy on Your Heirs 211
When to Revise Your Estate Plan 211
How to Pass Annuities on to Your Heirs 211
Don't Name IRA Beneficiaries Through Your Will ... 212
Protect Your Legacy from a Child's Divorce 212
Incentive Trusts and Your Heirs 212
Protect Pets After You're Gone 212
Joint Ownership Inheritance Trap 213

When There's Income Tax on an Inheritance 213
Rules of Proof for Charitable Contributions 213
Doubling Up on Tax-Free Gifts 213
Include Cost Records with Gifts 214
What It Means to Be a Health Care Proxy 214
Web Sites for Making End-of-Life Decisions 216
Power of Attorney vs. Durable Power of Attorney 216

14 • TRAVEL TIPS AND TRAPS

How to Get the Best Shopping Bargains on the Planet 217
Learn How Much to Bid at Priceline 219
Save Big on Last-Minute Travel 219
When to Buy Vacation Insurance 219
Convert Money Before You Go 219
Get Money Back When Traveling in Europe 220
Overseas ATMs Are No Longer Bargains 220
Tipping Guide 220
Last-Minute Airline Deals 220
Benefits of Travel Agents 221
Avoid Steep Airline Fees 221
Getting Bumped on Purpose 221
Faster Airline Check-In 221
Travel Warnings and Help Overseas 221
Savvier Flying 222
Better Airport Security 222
What's Even Worse Than Airline Food? 222
Recirculated Air Does Not Cause Colds 222
When You Shouldn't Get on a Plane 223
Refunds on Nonrefundable Tickets 223
How to Buy Frequent-Flier Miles 223
Don't Convert Hotel Points to Frequent-Flier Miles 223
New Baggage Fees 223
Tour Groups Beware of This Trap 224
Send Your Baggage Separately 224
How to Keep Airlines from Losing Your Luggage 224
The Fine Art of Travel 225
Pack a Whistle 225
Hotel Discounts If You're Over 50 225
Cheaper Hotel Rates 226
More on Getting the Best Hotel Rates 226
Free Hotel Rooms for Grandparents 226
Hotel Safety 226
Dance Your Way to a Discount Cruise 227
Cruise-Line Security 227
Self-Defense Against Viral Illness on Cruises 227
Healthier Food on Cruises 227
Smarter Cruising for First-Timers 228
Better Cruise Ship Cabins 228
For the Lowest Hotel Rates 228
Save an Expiring Bump Voucher 228
Protection Against Travel-Company Bankruptcies 228
Avoid Rental-Car Rip-Offs—Here and Abroad 229
Smarter Car Renting 229
Road Trip Know-How 229
Protect Your Health While Traveling 229
Don't Get Sick on Your Vacation 230
Stock Up Before You Go 230
Natural Treatment for Traveler's Diarrhea 231
How to Handle Illness After a Trip 231
Safer Adventure Vacations 231
Have Fun Traveling Solo 231
VIP Treatment in Las Vegas 232

PART FOUR: YOUR LEISURE

15 • JUST FOR FUN

How I Won More Than 500 Sweepstakes
   and Contests 233
Blackjack Tricks 234
Slot Machine Myths 236
Win at Baccarat 236
Casino Safety 237
How to Hook a Big One 238
Four Mistakes Even Golf Pros Make 239
Kite-Flying Secrets from a National Champ 239
Better Scrabble Strategy 240
Today's Hottest Collectibles 240
Baseball Cards Are Hot Again 242
How to Be an Extra in Movies or TV Shows 243
Write Your Memoirs 244
Better Autograph Collecting 244
Save a Pet via the Internet 244

16 • CAR CARE

The Biggest Mistakes Car Owners Make 245
Tire Blowout Smarts 246
Even Four-Wheelers Need Winter Tires 247
Tinted Glass Saves on Gas 247
Gas-Pump Alert 247
Don't Delay Fixing Your Windshield 247
Mold Danger in Your Car 247
Better Car Repairs 248
Avoid Hassles by Going On-Line to Buy a Car 248
Safer Cars 249
New-Car Checklist 250
Whiplash Protection 250
Dangerous Backseats 250
Better Driving with Your Spouse 250

17 • HOME AND FAMILY LIFE

How to Avoid the Biggest Dangers at Home 251
Allergic to Your Pet? 253
Little-Known Pet Danger 253
Drinking-Water Danger for Kids 253
Examine the Trees Around Your House 254
Mold Warning 254
Mr. Fix-It's Nine Things Every Home Owner
   Should Know 254
What You Must Know About Chimney Care 256
Weatherproof Your Home 257
Arsenic-Free Decks 258
Buying the Right Roof Gutters 258
Better Lawn Mowing 258
Keeping Deer Out of Your Garden 258
Disinfect with Your Microwave 259
Home Tricks for Do-It-Yourselfers 259
Decorating for Next to Nothing 259
Clutter Control 260
How to Make Much More at Your Yard Sale 261
Strategies for a Smooth Move 261
Dramatically Increase the Value of Your Home 261
Better Condominium Buying 263
Open House Trap 263
How to Price Your Home for Sale 264
Compare Available Homes On-Line 264

Check Zoning Rules Before Buying 264
Midlife Is the Right Time to Improve Your Marriage 264
Hope for Unhappy Marriages..266
"What Did I Just Say?" and Other Things
  Not to Say to Kids 266
The Right Ways to Spoil Grandchildren 267
Predict How Tall Your Child Will Grow 268

18 • WINNING WAYS

How to Say "NO!" When Others Ask Too Much..............269
Do Less, Achieve More 270
If You're a Perfectionist… 272
How to Get Much More Done with
  Much Less Stress..272
Stress-Free Problem Solving 274
How to Handle Difficult Conversations 274
Secrets of Letting Go of Painful Memories 276
Cures for Common Phobias..277
How to Defuse an Angry Confrontation 278
How to Talk to Those You Love.......................................279
Are Your Good Friends Good for You?.............................280
How to Stay Open-Minded..282
Boost Your Self-Esteem 282
How to Make People Like You in 90 Seconds or Less.....282
How to Feel More Comfortable at Parties 283
Rekindle Your Creative Spark at Work and Home...........283
How to Keep Your Mind Sharp at Any Age 285
Stop Misplacing Things...286
How to Keep Track of Kids in Crowds 286

PART FIVE: YOUR LIFE

19 • SMART BUSINESS MOVES

How to Succeed in Business Without
  Working So Hard..287
Stress Self-Defense...289
Better Hiring..289
Resolving Personality Conflicts at Work..........................289
Get People to Want What You Want 290
How to Be a Successful Leader...291
Six Special Ways to Reward Employees...........................293
If Asked to Evaluate Your Boss… 293
Are You a Layoff Candidate?..293
Make Time for Networking 294
Business Card Dos and Don'ts 294
What to Do When Your Computer Screen Freezes 294
Easy Ways to Control E-Mail Overload 294
Customer Service via E-Mail 295
How to Win a Business Award 295
Seven Steps to Increase Business in Tough Times 296
How to Create a Simple Web Site to
  Boost Your Business...297
Making the Most of Fringe Benefits 297
New Tax Deductions for Business...
  and Often Overlooked Old Deductions 299
How to Deduct a Home Office 301
Get a Bigger Refund on Your Business Tax Return 301
How Your Children Can Help the
  Family Business Cut Taxes..303
Get Top Dollar When You Sell Your Business.................305
When the Company You Work for Is in Trouble 305
How to Make the Most of a Job Loss...............................306

Losing Your Job Can Be Good for Your Health 308
Finding a Job in Tough Times 308
Check Your Credit Before a Job Search 309
Secrets for Getting Past the Receptionist.........................310
More Effective On-Line Résumés 310
Negotiating Know-How...310

20 • PLANNING FOR COLLEGE

How to Write a Winning College Essay...........................311
Don't Be Put Off by College Costs 312
Get the Inside Scoop on Colleges 312
Web Sites That Help Kids Choose Colleges 313
If Your Child Doesn't Want to Start College
  Right Away..313
College Savings Plans: Some Are Much
  Better Than Others..313
Look Beyond 529 Plans 315
College Savings to Use First..315
Tax Breaks to Help Pay for College 315
When Education Expenses Are Deductible 317
Financial Aid Basics 317
Where to Find Financial Aid for Adult Students 318
How to Use Life Insurance to Pay for College 318
Better Investing for College 318
If You're Falling Behind on Tuition… 319
Protect College Savings 319
What You Should Know About College Insurance.........319
Insurance for College Students...319
Save on College Textbooks 320
Parental-Control Credit Card 320
Smart Financial Aid Strategies 320

21 • SELF-DEFENSE FOR TRICKY TIMES

The Best Way to Protect Your Family
  Against Terrorism 321
How to Cope with the Threat of Terrorism.....................323
In Case of a Terrorist Attack… 324
Protect Yourself from Terrorist Bombs............................324
New Security Measures in Apartment Buildings.............324
The Smallpox Threat: What You Need to Know.............325
Fire Chief Reveals Most Common Causes of
  Household Fires 326
Protect Your Children 328
Choosing a Home-Security System 328
Is Someone Watching You?..329
Pickpocket Protection...329
What to Do When Pulled Over by the Police 329
How to Avoid Identity Theft…and What to Do
  If You've Been Victimized..329
New Twist on Identity Theft..331
New Identity Theft Scam Uses Phony Tax Notices..........331
Latest Scam Warnings 331
Daring New Scams and How to Avoid Them 333
Big Cons to Watch Out For..335
Protect Yourself On-Line 335
No More Spam 336
Better Cell Phone Protection 336
A Good Reason to Balance Your Checkbook 336
Index..337

Health News and Breakthroughs

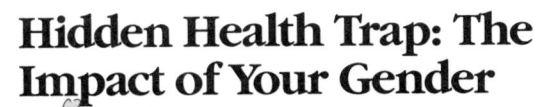

Hidden Health Trap: The Impact of Your Gender

Until just recently, medical researchers assumed that men and women were physiologically identical, save for their reproductive organs. But scientists have now uncovered vital differences in the ways in which men's and women's bodies function, experience illness and respond to treatments.

Much remains to be explored in the emerging field of gender-specific medicine. *However, new findings already show that common conditions can be treated much more effectively when gender is taken into consideration...*

PAIN IN WOMEN

Men and women have different physiological responses to intense pain.

For example, a man's blood pressure rises during intense pain. A woman's blood pressure remains stable or declines, but her heart rate accelerates. This difference has important implications after surgery, when anesthesiologists typically monitor blood pressure to assess a patient's need for painkilling analgesics.

Self-defense: A female surgical patient should request that heart rate be monitored along with blood pressure. If her heart rate increases, more pain medication needs to be administered.

SKIN CANCER IN MEN

More than one million adult Americans are diagnosed with skin cancer each year. Among these cases, white men age 45 or older are twice as prone as women to the most common skin cancers (basal and squamous cell carcinoma). Men are also more vulnerable to deadly melanoma, accounting for nearly two-thirds of the 7,000 deaths caused by this type of cancer each year.

Marianne J. Legato, MD, founder of the Partnership for Gender-Specific Medicine at Columbia University and a professor of clinical medicine at Columbia's College of Physicians and Surgeons, both in New York City. She is author of *Eve's Rib: The New Science of Gender-Specific Medicine and How It Can Save Your Life* (Harmony).

■ *Your Health* ■

Given that men just naturally have more protective *melanin*, or skin pigmentation, than women, their greater susceptibility to skin cancer is likely due to the fact that they typically spend more work and leisure time outdoors and are less inclined to wear sunscreen.

Self-defense: All adults age 40 or older should have a dermatologist perform a total-body examination annually to check for signs of skin cancer. The exam should include the scalp, toes, soles, even genitalia. Men's skin cancers occur most frequently on the ears and neck, two spots that are typically vulnerable due to their shorter hair. Women's skin cancers tend to appear on the legs and hips. But malignancies can strike even in unexposed areas. Both men and women should perform monthly self-exams and wear sunscreen with an SPF of at least 15 daily.

HEART DISEASE IN WOMEN

Long considered a man's problem, heart disease kills one in two women. Although male heart attack victims typically have chest pain, 20% of female heart attack sufferers do *not* experience this symptom. Instead, women experience pain or discomfort in the upper abdomen or back, shortness of breath, nausea or profuse sweating. Consequently, their condition is frequently misdiagnosed as indigestion or anxiety.

Other important facts...

• **Standard stress tests are inadequate for detecting coronary artery disease (CAD) in women.** This screening tool involves monitoring a patient on a treadmill for changes in blood pressure or cardiac electrical activity (measured with an electrocardiogram, or ECG).

These measurements are accurate indicators of heart disease in men. But an ECG is less valid in women because their cardiac electrical activity is likely to change during a treadmill test even with normal heart function.

Self-defense: Instead of a stress test, female heart patients should request a stress echocardiogram. This test uses an ultrasound probe to view your heart's motion at rest and during peak exercise.

• **Women with low levels of "good" HDL cholesterol are at increased risk for heart disease**—regardless of their "bad" LDL cholesterol levels. While both men and women should have HDL levels above 45, a level below 45 is especially dangerous in women.

Self-defense: Ask your doctor about boosting low HDL with cholesterol drugs (statins), hormone-replacement therapy (HRT) or niacin (a B vitamin).

OSTEOPOROSIS IN MEN

Before the age of 60, women lose bone mass faster than men. After this age, men and women lose bone at approximately the same rate. In fact, men account for one-quarter of diagnosed osteoporosis cases in the US.

While the "male" hormone *testosterone* helps maintain bone, particularly in the arms and legs, it's the "female" hormone *estrogen* that is key to a man's—and a woman's—bone density.

Self-defense: Excluding estrogen therapy (which men cannot take due to its feminizing effects), the best weapons against osteoporosis are bisphosphonate drugs, such as *alendronate* (Fosamax) and *risedronate* (Actonel). These drugs increase bone mass and reduce risk for fractures. Adequate calcium intake (1,500 milligrams (mg) daily for all adults over age 50... 1,000 mg to 1,200 mg for those who are under age 50) and weight-bearing exercises are also vital for bone density.

COLON CANCER IN WOMEN

Some people just assume that colon cancer affects far fewer women than men. That's false. Colon cancer afflicts the sexes nearly equally and is the third-leading cause of cancer deaths among women.

Caught early, colon cancer is highly treatable. But most colon malignancies are asymptomatic until the late stages. That makes regular screening essential.

Colon cancer tends to occur up to 20% higher in a woman's colon than it does in a man's colon. This makes malignancies undetectable with a sigmoidoscope—a device used to examine the beginning, or left side, of the colon.

Caution: Because the sigmoidoscopes don't access the right side, or ascending, colon, this test is of questionable value for both sexes. This is especially important because cancers are inexplicably occurring with greater frequency in this location.

Self-defense: All adults age 50 or older should have an annual occult blood test of stool to detect blood not visible to the naked eye. A confirmed positive finding should be followed with a colonoscopy, an outpatient procedure in which a long, flexible viewing tube is inserted through the rectum, to examine the entire colon. A routine colonoscopy every 10 years is recommended.

Studies also show that gallbladder removal (a surgery more common in women because they are more prone to gallstones) increases colon cancer risk.

If you've had colon polyps or gallbladder surgery or have a first-degree relative (parent or sibling) with colon cancer, consult your doctor. Although recent evidence has called into question the safety of HRT, postmenopausal women on HRT are 37% less likely to develop colon cancer than those not on HRT.

To decrease the risk of colon cancer, every adult should exercise regularly and eat a high-fiber, low-fat diet consisting of at least four vegetables and two fruits daily and 30% or less of calories from fat.

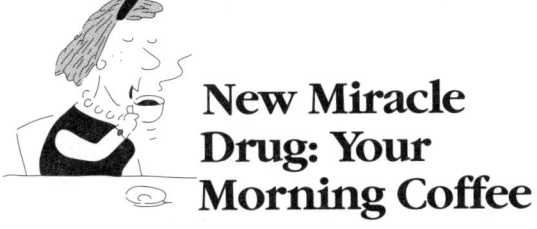

New Miracle Drug: Your Morning Coffee

Bennett Alan Weinberg and Bonnie K. Bealer, coauthors of *The Caffeine Advantage* (Free Press) and *The World of Caffeine* (Routledge). They have been researching caffeine for seven years, working with leading scientific and medical experts, and authored the chapter on caffeine for the textbook *Nutritional Impact of Foods and Beverages* (Humana). Based in Philadelphia, they develop continuing education programs that train physicians in the use of pharmaceuticals.

We all know that caffeine makes us more alert. But did you know that it can be a powerful drug with remarkable healing powers?

For decades, asthma sufferers have gotten relief from caffeine. Recent findings have shown that it also helps prevent Alzheimer's disease and Parkinson's disease...limits stroke damage ...and reduces the incidence of skin, colon and breast cancers. Mopping up damaging free radicals, it is a stronger antioxidant than vitamin C.

In addition to preventing illness, caffeine can help us in our day-to-day lives by doing everything from boosting mood to maximizing weight loss.

Is there a downside? Scientific studies looking at tens of thousands of people have shown that caffeine is not the villain it has been made out to be. For example, despite what many people think, it does not cause or exacerbate hypertension or heart problems.

Some people experience insomnia or "jitters" after having a lot of caffeine. These and other side effects usually disappear when it is consumed regularly or in smaller amounts. Pregnant women should limit caffeine. More than 300 milligrams (mg) a day raises risk of miscarriage. Check with your doctor.

HOW IT WORKS

Many of the day-to-day benefits we receive from caffeine stem from its effects on *neurotransmitters*, the chemicals that regulate communication between nerve cells. Caffeine boosts the effects of the neurotransmitters *dopamine* and *serotonin*, which improve mood. It also boosts levels of *acetylcholine*, a neurotransmitter that improves short-term memory.

Scientists at the National Addiction Centre in London studied more than 9,000 people and found that those who ingested caffeine scored higher on tests of reaction times, reasoning and memory. Other studies have shown that caffeine improves IQ test scores.

As little as 100 mg of caffeine—the amount in four ounces of drip-brewed coffee—boosts mood and memory. Larger amounts—200 mg or more—are needed for optimal mental or physical performance.

You won't develop a tolerance to the beneficial effects of caffeine. If 300 mg helps you run faster the first time you take it, the same dose will deliver the same benefit even after taking caffeine for years.

It takes about 15 minutes for caffeine to kick in. The effects usually last three to four hours,

■ *Your Health* ■

but this varies from person to person. Women who take oral contraceptives metabolize caffeine more slowly and may feel the effects twice as long. Smokers metabolize caffeine more quickly and experience a shorter "buzz."

The amount of caffeine that is "right" for you also varies by the individual. A small number of people can barely tolerate a 50-mg dose of caffeine, while many others can have 500 mg or more every day with no problems. Start with about 100 mg in the morning, and gradually increase your dose until you experience the benefits without side effects.

Also, determine your personal "caffeine cutoff point," the time after which consuming caffeine interferes with your sleep. This is different for each person. Some people find they can't have caffeine after noon, while others can consume it right before bed and sleep soundly. The cutoff point for many people is five to six hours before bed.

Helpful: Caffeine pills, such as NoDoz, give a better boost than coffee or tea. One of the chemicals in coffee and tea, *chlorogenic acid,* partially dampens the effects of caffeine. Caffeine pills don't work any faster, but the effects are more dramatic and predictable.

Here are five ways in which caffeine can enhance your life…

RELIEVE HEADACHES

Caffeine is an active ingredient in some over-the-counter painkillers, such as Anacin and Excedrin, and prescription painkillers, such as Darvon Compound-65.

It is particularly helpful for tension and migraine headaches because it stimulates the body's natural painkilling mechanisms. Studies at Chicago's Diamond Headache Clinic showed that caffeine eliminated headaches in nearly two-thirds of participants—and took effect 30 minutes faster than *ibuprofen.*

Caffeine Rx: Take 200 mg of caffeine at the first sign of a tension headache or migraine… and continue to take 100 mg every two to three hours, as needed. For additional relief, take caffeine with 200 mg to 400 mg of ibuprofen. This combination increases the analgesic effects, without risk.

LOSE WEIGHT

Caffeine stimulates the release of *cholecystokinin* (CCK), a hormone that suppresses appetite, delays the onset of hunger and promotes a feeling of fullness. In addition, caffeine promotes efficient fat-burning (lipolysis) and increases metabolism.

Caffeine Rx: A daily 200-mg dose helps burn 50 to 100 extra calories. That means a loss of five to 10 pounds a year. You will eat less if you consume caffeine 15 minutes *before* a particularly tempting meal.

MAXIMIZE WORKOUTS

Caffeine enhances nearly every aspect of physical activity, including endurance, speed and lung capacity. It also helps damaged muscle cells recover.

Caffeine Rx: A 200-mg dose will improve endurance by as much as 20% when riding an exercise bike, running on a treadmill or doing other moderately strenuous workouts. Prior to more strenuous exercise—like running a marathon—take 300 mg to 400 mg of caffeine.

DRIVE SAFELY

Driver fatigue is the leading cause of highway fatalities. A study by the US Department of Health, Education and Welfare showed that drivers who consumed 200 mg of caffeine had significant improvements in alertness and reaction times as compared with people who were not given caffeine.

Caffeine Rx: If you feel sleepy while driving, pull off the road…drink coffee or take a caffeine pill…and take a nap for 15 minutes. The caffeine enters your bloodstream while you rest, making you more alert when you're back on the road.

Warning: Most people rest, *then* drink coffee when they resume driving. That's dangerous—you are groggy from the nap, and the caffeine hasn't had time to take effect.

FIGHT JET LAG

About 94% of long-distance travelers suffer fatigue, irritability, headaches and/or gastrointestinal discomfort due to jet lag. Your body needs one day to adjust for every time zone you cross.

Caffeine Rx: Before your trip, avoid caffeine to increase its effects later. But don't stop using caffeine suddenly. This can result in withdrawal symptoms, such as headaches and anxiety. Instead, taper off, reducing your intake by about 150 mg a day—for example, by eliminating one cup of coffee. By the time you leave for your trip, you should have stopped having caffeine entirely for a day or two.

Take one 200-mg caffeine pill or drink about one and a half cups of coffee immediately after arriving at your destination. You can repeat the dose every three hours until you reach your personal caffeine cutoff point. The boost in energy will help you stay awake and shift your body clock to the new time zone.

Best Home Medical Tests

Steven I. Gutman, MD, director of the US Food and Drug Administration's Division of Clinical Laboratory Devices in Rockville, MD, *www.fda.gov.*

Home medical testing kits and devices sold at pharmacies and on the Internet allow anyone to conveniently test for illnesses and other medical conditions in the privacy of his/her own home.

Home-test manufacturers must prove to the Food and Drug Administration that their products are as accurate as the laboratory tests used by medical offices.

None of the tests requires a doctor's prescription, but they aren't substitutes for doctor visits. These tests are not covered by insurance.

Important: Carefully read the instructions that come with any test. Doing a test improperly —taking urine at the wrong time of day, for example—can invalidate the results.

Editor's note: Home medical tests are available at retail and on-line pharmacies and from such Web companies as *www.home-health testing.com* and *www.homeaccess.com.*

Some of the best home tests…

CHOLESTEROL

High cholesterol is a leading risk factor for stroke, heart disease and other cardiovascular conditions.

How the test works: Place some blood from a finger prick on a chemically treated strip. Cholesterol readings will appear on a thermometer-like scale in about 10 minutes or so. Some tests provide separate breakdowns for LDL (bad) and HDL (good) cholesterol. For this, you must send the blood sample to the manufacturer and wait several weeks for the results.

Average cost: $20 to $25 for a package of two tests.

COLON CANCER

Fecal occult blood tests (FOBTs) can detect small, often invisible amounts of blood in the stool—an early sign of colon cancer.

How the test works: Traditional FOBTs require you to take stool samples at home, then bring them to a lab for analysis. A newer FOBT doesn't require stool samples. You drop a chemically treated tissue into the toilet after you've had a bowel movement. A color change indicates blood is present. If so, you need additional tests, such as a colonoscopy, to check for cancerous or precancerous growths.

To ensure accuracy: You must repeat the test for three consecutive bowel movements. Do not take aspirin, *ibuprofen* or other non-steroidal anti-inflammatory drugs for one week prior to testing. They may cause bleeding that can skew the results.

For three days prior to the test, avoid eating red meat and don't take vitamin C supplements in excess of 250 milligrams (mg) daily. Don't use this test if you have bleeding hemorrhoids or anal fissures.

Average cost: $10 for a five-pad test kit.

DRUG USE

Parents who suspect their children of drug use may want to do a home test. Some tests check for a specific drug, such as marijuana. Broader tests detect multiple drugs—including cocaine and amphetamines.

How the test works: Some urine is dropped in a test cassette. Markings or color changes show if drugs are present. Marijuana generally can be detected within two to 30 days after use.

Important: About 5% of all urine drug tests result in false positives—the tests indicate that

■ *Your Health* ■

drugs are present when they're not. A positive home test should be confirmed with a laboratory drug test, such as a gas chromatography.

Average cost: $10 for one test.

Drugs can also be detected in hair clippings, which are sent to a laboratory for analysis.

Cost: About $60.

HIV

Privacy concerns prevent many people from getting tested for HIV, the virus that causes AIDS. Home-test manufacturers that analyze results follow strict confidentiality guidelines.

How the test works: Prick your finger, and apply the blood to special paper. Call a toll-free number to activate your personal code. Mail the blood sample and an anonymous personal identification number to a laboratory. To get the test results, you call a toll-free number and give your personal code.

Average cost: $44 for one test.

MENOPAUSE

Women in their 40s and 50s commonly experience hot flashes, mood swings or other menopause-like symptoms. They can confirm that they are entering menopause with a simple home test.

How the test works: Place a few drops of urine on a test strip. Premenopausal levels of follicle-stimulating hormone are lower than 25 IU/L. Readings that are above 25 indicate a woman has entered menopause.

Home-test manufacturers advise women to repeat the test every six to 12 months when the symptoms of menopause occur.

Average cost: $60 for two tests.

OVULATION

The home-test kits have taken much of the guesswork out of when women may be able to get pregnant.

How the test works: Wet a test strip with urine to measure luteinizing hormone. Levels peak 24 to 36 hours prior to ovulation, which is the optimal time to try to conceive.

Average cost: $10 for five tests.

URINARY TRACT INFECTIONS (UTIs)

With a home test, you can confirm that you have an infection. Then your doctor may prescribe antibiotics for you over the phone.

How the test works: Wet a plastic strip with urine. Part of the strip will change color if a UTI is present.

These tests are recommended only for people who get recurrent UTIs and are familiar with the symptoms, including frequent and/or painful urination.

If you have not experienced a UTI before, you should see your doctor to rule out any other possible conditions, such as chlamydia or kidney stones.

Important: The test fails to detect infections about 30% of the time. See your doctor if the test is negative but you have symptoms.

Average cost: $20 for six test strips and collection cups.

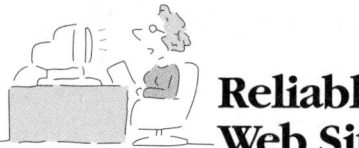

Reliable Health Web Sites

Looking to do some health research on the Internet? *Try out some of these helpful Web sites...*

•**www.clinicaltrials.gov.** A database of clinical trials in the US. Searchable by disease.

•**www.emedicine.com.** Provides a searchable database of information on diseases and conditions. Content is written by physicians.

•**www.healthfinder.gov.** Provides links to hundreds of other reliable health-related sites. Click on "Directory of Healthfinder Organizations" to look for approved organizations.

•**www.medem.com/medlb/medlib_entry.cfm.** Medem is an organization that provides health care information from major health organizations, such as the American Medical Association and the American Academy of Pediatrics. This site gives you access to Medem's on-line medical library.

•**www.nlm.nih.gov/medlineplus.** From the US National Library of Medicine and the National Institutes of Health. Provides health information and a medical dictionary. Click "Other Resources" to find links to other sites, including the Medline database, which can be used to search for medical journal abstracts.

Full-Body CT Scan Hype

E. Stephen Amis, MD, chairman of radiology, Albert Einstein College of Medicine and Montefiore Medical Center, Bronx, NY.

Full-body CT scans, in which a symptom-free person gets scanned in an effort to detect early-stage cancer, heart disease or some other illness, have become increasingly popular.

Are full-body CT scans a good idea? The American College of Radiology, the American Cancer Society and the American Heart Association do *not* recommend them. *Here's what consumers should know...*

•**There's no scientific evidence to support the use of full-body CT scans** as a screening technique for people without symptoms. However, the targeted CT scans, such as chest scans to detect lung cancer in smokers and former smokers, are effective.

•**Early-stage cancer can be missed.** Although full-body CT scans examine the entire torso, from neck to pelvis, they are unlikely to detect small malignancies of the colon, breast or prostate.

Better: Colonoscopy, mammography or a prostate-specific antigen (PSA) test.

•**Radiation doses are high.** A full-body CT scan delivers up to 300 times the amount of radiation of a chest X ray. Because radiation risks are cumulative, people who get full-body CT scans regularly increase their risk for radiation-induced cancer.

To learn more, visit the American College of Radiology Web site at *www.acr.org*.

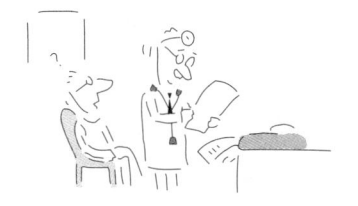

The Miracle Heart Drugs 13 Million Americans Take

Steven Nissen, MD, vice chairman, department of cardiovascular medicine, Cleveland Clinic Foundation, and medical director, Cleveland Clinic Cardiovascular Coordinating Center.

Everyone knows that too much cholesterol is bad. High levels of this fat-like substance in the blood raise the risk of heart attack and sudden death.

But how much is too much? And what's the best way to reduce cholesterol levels? The answers have changed recently, largely because of cholesterol-lowering drugs called *statins*. Already, 13 million Americans take them...and each study seems to enlarge the circle of people who may benefit from statin therapy. How about you?

LATEST GUIDELINES

In 2001, the National Cholesterol Education Program issued new guidelines to help people decide if they need to lower their cholesterol levels.

Healthy people should keep LDL cholesterol (the kind linked to heart disease) below 130 milligrams per deciliter (mg/dl). Those who have had a heart attack or stroke or who have diabetes or cardiovascular disease should aim for an LDL level of 100 mg/dl. The same is true if you smoke cigarettes or have a family history of heart disease.

If a low-fat, high-fiber diet doesn't reduce cholesterol enough within three months, you may need drug therapy to bring down levels.

SURPRISING FINDINGS

Recent data suggest that these guidelines do not go far enough. The British Heart Protection Study, released in November 2001, was the largest clinical trial of statins ever done. Over 20,000 people with cardiovascular disease or diabetes were randomly selected to take either *simvastatin* (Zocor) or a placebo for five years.

The results were striking. People who were given simvastatin had 33% less heart attacks and strokes than those who were given the placebo. They also required significantly fewer heart surgeries, angioplasties and amputations.

■ *Your Health* ■

Most important: The benefit was not limited to people with high cholesterol. Simvastatin appeared to prevent heart attacks and strokes even in those whose LDL cholesterol levels were *below* the recommended level.

WHAT DOES IT MEAN FOR YOU?

If you have had a heart attack or stroke or have been diagnosed with cardiovascular disease or diabetes, you would probably benefit from statin therapy. This is true even if your cholesterol levels are in the healthy range.

If you don't fit into these categories but have several *risk factors* for heart disease—you are male, middle-aged, smoke cigarettes, have high blood pressure or a family history of heart attacks—you are in a gray zone. But I generally recommend statins for such individuals.

Statin medication does not mean you can become complacent. Lifestyle still counts. You should take steps to lower your heart attack risk—exercise, improve your diet and maintain a healthy weight.

CHOOSING THE BEST STATIN

Statins are usually taken to lower cholesterol. *Atorvastatin* (Lipitor) and simvastatin (Zocor) seem to be the most effective. *Rosuvastatin* (Crestor), which was recently released, should be just as effective.

While statins are usually the most effective medications for lowering LDL cholesterol, other drugs are sometimes more suitable for people with certain cholesterol problems…

•Your HDL cholesterol level is too low. If this "good" cholesterol that removes fatty deposits from the arteries is too low, your doctor may prescribe niacin. Niaspan, a prescription-only, sustained-release formulation, has minimal side effects.

•Your level of triglycerides—another blood fat—is high. Your doctor may advise you to take a fibric acid derivative, such as *gemfibrozil* (Lopid) or *fenofibrate* (Tricor). These also raise HDL cholesterol levels.

Both niacin and fibric acid drugs may be taken along with a statin for double-barreled action against heart disease.

HOW SAFE ARE STATINS?

Several years ago, *cerivastatin* (Baycol) was pulled off the market. The drug was linked to more than 100 deaths from *rhabdomyolysis,* a serious condition marked by severe muscle pain and weakness. The risk with other statins is exceedingly low—an estimated one person in three million has a fatal reaction.

A minority of people experience muscle aches. They usually feel better when they switch to a lower dose or a different statin.

Some people may worry that their cholesterol levels will drop too low. The body does need some cholesterol for such biological functions as the formation of cell membranes. But the amount needed is very small.

TWO MORE POSSIBLE BENEFITS

According to a study presented at the American Academy of Neurology meeting in Denver in April 2002, more than 2,500 people who took statins were far less likely to develop Alzheimer's disease, the leading cause of dementia.

More research needs to be done on this front, but brain protection could turn out to be another compelling reason to consider statins.

There is also preliminary evidence that statins may help reduce the risk of colon cancer, especially when they are taken in combination with the nonsteroidal anti-inflammatory drugs, such as aspirin. But, again, more research needs to be conducted.

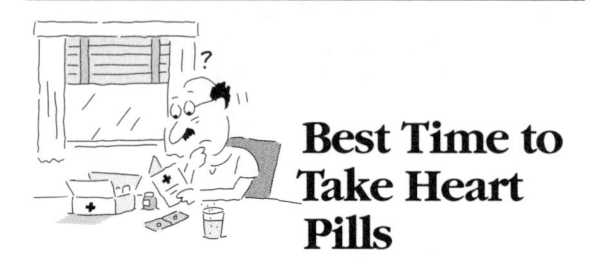

Best Time to Take Heart Pills

The best time to take heart medication is in the morning. Cardiac medicines (beta blockers, ACE inhibitors) taken in the morning take effect when you are up and about, and therefore putting greater demands on your cardiovascular system.

Exception: Take statins at bedtime because they work in conjunction with cholesterol synthesis, and the liver makes more cholesterol at night.

Thomas H. Lee, MD, editor in chief, *Harvard Health Letter,* 10 Shattuck St., Boston 02115.

Ibuprofen Linked to High Blood Pressure?

Gary C. Curhan, MD, ScD, associate professor of medicine, Harvard Medical School, Boston. His study of medical data of 80,020 women was published in the *Archives of Internal Medicine.*

Heavy use of nonaspirin pain relievers does increase risk for high blood pressure. In one groundbreaking study, women who took nonsteroidal anti-inflammatories (NSAIDs), such as *ibuprofen,* 22 times a month or more were 86% more likely to have high blood pressure than those who did not take NSAIDs. Those taking acetaminophen were twice as likely to be hypertensive. Aspirin did not increase risk.

Theory: NSAIDs inhibit the production of fatty-acid derivatives known as *prostaglandins,* which dilate blood vessels, cause sodium retention and increase production of *endothelin 1,* a compound that constricts blood vessels.

If you are at risk for high blood pressure or already have the condition, ask your doctor which pain reliever is appropriate for you.

When to Take Your Daily Aspirin

Nighttime is the best time to take a daily aspirin to protect your heart. In a recent study, people with mild hypertension who waited until bedtime to take an aspirin tablet lowered their systolic blood pressure by an average of seven points after three months. Those who did not take aspirin or who took aspirin in the morning showed no change in blood pressure. Check with your doctor.

Ramon C. Hermida, PhD, director, bioengineering and chronobiology labs, University of Vigo, Spain.

Aspirin and Heart Attack Risk

Aspirin does not always reduce heart attack risk...and its failure may be related to high cholesterol. Daily aspirin therapy fails as a blood thinner in 20% of people whose cholesterol levels are 180 milligrams per deciliter (mg/dl) or lower...and fails in 60% of people whose levels are 220 mg/dl or higher.

If you have high cholesterol: Ask your doctor if you should take medication to lower cholesterol in addition to aspirin.

Michael Miller, MD, director of the Center for Preventive Cardiology, University of Maryland Medical Center, Baltimore, and leader of a study of 63 heart disease patients, presented at an annual meeting of the American Heart Association.

Trans Fatty Acids Are Worse Than Butter

Trans fatty acids are even worse for your health than the saturated fats in sour cream, butter and lard. According to the National Academy of Sciences, trans fatty acids increase your risk of heart attack by raising "bad" LDL cholesterol and lowering levels of protective HDL cholesterol as much or more so than do saturated fats. There is no safe level of intake. Besides being present in high-fat dairy products, trans fats are in foods containing hydrogenated or partially hydrogenated vegetable oils, such as cakes, pies and cookies...and fast-food french fries, chicken and other deep-fried foods.

Suzanne Havala Hobbs, DrPH, RD, registered dietitian and adjunct assistant professor in the School of Public Health at the University of North Carolina in Chapel Hill. She is author of several books, including *Being Vegetarian for Dummies* (Wiley).

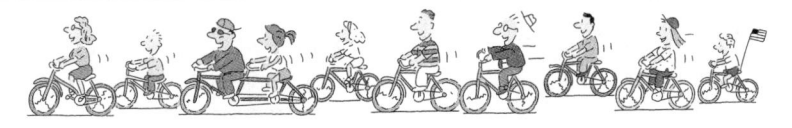

Your Health

The Right Waist Measurement

Waist measurement predicts risk of cardiovascular disease. To keep risk down, men should have a waist measurement of 40 inches or less...women, 35 inches or less.

Sidney C. Smith, Jr., MD, chief science officer, American Heart Association, Dallas, *www.americanheart.org*.

Hypertension and Rosacea May Be Linked

In a study, 21% of patients with rosacea—an acne-like skin condition—had hypertension. Rosacea, whose cause is unknown, may be part of a disorder of the blood vessels. If you have rosacea, ask your doctor to check your blood pressure.

Aditya Gupta, MD, PhD, associate professor, department of medicine, University of Toronto, and leader of a study of 1,950 patients who visited a dermatology clinic, results of which were presented at a meeting of the American Academy of Dermatology.

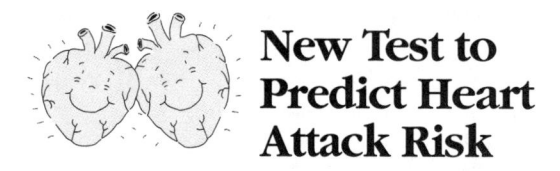

New Test to Predict Heart Attack Risk

A new blood test is a better predictor of heart attack than cholesterol or homocysteine levels. The *C-reactive protein (CRP) test* measures a protein in the body, elevations of which have been correlated with both heart attack and stroke. The test generally costs $65 and may not be covered by insurance.

Good news: Diet, exercise and statin drugs can reduce CRP significantly.

Richard Milani, MD, director of Cardiovascular Health Center and vice chairman of the department of cardiology at Ochsner Clinic Foundation, New Orleans.

Faster Test for Heart Attack Now in the ER

Only 15% of the emergency room patients who complain of heart pain are having heart attacks—but ruling one out can take 24 hours. The *Triage Cardiac System* takes only 90 minutes. The cost is about $100 and is usually covered by insurance. It measures levels of enzymes released during a heart attack.

Recent study: This test was 100% accurate when combined with an electrocardiogram and a patient history.

Alan Maisel, MD, director of coronary care, VA San Diego Healthcare System, and professor of medicine, University of California, San Diego. His study of 1,285 emergency room patients was published in *The American Journal of Cardiology*.

Bypass Surgery Danger for Women

Viola Vaccarino, MD, PhD, associate professor of medicine, Emory University School of Medicine, Atlanta, and leader of a study of more than 57,000 bypass-surgery patients, reported in *Circulation*.

Women between the ages of 50 to 59 are three times more likely to die after coronary-artery bypass surgery than men who are the same age.

Possible reasons: Since doctors are less inclined to suspect heart disease in younger women, women are referred for surgery only when heart disease is advanced.

Also: Women have smaller arteries, making bypass surgery more difficult.

But women shouldn't avoid this potentially lifesaving surgery.

Self-defense: Undergo regular screening for heart disease risk factors, such as high blood pressure, high blood sugar and high cholesterol, beginning in young adulthood. If any of these levels is elevated, seek prompt treatment to reduce risk.

Heart-Bypass Surgery Side Effect

Heart-bypass surgery can be hard on the brain. In one study of 300 patients, 39% showed a decline in thinking skills six weeks after surgery. The greatest decline occurred in patients with the highest fevers in the 24 hours after surgery.

Self-defense: Ask your surgeon what steps will be taken to protect the brain.

Examples: Slow postoperative rewarming…temperature monitoring…arterial line filters, which remove harmful debris…cell-saving devices that recycle a patient's blood and decrease debris in the bypass circuit.

Hilary Grocott, MD, associate professor of anesthesiology and critical-care medicine at Duke University Medical Center in Durham, NC. His findings were published in *Stroke*.

Falling Blood Pressure Alert

Falling blood pressure can be a sign of failing health.

Background: Blood pressure very slowly increases with age. But a new study shows that adults age 65 or older who had a decline in systolic blood pressure of 20 points or more or a decline in diastolic blood pressure of 10 points or more over a three-year period had a 60% higher chance of dying from heart disease during the succeeding three years than those people who had no change in their blood pressure.

Speak with your physician if your blood pressure declines by more than 20 points without any blood pressure–lowering medications.

Shiva Satish, MD, MPH, professor of internal medicine, University of Texas, Galveston.

Health News and Breakthroughs

Hot Tub Health Risk

Thomas Allison, PhD, cardiovascular disease specialist, Mayo Clinic, Rochester, MN.

People who have low blood pressure—as well as those taking blood pressure medications—may pass out in hot tubs. Heat dilates blood vessels, lowering pressure suddenly when you stand. Blood rushing from your brain can cause dizziness or fainting.

Self-defense: Limit time in a hot tub to 20 minutes. Immediately get out of the hot tub if you feel overheated, short of breath or light-headed. Do not drink alcohol before entering the hot tub or while you are in it. Emerge slowly, using handrails.

If you feel dizzy after getting out: Sit or lie down. Drink cold water.

Even better: If you have low blood pressure or take blood pressure medication, do not get in a hot tub.

Don't Stand Up Quickly After a Meal

Standing up too quickly after a meal may set you up for a fall. In a recent study of 50 people, 22% of those who stood after eating had a precipitous drop in blood pressure. This can cause dizziness and light-headedness, increasing the likelihood of a fall—especially among those age 50 and older.

Self-defense: If you experience dizziness upon standing after a meal, see your doctor for blood pressure monitoring.

M.S. Maurer, MD, assistant professor of medicine, division of circulatory physiology, College of Physicians and Surgeons, Columbia University, New York City. His study was published in the *Annals of Internal Medicine*.

■ *Your Health* ■

Better Stroke Prevention

Two types of surgery are used to clear out clogged carotid (neck) arteries, a common cause of stroke. Carotid endarterectomy involves cutting open the affected artery to remove fatty deposits. Angioplasty—in which a balloon-tipped wire is inserted into the groin and threaded through clogged arteries—also can be used to clear the blockage. The two procedures are comparable in effectiveness and complications.

Now: A tiny filter, placed in the carotid artery during angioplasty, catches fatty deposits that can become dislodged and trigger a stroke. In a recent study, patients undergoing angioplasty with the new filter had *half* the complications, such as stroke or heart attack, as those who underwent carotid endarterectomy. The filter should be available in Spring 2004.

Jay S. Yadav, MD, director, vascular intervention, Cleveland Clinic Foundation, OH.

Warning for Women Smokers

Women who smoke are three times more likely to develop lung cancer than men who smoke.

Theory: A woman's cells are less able to repair DNA damage.

If you smoke or once smoked: Ask your doctor about having an annual spiral CT scan. It is better than a chest X ray at detecting lung cancer when it's still most treatable. Few insurance companies pay for the test. But it's worth the cost, generally $300 to $1,000.

Signs of lung cancer include persistent cough, shortness of breath, hoarseness, bloody phlegm, recurrent respiratory infections, chest pain, unexplained weight loss and/or loss of appetite.

Claudia Henschke, MD, PhD, chief, division of chest imaging, Weill Medical College of Cornell University, New York City.

Flu Vaccine Cuts Stroke Risk

The flu vaccine cuts stroke risk in half—and even more in people who have been vaccinated for five consecutive years. The vaccine helps prevent influenza and resulting secondary infections, which cause inflammation. Inflammation is associated with atherosclerotic plaque buildup in the arteries, and a rupture of this plaque leads to stroke.

However: The flu vaccine does *not* prevent stroke in people age 75 or older, perhaps because high blood pressure and other conditions override this protective effect.

Self-defense: Speak to your doctor about receiving the flu shot every October.

Pierre Amarenco, MD, chairman, Neurology and Stroke Center, Denis Diderot University, Paris. His study was published in *Stroke*.

Another Secondhand Smoke Warning

Passive smoking is already known to cause respiratory and behavior problems in kids. But now, secondhand smoke has been shown to lower children's intelligence as well.

In a recent study of more than 4,000 children ages six to 16, the higher a child's blood levels of *cotinine,* a by-product of nicotine, the worse they performed on intelligence tests. One parent smoking even less than a pack a day could raise a child's blood levels enough to reduce intelligence quotient (IQ) by about two points.

Self-defense: Parents should stop smoking. Also, do not take children to cigarette-smoke-filled restaurants or other settings.

Kimberly Yolton, PhD, research associate, General and Community Pediatrics Research, Cincinnati Children's Hospital Medical Center.

Quit Smoking Without Gaining Weight

Michael F. Roizen, MD, professor of anesthesiology and medicine, Upstate Medical University of the State University of New York, Syracuse, and author of *RealAge: Are You as Young as You Can Be?* (HarperResource).

Within six months of kicking the smoking habit, men gain an average of 10 pounds, while women put on eight. *Here's how you can prevent the weight gain...*

- **Chew sugarless gum** to ease oral cravings.
- **Snack on low-fat foods**—raw vegetables, fruit and popcorn without butter.
- **Exercise.** Walk for a minimum of 30 minutes each day.
- **Wait until after the holidays to quit smoking.** Rich holiday foods and treats are just too tempting.
- **Purchase some desk gadgets** and other objects to help keep your hands occupied while at work.
- **Whenever you feel the urge to smoke,** close your eyes and take several deep breaths. Tell yourself the reasons that you have quit.
- **Don't downplay your accomplishment.** Quitting is a big deal.

Diabetes Drug Danger

A recent survey of 100 patients taking the popular diabetes drug Glucophage (*metformin*) found that 22% should not have been taking it. Glucophage may be associated with *lactic acidosis* in people with diabetes and congestive heart failure or kidney dysfunction. This sharp increase in blood levels of lactic acid has a mortality rate of nearly 50%. Symptoms include muscle cramps, stomach pains and confusion.

Self-defense: Consult with your physician to confirm that Glucophage is safe for you or to inquire about alternatives. Do not stop taking it without a doctor's supervision.

Russell Rothman, MD, assistant professor of internal medicine and pediatrics, Vanderbilt University School of Medicine, Nashville. His report was published in *The Journal of the American Medical Association*.

Knee Surgery May Not Help Arthritis

Arthroscopic surgery for an arthritic knee may not be effective. This surgery involves removing injured cartilage. In a recent study, some patients underwent real arthroscopic surgery and others a placebo surgery (small incisions were made, but cartilage was not removed). During the following two years, patients who had the placebo surgery consistently reported the same improvement as patients who underwent the real thing.

Nelda Wray, MD, chief of general medicine, Houston VA Medical Center, and professor of medicine, Baylor College of Medicine, Houston. Her study of 180 patients was published in *The New England Journal of Medicine*.

New Alzheimer's Test

A new Alzheimer's test is as easy as picking out playing cards on a computer screen. The 15- to 18-minute test measures attention, memory and other mental functions, and may detect pre-Alzheimer's cognitive impairment years sooner than current neurological tests. For more information, go to the manufacturer's Web site, *www.cogstate.com*.

New Scientist, Reed Business Information Limited, 151 Wardour St., London.

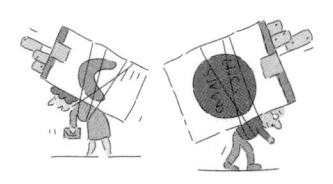

■ *Your Health* ■

Don't Believe the HGH Hype

Despite the hype, human growth hormone (HGH) does *not* slow aging. This is true whether HGH is taken orally or injected. Taken orally, HGH is inactivated by stomach acid, making it valueless. And, the same is true for *growth hormone releasing factor*, which also is being advertised. By injection, HGH is only for patients with HGH deficiency caused by a disease of the pituitary gland, which produces HGH.

Caution: HGH may cause tumors to grow. Side effects include diabetes and arthritis.

Paul S. Jellinger, MD, clinical professor of medicine at University of Miami, FL, and past president of American Association of Clinical Endocrinologists.

No More Snoring

Injection snoreplasty is a new treatment that cuts snoring in half. The procedure, which costs $400 and up, involves injecting the soft palate with *3% sodium tetradecyl sulfate,* a sclerosing agent which causes the palate to stiffen and shorten. The no-longer-floppy palate is then less likely to vibrate during sleep, quieting the snoring. The procedure takes up to six weeks to bring relief. It causes some pain from the injection.

If you suffer from snoring: Ask your doctor if this procedure is appropriate for you.

Kathleen Yaremchuk, MD, vice chair, department of otolaryngology, head and neck surgery at the Henry Ford Health System, Detroit.

Aspirin for a Healthier Colon

Aspirin therapy reduces colon cancer risk in people at high risk for the disease. In a recent study, daily use of baby-strength aspirin —81 milligrams—decreased the recurrence of colon polyps by 19% in people who had polyps removed. Polyps can become cancerous.

If you have a family history of colon cancer: Ask your doctor whether you should take a daily low-dose aspirin.

Caution: Don't start aspirin therapy if you are allergic to aspirin or have bleeding problems.

John Baron, MD, professor of medicine, Dartmouth Medical School, Hanover, NH, and leader of a study of 1,121 people who had polyps removed during routine cancer screening, presented at a meeting of the American Association for Cancer Research.

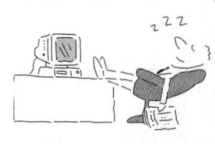

Thyroid Disease Could Be the Cause of Your Symptoms

Richard L. Shames, MD, thyroid specialist who maintains a private practice in San Rafael, CA, *www.thyroidpower.com*. He is coauthor of *Thyroid Power: 10 Steps to Total Health* (HarperResource).

America is in the grip of an energy crisis. Millions of men and women drag themselves around from day to day, feeling fatigued, unable to work productively or enjoy life. Many suffer additional ills, such as depression, anxiety, digestive misery, headaches and muscle pains.

What is their problem? Low levels of thyroid hormone.

Trouble with the butterfly-shaped gland at the base of the throat is surprisingly common —and since the symptoms of hypothyroidism are vague and nonspecific, thyroid disorders often go undetected.

THE MASTER GLAND

The thyroid functions much like a gas pedal for the entire body. Its hormones penetrate every cell to regulate the body's energy-producing "machinery." Too little thyroid hormone, and your organs can slow down—with consequences that range from irritating to devastating.

According to estimates, 5% of adult Americans have hypothyroidism. But recent surveys show that actually double that number—one in 10 Americans—have the problem. Among

Health News and Breakthroughs

women who are in menopause, *one in five* has hypothyroidism.

Why the epidemic? No one knows for sure. But some endocrinologists theorize that the thyroid is affected by air pollution, pesticides and other chemical pollutants...increased radiation exposure from power plants, microwaves and cell phones...and chronic psychological stress.

Regardless of the reason, hypothyroidism can cause symptoms as diverse as the body systems the gland regulates.

In addition to the fatigue, low energy and mild depression that occur so frequently, many people with the condition have difficulty controlling their weight because their metabolism is sluggish. They may also feel cold when others are comfortable.

Additional problems that may point to thyroid disorder include allergies...dry skin, eczema or adult acne...poor concentration or forgetfulness ...difficulty swallowing...or recurrent infections.

GETTING DIAGNOSED

Because the symptoms can have a number of causes, doctors* often mistake thyroid problems for another condition, such as menopause, irritable bowel syndrome or rheumatoid arthritis.

To avoid misdiagnosis, blood tests to assess thyroid function should be a routine part of any physical checkup—especially for people over age 35.

Make even more sure to have your thyroid checked if anyone in your family (even an aunt or a cousin) has had thyroid problems or a condition, such as diabetes or prematurely gray hair, which often suggests thyroid malfunction.

Caution: The most common test, which measures levels of thyroid-stimulating hormone (TSH), sometimes gives a "false negative" (a normal reading even when there is thyroid trouble).

It's wise to follow up an all-too-frequent negative result with tests that can detect levels of the thyroid hormone *thyroxine* (T-4), which the body converts into *thyronine* (T-3).

Ask for: Free T-3 and free T-4 tests.

*To locate a thyroid specialist in your area, contact the Thyroid Foundation of America (800-832-8321 or *www.allthyroid.org*).

TREATMENT—THE HORMONE GAME

Standard treatment for low thyroid levels is a daily dose of T-4. But getting good results sometimes requires a little fine-tuning.

There are four brands of synthetic T-4, or *levothyroxine*—Synthroid, the largest seller and one of the most prescribed drugs in America ...Levothroid...Levoxyl...and Unithroid. These formulations are *not* always equivalent. Some people fare much better on one than another. Unfortunately, it's impossible to tell in advance which will be best for you.

If symptoms persist for six months despite T-4 treatment, ask your doctor about switching brands. Generic T-4 is available. But its quality control may be less reliable than that of brand-name products, and potencies may vary.

It may be that *no* brand of T-4 hormone will do the job because your body can't convert it into T-3 properly. In this case, doctors often recommend adding a synthetic form of T-3, called *liothyronine* (Cytomel). This more active hormone works on its own and boosts the effectiveness of T-4 to help your body restore normal function. In many instances, a better approach is a natural thyroid extract containing both T-3 and T-4.

Bonus: Brands of natural thyroid hormone, such as Armour Thyroid and Westhroid, cost less than synthetic preparations.

WATCH YOUR DIET

Even the best medical regimen needs nutritional help. To keep your thyroid healthy, minimize exposure to chemicals found in processed foods. Eat natural foods—without preservatives, additives or artificial sweeteners. *Also take daily supplements that contain...*

- **Vitamin A.** 10,000 international units (IU)
- **Vitamin C.** 500 milligrams (mg)
- **Vitamin E.** 400 IU
- **Vitamin B complex.** At least 50 mg each of B-1, B-3, B-5 and B-6.
- **Folic acid.** 800 micrograms (mcg)
- **Zinc.** 25 mg
- **Selenium.** 200 mcg
- **Manganese.** 20 mg

The thyroid needs iodine to function, but deficiencies of this mineral are largely a thing

Your Health

of the past due to our high consumption of iodized salt. Especially if you live near a coast, you may be getting too much iodine, which is harmful to the thyroid.

To reduce iodine intake: Buy noniodized salt and minimize sodium intake by avoiding salty snacks and other high-sodium foods.

Fluoride is highly toxic to the thyroid. Don't use fluoridated toothpaste. If your water supply is fluoridated, drink bottled water.

Better Lyme Disease Test

An improved Lyme disease test reduces the need for unnecessary antibiotics. That's because the new blood test, named PreVue, identifies antibodies to the bacterium that causes Lyme disease in 20 minutes, instead of the seven days required for previous tests. This allows doctors to determine more quickly whether antibiotics should be prescribed and if follow-up testing is needed to confirm the diagnosis.

Raymond Dattwyler, MD, professor of medicine, State University of New York at Stony Brook. His study was published in the *Archives of Internal Medicine*.

Most Common Sites For Melanoma

Don't forget the backs of your legs and your back when applying sunscreen. These are the most common sites for melanoma—the deadliest form of skin cancer.

Other often overlooked spots: Hair part and the tops of ears.

Use a waterproof, broad-spectrum sunscreen—meaning it blocks out UVA and UVB rays—with an SPF of at least 15. Apply it 20 minutes before going outside. Reapply every two hours—more often if swimming or exercising.

Andrew Kaufman, MD, assistant clinical professor of medicine at the University of California, Los Angeles, School of Medicine, and dermatologist in private practice in Thousand Oaks, CA.

New Medications For Psoriasis

Psoriasis patients often suffer without need. That is because many primary-care doctors continue to prescribe the corticosteroid creams despite the availability of new medications that are safer and equally effective. The old standbys—*betamethasone* (Diprosone) and *diflorasone* (Florone)—can cause permanent damage, such as skin thinning and unsightly blood vessels. They can also interfere with hormone production, resulting in adrenal insufficiency or Cushing's syndrome (caused by excessive steroid production). The only significant side effect of newer creams, such as *calcipotriene* (Dovonex) and *tazarotene* (Tazorac), is minor skin irritation.

Daniel Federman, MD, associate professor of medicine, Yale University School of Medicine, New Haven, CT.

Ultrasound Speeds Healing of Broken Bones

In a recent review of studies involving hand, wrist and shin fractures, a low-dose ultrasound decreased healing time by up to 35%. Patients use portable, FDA-approved equipment for 20 minutes each day to stimulate bone growth at the site of the fracture. While high-dose ultrasound can harm bone, *low-dose* treatments carry no known risk. This procedure has not yet been tested on fractures resulting from osteoporosis.

To find a practitioner: Contact Smith & Nephew, manufacturer of the Exogen machine, at 800-836-4080. Ask your health insurer if it provides coverage.

Jason Busse, DC, vice president, chronic pain division, Oncidium Health Group, Burlington, Ontario. His analysis of studies involving 158 fractures was published in the *Canadian Medical Association Journal*.

Screening for Osteoporosis

Routine osteoporosis screening should be part of normal medical care for women over age 65. Women 60 to 64 with higher-than-average risk factors for bone thinning—such as thin women or women not taking estrogen—should also be screened routinely.

Best procedure: The dual-energy X-ray absorptiometry (DEXA), a painless scan.

Janet D. Allan, PhD, RN, dean of nursing, University of Maryland School of Nursing, Baltimore, and vice-chair of the US Preventive Services Task Force.

Vitamin A Warning

Diane Feskanich, ScD, assistant professor of medicine at Harvard Medical School, Brigham & Women's Hospital, Boston, and leader of a study of 72,337 postmenopausal women, reported in *The Journal of the American Medical Association.*

Too much vitamin A in the form of *retinol* after menopause can harm bones. The upper limit dosage of 3,000 micrograms (mcg) daily may be too high.

Recent finding: Women who consumed more than 2,000 mcg per day of retinol—vitamin A's active form—were twice as prone to hip fractures as those who consumed just 500 mcg a day.

Caution: Most multivitamins contain 1,500 mcg of retinol, and it is easy to get 500 mcg more from fortified foods, such as milk, margarine and cereals.

Self-defense: Monitor the amount of retinol in your diet. Check the amount of vitamin A on multivitamin and food labels. Choose a multivitamin that provides some vitamin A in the form of beta-carotene, which is less potent.

Painkiller Trap for Broken Bones

Some painkillers may impede the healing of fractured bones. In animal studies, broken bones failed to heal fully when treated with Cox-2 inhibitors—prescription nonsteroidal anti-inflammatory drugs (NSAIDs), including *rofecoxib* (Vioxx) and *celecoxib* (Celebrex). Older NSAIDs, such as *ibuprofen* (Advil) and *indomethacin* (Indocin), also appear to delay healing. NSAIDs inhibit the activity of an enzyme essential for fracture healing.

Better: Aspirin and mild narcotics, such as Percocet (*acetaminophen* combined with *oxycodone*), do not have this effect.

J. Patrick O'Connor, PhD, assistant professor of orthopaedics, University of Medicine and Dentistry of New Jersey, New Jersey Medical School, Newark.

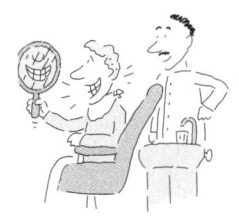

Should You Have Your Fillings Removed?

Some people have been concerned that silver-colored, mercury-containing amalgam fillings may cause multiple sclerosis and Alzheimer's disease. But there's no proof to support these fears. The mercury the fillings contain is mixed with other metals, such as silver, to form a stable alloy. Removing fillings can weaken teeth, since the replacement filling must be made larger. If a dentist wants to remove an amalgam filling, ask if there are other options.

Frederick C. Eichmiller, DDS, director, Paffenbarger Research Center, Gaithersburg, MD.

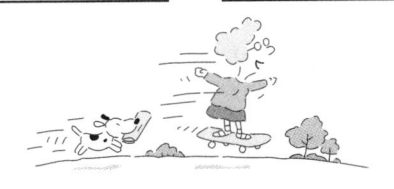

■ *Your Health* ■

Better Than Novocaine

If you find novocaine shots really painful, ask your dentist about the DentiPatch. Approximately half the size of a postage stamp, the patch adheres to the gum and numbs it by releasing the anesthetic *lidocaine*. Patients who received the patch reported half as much pain during needle sticks than when conventional gel was applied to the gum first.

Michelle Carr, registered dental hygienist and assistant professor of primary care at Ohio State University, Columbus.

Let Your Dentist Know If You Have Heart Problems

If you've had heart problems, be sure to tell your dentist. Blood pressure levels of heart patients undergoing tooth extraction can rise high enough to increase risk for an episode of heart failure. An informed dentist can take steps, such as early-morning appointments and appropriate local anesthesia, to relieve anxiety and pain.

Lucio Montebugnoli, MD, DDS, professor of dentistry, University of Bologna, Italy.

Booster Shots for Adults

Adults need regular booster shots to remain protected against diphtheria and tetanus.

Problem: Many people view these boosters as childhood immunizations. Only 60% of US adults have immunity against diphtheria...and only 72% against tetanus.

Boosters should be given once every 10 years. If you can't remember when you last had one, it is probably time. For information and an adult immunization schedule, contact the Immunization Action Coalition (651-647-9009 or *www.immunize.org*).

Geraldine M. McQuillan, PhD, senior infectious epidemiologist, National Center for Health Statistics, Hyattsville, MD, and leader of the third National Health and Nutrition Examination Survey of 18,045 adults, reported in the *Annals of Internal Medicine*.

Adieu to the Flu

People who experience a sudden onset of body aches, fever and chills during winter should consult a physician right away. If an antiviral prescription drug—such as *oseltamivir* (Tamiflu) or *zanamivir* (Relenza)—is started within 48 hours, patients recover much faster.

Best defense against the flu: An annual vaccination. Call your local health department to learn where flu shots are administered in your community.

Frederick Hayden, MD, professor of internal medicine and director of the respiratory disease study unit, University of Virginia School of Medicine, Charlottesville.

When to Treat a Fever

Treat a fever, when it makes you very uncomfortable. If you have mild to moderate fever and can tolerate it, do not treat it—reducing fever can undermine your body's natural defenses against disease. But if fever rises above 102°F, most people need drugs to reduce it.

Call a doctor if fever lasts longer than three days or if you also have frequent, burning or bloody urination...pain focused in one area of the abdomen...chills...severe diarrhea lasting more than one day...severe or unusual headache...a rash.

Bruce H. Yaffe, MD, internist and digestive disease specialist in private practice in New York City.

Vitamin E Makes Colds And Flu Worse

In a recent study, 652 healthy people age 60 or older were given either a daily supplement of vitamin E or a placebo. Of those who contracted a cold or the flu, the vitamin E takers suffered illness for an average of 19 days versus only 14 days for those who took placebos, and they suffered from an average of six symptoms rather than four. This rigorous trial contradicts earlier suggestions that vitamin E might boost immunity in seniors.

Nutrition Action Healthletter, 1875 Connecticut Ave. NW, Washington, DC 20009.

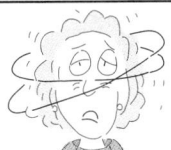

Sinus Relief

Harvey Plasse, MD, associate professor of otolaryngology at New York University School of Medicine and director of otolaryngology at NYU Downtown Hospital, both in New York City. He is coauthor of *Sinusitis Relief* (Owl).

Don't assume that sinus inflammation is harmless. Left untreated, this annoying condition eventually causes permanent scarring of the sinuses—and may, in rare cases, even lead to blindness or brain abscess.

AN ACCURATE DIAGNOSIS

Because sinusitis often begins as a common cold, the condition frequently goes undiagnosed and untreated.

Anyone who experiences a cold for more than 10 days should be checked for the presence of sinus infection.

Other symptoms...

- **Thick or discolored nasal discharge** (yellow or green).
- **Fever.**
- **Bad breath.**
- **Facial pain or pressure in the forehead and over the eyes,** between the cheek and nose, in upper teeth or between the eyes.
- **Reduced or absent sense of smell.**
- **Ear pain.**

Symptoms that subside within four weeks are diagnosed as acute sinusitis...subacute sinusitis lasts for four to 12 weeks. If not treated effectively, this condition can turn into chronic sinusitis, in which symptoms persist for more than 12 weeks.

ACUTE SINUSITIS

Antibiotics are the primary treatment for acute sinusitis. The main goal is to eradicate the infection and prevent the development of chronic sinusitis.

The effective antibiotics include *amoxicillin* (Amoxil)...*amoxicillin* and *clavulanate* (Augmentin)...*cefpodoxime* (Vantin)...and *cefuroxime* (Ceftin).

Important: Many people make the mistake of discontinuing the antibiotic once symptoms subside. But the drug should always be taken for the full course—typically 10 days—to ensure that the bacteria are eliminated. If symptoms are unchanged after three days, your doctor should reevaluate your condition and possibly switch antibiotics.

In addition to taking antibiotics, sinusitis sufferers should drink at least eight 8-ounce glasses of water daily. It's also important to avoid alcohol, sugary drinks and caffeinated beverages. *Other strategies to consider...*

- **Fill a bowl to one-third full with hot water,** drape a towel over your head and the bowl and inhale the steam for several minutes. The moisture helps loosen secretions in the nose, throat and lungs, making them easier to clear.
- **Use an over-the-counter (OTC) mucous thinner,** such as *guaifenesin* (Robitussin).
- **Take an OTC oral decongestant,** such as *pseudoephedrine* (Sudafed).
- **Try out an OTC spray decongestant,** such as *naphazoline* (Privine) or *oxymetazoline* (Afrin).

Caution: Never use a spray decongestant for more than three consecutive days. Doing so often triggers rebound swelling of the nose.

The saline nasal sprays are also very helpful. They clear the nose of secretions and irritants. Saline sprays can be used as frequently as every two hours.

■ Your Health ■

CHRONIC SINUSITIS

If chronic sinusitis develops, a longer course of antibiotics—typically from three to six weeks—should be taken.

Reason: Chronic sinusitis has been linked to anaerobic bacteria, especially hardy microorganisms that can survive without oxygen.

The condition is also more likely to involve multiple types of bacteria. A long-term course of antibiotics is the most effective treatment against these bacteria.

Inflammation and swelling can be reduced by using a nasal steroid spray, such as *beclomethasone* (Beconase)...or an oral steroid, such as *prednisone* (Deltasone) or *dexamethasone* (Decadron).

Oral or spray decongestants eliminate congestion. Mucous thinners promote drainage. Anticholinergic nasal sprays, such as *ipratropium bromide* (Atrovent), may help with dry secretions.

To determine if allergies are involved, your doctor should perform a skin or blood test measuring your reaction to different allergens.

Nasal fungus is also being identified in an increasing number of chronic sinusitis cases. Clinical trials are under way of two medications, *itraconazole* and *amphotericin B,* for use in sinus fungal infections.

WHEN TO SEE A SPECIALIST

If sinusitis symptoms persist longer than four weeks or if you suffer recurrent bouts of acute sinusitis, see an otolaryngologist (ear, nose and throat specialist) for a thorough exam. This should include a nasal endoscopy, in which an endoscope is passed through the nose into the sinuses to check for blockages and to collect a sample of mucus.

A CT scan of the sinuses should also be performed to check for nasal polyps, thickening of the mucous membrane, changes in bone structure or increased bone thickness.

SINUS SURGERY

If drug treatment doesn't help, sinus surgery may be your best option. New, less-invasive techniques have made sinus surgery easier and safer than ever before.

The surgical method of choice is functional endoscopic sinus surgery (FESS), in which an endoscope inserted through the nose into the sinuses is used to clean and drain the sinuses...remove an obstructive growth, such as a polyp, tumor or cyst...or to reopen or enlarge the natural openings of the sinuses to allow drainage and ventilation.

Best Time to Give Antihistamines To Children

Over-the-counter (OTC) allergy medicines can be given anytime, but allergy symptoms often peak at night or in early morning, so doses given at night do the most good. Most OTC products make kids sleepy as well, so a nighttime dose helps them get to sleep despite allergy symptoms.

Caution: Avoid products that contain a decongestant, such as *pseudoephedrine.* This is a stimulant that can override the sedating properties of the antihistamine and result in sleep problems.

Michael Smolensky, PhD, professor of environmental physiology, Houston School of Public Health at the University of Texas, and coauthor of *The Body Clock Guide to Better Health* (Henry Holt & Company).

Migraine/Bacteria Connection

Headaches can be triggered by bacteria. About 50% of chronic migraine sufferers are infected with the ulcer-causing stomach bug *Helicobacter pylori* (H. pylori).

Recent finding: Treating the infection with antibiotics reduced the frequency of migraine attacks. Among migraineurs who were also treated with supplements of the friendly bacterium *Lactobacillus,* 80% were headache-free for one year. Lactobacillus has been shown to inhibit growth of H. pylori.

If you suffer from recurrent headaches: Ask your doctor if you should be tested for H. pylori—and if treatment with antibiotics and/or Lactobacillus is right for you.

Maria Rita Gismondo, MD, professor of clinical microbiology and head of the clinical microbiology laboratory, both at the University of Milan School of Medicine, Italy.

Some Migraine Drugs Worsen the Pain

Migraine wafers, such as *rizatriptan* (Maxalt-MLT) and *zolmitriptan* (Zomig-ZMT), contain trace amounts of the artificial sweetener *aspartame* to make them more palatable when they melt on the tongue. Some people find this form of medication more convenient and easier to swallow. But aspartame triggers headaches in a small number of migraine sufferers.

If you find that aspartame triggers your headaches: Request the drug in tablet form.

Lawrence C. Newman, MD, director of The Headache Institute at St. Luke's–Roosevelt Hospital Center in New York City.

Acetaminophen/Alcohol Alert

Alcohol and *acetaminophen* do not mix. Acetaminophen—in Darvocet, Tylenol, Vicodin and other products—causes 70 to 100 deaths per year from acute liver failure, usually due to overdoses or use in combination with alcohol.

Self-defense: Never take more than eight 500-milligram acetaminophen tablets in one day. Don't take it within 48 hours of drinking alcohol. And, never use acetaminophen to treat a hangover.

Peter Draganov, MD, assistant professor of medicine, division of gastroenterology, hepatology and nutrition, University of Florida College of Medicine, Gainesville.

Health News and Breakthroughs

Pill Dosage Danger

Tablet splitting may result in inaccurate dosing. Talk to your physician or pharmacist before splitting any drug. In a recent study, when older patients used one of two commercially available tablet splitters, doses varied from 9% to 37% of the intended 50-50 split. Patients split tablets more accurately depending on the splitter used, the shape of the tablet and whether they received instructions beforehand.

Brian T. Peek, PharmD, clinical pharmacy specialist, Ambulatory Care at the Veterans Affairs Medical Center in Asheville, NC.

Don't Mix Bananas and These Antidepressants

Don't eat bananas if you take a *monoamine oxidase inhibitor* (MAOI), such as Nardil or Parnate, for depression. Bananas contain *tyramine*, an amino acid that can interfere with MAOIs and cause serious side effects, such as dangerously high blood pressure. This can lead to stroke or heart attack.

Thomas Brunoski, MD, specialist in food and environmental allergies and nutritional medicine, Westport, CT.

How Long to Keep Foods

Unsure about whether it's time to toss the lunch meat or milk? *FDA guidelines on how long it's safe to keep various foods...*

- **Ground beef.** Up to two days refrigerated...four months frozen.
- **Lean fish**—such as cod or flounder. Up to two days refrigerated...six months frozen.
- **Fatty fish**—such as bluefish or salmon. Up to two days refrigerated...two to three months frozen.
- **Whole chicken.** Up to two days refrigerated...12 months frozen.

■ *Your Health* ■

- **Luncheon meat.** Up to five days refrigerated...one to two months frozen.
- **Milk.** Five days refrigerated...one month frozen.

FDA Consumer, US Government Printing Office, Box 37195, Pittsburgh 15250.

Does Bottled Water Spoil?

According to the US Food and Drug Administration, which regulates bottled water, properly bottled and sealed water should last indefinitely. But it may pick up an unpleasant odor and taste when stored in certain sites, such as a garage, where gasoline fumes can be absorbed through the plastic bottle.

The International Bottled Water Association recommends that bottled water be kept in a cool, dry location. Be sure to store it far away from toxic substances that may be absorbed through the bottle.

Note: The expiration date printed on bottles is meant to serve as a guideline to stores for rotation of stock, not as an indication to consumers that the water is unhealthful after that date. Bottled water that has already been opened should be consumed as soon as possible.

US Food and Drug Administration, College Park, MD, *www.fda.gov*, and International Bottled Water Association, Alexandria, VA, *www.bottledwater.org*.

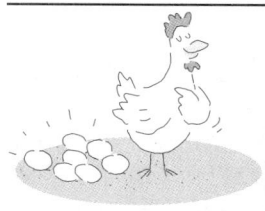

Superbugs In Poultry

A recent study of 484 broiler chickens found 42% contained *campylobacter* and 12% *salmonella*. These bacteria can cause diarrhea, fever, abdominal pain—even death. Of the bacteria tested, 90% of the campylobacter and 34% of the salmonella were resistant to one or more antibiotics. This means that people who are sickened by tainted or undercooked chicken may stay sick longer with possibly more serious illness...and doctors may have to prescribe several antibiotics before finding one that works.

Self-defense: Cook chicken to about 180°F —until the meat has no pink traces and juices run clear.

R. David Pittle, PhD, senior vice president for technical policy at *Consumer Reports*, 101 Truman Ave., Yonkers, NY 10703.

Deli Meat Danger

Precooked chicken and turkey deli meats may be contaminated with deadly *Listeria monocytogenes* bacteria. The bacteria can cause a variety of health problems, including flulike symptoms, meningitis or even miscarriage. Seven people died in a recent listeria outbreak.

Self-defense: All individuals at high risk—including young children, the elderly, pregnant women and people with impaired immunity—should eat precooked poultry products only if they have been reheated until they steam.

Caroline Smith DeWaal, JD, director of food safety, Center for Science in the Public Interest, Washington, DC, *www.cspinet.org*.

Organic Food Trap

Advertisers may claim that organic produce is grown without pesticides. But a new study has found that 23% of these fruits and vegetables contain trace amounts of pest-fighting chemicals. That's because long-lived pesticides, such as DDT, which has been banned in the US, can remain in the soil for years. Seventy-three percent of nonorganic produce contains pesticide residue, according to recent research. To be safe, wash *all* fruits and vegetables thoroughly.

Edward Groth III, PhD, senior scientist at Consumers Union, 101 Truman Ave., Yonkers, NY 10703.

■ Your Health ■

2

Getting the Very Best Medical Care

How to Survive a Trip to the ER

Each year, Americans make 100 million visits to hospital emergency rooms (ERs).* It's not news that overburdened hospital personnel are often rushed and tired, and the environment is noisy and chaotic. And because new doctors often train in emergency rooms, the person caring for you may have little or no experience treating your complaint.

To get the best possible care...

●**Speak up.** You must be as assertive in the ER as you are in all other health care situations.

Few people realize that they can request a specialist or more senior ER physician. If he/she practices in that hospital and is available, you have a good chance of being seen by the physician of your choice.

Smart idea: If you have a chronic condition, such as heart disease or emphysema, keep a list in your wallet of specialists recommended by your physician to request in case of an emergency.

At the very least, call your family doctor from the waiting room or while en route to the hospital. He may be able to meet you there—or at least make a phone call—to expedite your treatment.

●**When you are evaluated by a doctor,** focus on your main complaint. Stick to the one or two most important and distressing symptoms. Listing multiple symptoms may make diagnosis more difficult.

●**Check credentials.** You also have the right to ask about the experience levels of the doctors who treat you in the ER. Before you

---

*In the event of a life-threatening emergency, call 911. This includes uncontrolled bleeding, chest pain, shortness of breath, fainting, a sudden unexplained weakness or paralysis, falling for no apparent reason, seizure, severe abdominal pain, a worst-ever headache or change in mental function.

Joel Cohen, MD, physician practicing in Mesa, AZ. Dr. Cohen has practiced emergency and urgent-care medicine for 11 years and is author of *ER: Enter At Your Own Risk* (New Horizon).

23

■ *Your Health* ■

agree to any risky test, procedure or operation, ask how long the doctor has been practicing.

There is no single "correct" answer. But if you feel uncomfortable with the experience level of your ER doctor, ask to see the physician in charge or get a specialist consultation for a second opinion.

Helpful: If possible, bring a friend or family member with you to act as your advocate. This is especially important if you are too sick or weak to be assertive.

•**Avoid unnecessary tests and treatments.** Do *not* agree to any test unless you know the risks involved...what the test will show...and how the results will change your course of treatment.

Before allowing yourself to be treated, find out if the treatment is necessary or just a precaution...and whether treatment can wait until you've had a chance to talk with your primary-care physician. Your goal is to participate fully in the decision-making process.

Caution: Do *not* leave the hospital if you don't feel better or if you feel worse than when you first arrived. Tell the doctor that you feel just as sick...and that you would like a second opinion.

THE RIGHT DIAGNOSIS

If you're experiencing unexplained symptoms, here are the emergency tests you will need to ensure a proper diagnosis...

•**Chest pain or indigestion.** An electrocardiogram (ECG) to rule out heart disease.

•**Abdominal pain.** A complete blood count (CBC) and urinalysis to check for infection. A sonogram may be given if a physical problem, such as gallstones, is suspected. Follow up with your physician within 24 hours.

•**Shortness of breath.** An ECG, chest X ray and simple blood oxygen test to determine if there is enough oxygen in your system and to rule out a collapsed lung or heart problem.

•**Numbness or paralysis of the face or limbs, unexplained dizziness or falling.** Each of these symptoms may signal a stroke. A magnetic resonance imaging (MRI) scan provides the most detailed picture of the brain. At a minimum, a computed tomography (CT) scan should be performed to determine if a stroke has occurred. If so, these tests will identify the type of stroke, so doctors can prescribe appropriate treatment.

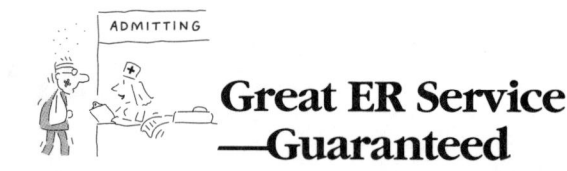

Great ER Service —Guaranteed

Emergency room guarantees are being provided by some hospitals to attract patients. They promise that patients will be seen within 30 minutes. Those who must wait longer get personal apologies, gifts, such as movie tickets, or even free care for that visit. Hospitals giving the guarantees say it makes them more efficient in treating patients. Some doctors worry that the guarantees might compromise medical care —but it is too soon to tell.

Charles Inlander, president, People's Medical Society, Box 868, Allentown, PA 18105, and author of *Take This Book to the Hospital with You* (St. Martin's).

More from Charles Inlander...

Don't Be Afraid to Visit a Hospital Patient

Hospital visitors need not worry about picking up a bug from patients. Visitors are more likely to bring in germs that would affect patients—whose immune systems are weakened—than to get sick themselves. Most visitors do not stay in the hospital long enough to be exposed to anything infectious. Patients who are highly infectious often can't have visitors at all. Use common sense when visiting so you do not bring in a minor infection, such as a cold, that could be dangerous to hospital patients. Be particularly careful when visiting the maternity ward.

Also from Charles Inlander...

Older Drugs May Be Better Than Newer Versions

Updated—and more expensive—versions of old drugs may not be much better for you. Some drug companies will make small changes to existing medications and apply for new patents. The new products typically are only 3% to 5% more effective than the older ones. But they can cost 40% to 50% more.

Example: Clarinex is a slightly stronger form of Claritin, which is now available over the counter.

Self-defense: Ask your doctor about drug options. Don't switch blindly.

Finally from Charles Inlander...

How to Get Drugs Not Yet FDA Approved

Medicines not yet FDA approved may be available for patients who demonstrate real need. The patient's doctor has to recommend the patient, and the drug has to be in the human-testing stage or beyond. Find out about *compassionate use* programs, for conditions ranging from lung cancer to obesity, at drug manufacturers' Web sites or search for "Expanded Access" at *www.clinicaltrials.gov*.

How Dangerous Medication Mistakes Can Be Avoided

Netra Thakur, MD, practicing physician and clinical assistant professor of family medicine, Jefferson Medical College of Thomas Jefferson University Hospital, Philadelphia. She is a member of the American Academy of Family Physicians.

Medication mistakes—such as forgetting to take drugs at the proper times or taking more or less than the prescribed amounts—account for about 10% of all hospital admissions.

Here are the most common mistakes—and how to prevent them...

Mistake #1: **Ignoring directions on the label.** Check the label for the right dosage. Taking the wrong dose of a medication can be very dangerous.

Example: Taking too much of a blood thinner can cause internal bleeding. Labels also state other directions. For example, you may need to take painkillers with food to prevent stomach upset.

What to do: Every time you get a new drug or a refill, review the label and the pharmacy drug summary.

Mistake #2: **Missing doses.** It's easy to forget to take your medications at the appropriate times.

What to do: Keep bottles where you will see them, such as on your desk or next to your toothbrush. If you take multiple medicines, use a pillbox that has a compartment for each day.

Important: If you forget to take a dose, read the package insert for directions or ask your doctor or pharmacist. For some drugs, such as antibiotics, you can usually take a double dose at the next scheduled time. For others, such as blood pressure drugs, it is safer to skip the missed dose and then take your usual amount at the next scheduled time.

Mistake #3: **Not knowing which drugs you take.** If you don't know the names of all the drugs you're taking—and you aren't sure why you're taking them—there is no way to know if your doctor or pharmacist accidentally gives you the wrong ones.

Different drugs will sometimes have similar names. For example, the cough medicine Benylin can be very easily confused with the antihistamine Benadryl.

If you don't know what drugs you're taking, you also won't be able to alert doctors in an emergency. You could be given the wrong treatment in a hospital emergency room.

Example: Beta-blockers, which are often used to control high blood pressure, can cause severe asthma-like symptoms.

What to do: Before leaving your doctor's office with a prescription, ask him/her to write down the medication's name and why you need to take it. Review this information with the pharmacist.

Mistake #4: **Failing to recognize side effects of the drug.** Patients do not always make the connection between a drug and symptoms that are actually side effects.

■ *Your Health* ■

Example: Blood pressure drugs called ACE inhibitors can cause a dry cough that may be dismissed as a sign of a cold or allergy.

What to do: Tell your physician about any symptom that begins after starting a new drug, even if it seems unrelated. Most side effects can be reduced or eliminated by switching drugs or adjusting the dose, with medical supervision.

Mistake #5: **Insisting on new drugs.** Both patients and doctors can be influenced by magazine and TV advertisements for "new and improved" drugs. The vast majority of new drugs have few or no advantages over older ones. They also may be riskier because they haven't been on the market long enough for doctors to know much about side effects or complications, some of which might not emerge until years later.

What to do: Ask your doctor if the new drug he/she is prescribing is clearly superior to older available medication.

Mistake #6: **Combining prescription drugs with supplements.** The risk of side effects rises sharply when you combine prescription drugs with herbs, dietary supplements or over-the-counter (OTC) medicines.

Examples: Garlic supplements increase the risk of internal bleeding when combined with the blood-thinner *warfarin* (Coumadin) ...vitamin C may increase iron absorption, which can be dangerous for some people... and the herb ephedra may interact with many cardiac drugs.

What to do: Tell your doctor about all supplements and OTC drugs you take.

Mistake #7: **Stockpiling drugs.** No one wants to throw away expensive drugs that might be useful in the future. Keeping drugs that you are not using, however, increases the chance that you will take the wrong one by mistake.

What to do: Throw out any drug that you are no longer using or is well beyond the expiration date.

Mistake #8: **Poor communication.** People with multiple health problems usually receive drugs from different specialists—rheumatologists, cardiologists, internists, etc. It is unlikely that any one of the doctors knows exactly what medications the others are prescribing. Patients can even get prescriptions for the same drug from two different doctors. The same drug may be sold under different names...or different drugs may be prescribed for the same purpose.

What to do: Ask your primary doctor to review all your prescriptions. Put the drugs in a paper bag, and take them to the doctor. Or e-mail, fax or mail a list to your physician. A "brown-bag review" ensures that you aren't taking drugs unnecessarily...you are getting the right dosages...and the drugs aren't interacting in harmful ways.

Buy all prescription drugs at the same pharmacy. Most pharmacies use computers to track prescriptions and can alert you to duplications or potential interactions.

Self-Defense Against Prescription Mistakes

To avoid prescription mistakes, take time at your doctor's office to write down the generic and brand names of the medicine and its purpose and proper dosage. Also, remind your doctor and pharmacist of any drug allergies you have and other medicines you are taking—including over-the-counter or herbal medicines and vitamins. Check refills to be sure pills are the same color and size as before. Call in refills a day or two ahead so the pharmacist doesn't rush to fill them. Finally, avoid ordering prescriptions on Monday—pharmacists' busiest day.

Rosemary Soave, MD, associate professor of medicine, Cornell University Medical College, New York City.

Drug Overdosing Danger

Larry Sasich, pharmacist and drug analyst at the Washington, DC–based health watchdog group Public Citizen.

According to recent findings published in *Pharmacoepidemiology and Drug Safety,* more than one in five new drugs are initially marketed at the wrong dosage. In fact, researchers report that some recommended dosages are *twice* as high as they should be.

Drugs are typically tested in men ages 20 to 50. Yet a dosage that's appropriate for a 30-year-old man might be dangerously high for women and children. Adults over age 60 are particularly at risk because they don't eliminate drugs from their bodies as efficiently as younger people.

Higher drug dosages are among the main causes of side effects.

Examples: Sexual dysfunction from *fluoxetine* (Prozac)...or muscle pain from *atorvastatin* (Lipitor).

To protect yourself...

•**Avoid new drugs.** If possible, don't take any new drug until it's been on the market for a minimum of seven years. It could take that long for doctors to identify the optimum dosage—and for any serious problems to emerge.

•**Ask your doctor for the lowest possible dosage.**

Best advice: Start low, go slow.

•**Monitor for side effects.** Assume that any new health problem may be caused by a drug you've recently started taking—even if it seems unrelated.

New-Drug Dangers

One-fifth of the 548 drugs approved by the Food and Drug Administration over the past 25 years turned out to have serious side effects that were not known when they were approved. Seven of the drugs, which were later withdrawn from the market, had side effects so severe that they may have contributed to more than 1,000 deaths.

Self-defense: Avoid drugs that have been on the market for fewer than five years. If your doctor prescribes a new drug, ask whether there are older, time-tested alternatives.

Karen Lasser, MD, instructor in medicine, Harvard Medical School, Boston, and leader of a study published in *The Journal of the American Medical Association.*

All About Generics

A generic drug is the chemical equivalent of a brand-name drug. *Ibuprofen,* for example, is the generic version of Motrin IB. The Food and Drug Administration (FDA) requires generics to have the same active ingredients, strength, purity and stability as their brand-name counterparts—that's called being "bioequivalent." Yet they cost considerably less—generics save consumers an estimated $8 million to $10 million a year at retail pharmacies. The only difference between the two may be in the inactive ingredients, such as the dyes and coatings used.

To find out if a brand-name drug that you take regularly has a generic equivalent, contact the FDA/Center for Drug Evaluation and Research at *www.fda.gov/cder/ogd* (click on "Drug Information") or call 888-463-6332.

Nancy Dunnan, financial adviser and author in New York City. Her latest book is *How to Invest $50–$5,000* (HarperCollins).

Has Your Medication Been Switched?

Health insurers often switch patients to a different prescription drug based on the drug formulary (a listing of prescription drugs covered by an insurance company).

But, according to recent research, 22% of patients who were switched to another prescription drug reported side effects from the new medication.

In addition, switching drugs can cost patients an average of $58.50 more in out-of-pocket expenses, including extra trips to their health care providers, additional medications and/or hospital visits.

Self-defense: If your health insurer changes your prescription based on a drug formulary, check with your doctor.

David Chess, MD, chairman and president, Project Patient Care, a Stratford, CT–based nonprofit organization dedicated to improving patient care.

■ *Your Health* ■

Check Your Medication Dosage

Do the antihistamines make you extremely tired—more than they do other people? Do you have paradoxical reactions, in which a medicine does the opposite of what it is supposed to do? Standard drug dosages are too high for up to 20% of patients.

When prescribed a new medication: Ask your physician if you can halve the recommended dose, then work up to the standard dose over a few days or weeks.

Richard N. Podell, MD, chronic fatigue expert and clinical professor, Robert Wood Johnson Medical School, New Brunswick, NJ.

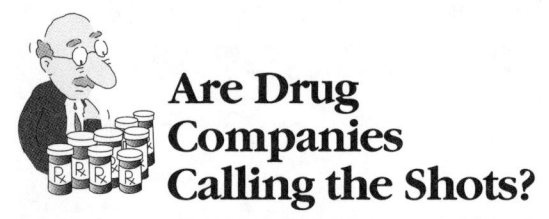

Are Drug Companies Calling the Shots?

Timothy McCall, MD, Boston internist, medical editor of *Yoga Journal* and author of *Examining Your Doctor: A Patient's Guide to Avoiding Harmful Medical Care* (Citadel).

Drug companies spend an enormous amount of time and money trying to influence the prescribing habits of physicians. And they do it for one reason—it works. Millions of dollars spent in swaying physicians can result in billions of dollars of revenue from exorbitantly priced "blockbuster" drugs.

Unfortunately, this practice is usually not in the best interest of the patient. This point was recently driven home by a major new study showing that old-fashioned diuretics—"water pills" costing pennies a pill—were more effective for high blood pressure than heavily promoted drugs costing a buck or more a pill.

As a patient, you simply want the best medical care you can get. You'd like your doctors' recommendations to be based on science and common sense—not on the marketing efforts of the drug companies.

How can you tell if your doctor is overly influenced by the drug companies? Here are a few warning signs. (Keep in mind, however, that it's a pattern—not an individual transgression—that most suggests a problem.)

• **The doctor prescribes drugs promoted with freebies.** Be careful if the name on your prescription matches the name on the pens, notepads, posters or other drug company freebies littering your doctor's office. Personally, I don't think doctors should accept any such promotional materials. It can subtly influence their prescribing behavior, and the expense contributes to the high cost of drugs.

• **The doctor never prescribes generics.** For most drugs, generics are every bit as effective as the name brand. Doctors who prefer a name brand ought to have a good reason why and be able to articulate it if you ask. Similarly, if there is *never* a generic version of the drugs your doctor recommends, it means that he/she is favoring the newer, more expensive drugs. (Generics become available only after the patent expires on brand-name drugs.)

• **The doctor gives "a pill for every ill."** Handing a patient a prescription is one way some busy doctors signal that your appointment time is up. But often, what's best is to explore nondrug options, such as exercise, dietary changes and stress-reduction strategies, before resorting to drugs. It takes longer to explain nondrug options, however, so this route is increasingly a thing of the past for too many doctors.

• **The doctor is always willing to prescribe drugs you request.** In recent years, drug companies have realized that another way to manipulate doctors is to advertise directly to patients, who then ask their doctors for specific medications. But often, direct-to-patient ads are for drugs that you don't need or that may not be the best choice for your condition. Good doctors refuse to go along—at least some of the time—with patient requests. They may suggest a better alternative or explain why no drug is needed. Some patients may be disappointed, and it can be bad for business. But the best doctors know when to just say, "no."

Getting the Very Best Medical Care

More from Timothy McCall...

Why You Really Need to Have an Annual Physical

Though most people seem to value the ritual of an annual checkup, much of what happens in those exams—listening to the heart and lungs, doing a urinalysis, an electrocardiogram (ECG) and routine blood tests—is not very useful for people who are feeling fine. Those tests aren't likely to find anything wrong if you don't have symptoms.

Other tests that typically occur during annual exams are of proven value. These include cholesterol measurement, Pap smears and, for those over age 50, colon and breast cancer screening. Experts are still debating whether women in their 40s should have mammograms. Prostate-specific antigen (PSA) testing has also been controversial. Recent evidence suggests, however, that the test, administered annually, may be worthwhile for men between the ages of 50 and 70.

Still, the value of an annual physical exam isn't based primarily on tests. Much of what really matters in good preventive medicine is talking with the doctor. That's why I still think the annual exam is worthwhile. Advice about diet, quitting smoking, stress reduction and the like are among the most powerful preventive tools a doctor has. The longer the doctor spends talking with you and answering your questions, the better.

An annual exam might not be necessary if your doctor incorporates prevention into the course of the normal medical care you receive for, say, a cold or a bum knee. The problem is that doctors are so rushed these days that they barely have enough time to treat the problems you're there for—much less advise you on how to start an exercise program or lower your risk for heart attack. Studies confirm that skipping the annual physical often means some worthwhile preventive services—such as updating your vaccinations, doing a careful breast exam or checking your entire body for skin cancer—get overlooked.

Another benefit of an annual physical is that it provides a chance to get to know your doctor. In this age of managed care, many people have changed insurers and been forced to give up long-standing relationships with their physicians. As a result, many of us hardly know our primary-care doctors.

Since topflight medical care can depend on the doctor knowing you—as well as you trusting the doctor—the annual exam provides a chance to solidify the relationship. An expert might tell us that tapping on your knees is a waste of time and money. But, if while checking your reflexes, the doctor ends up asking you about your job, family or sources of life stress, the information could allow him/her to serve you better down the road.

The annual exam also gives you an opportunity to evaluate your doctor. Is he talking to you about prevention? Reviewing all your medications, including vitamins and supplements? Making a real effort to get to know you as a human being? Clues you pick up during an annual exam about the physician's competence, values and communication style should help determine whether this is someone you would like to have in your corner the next time you really need a doctor.

Why You Must Know The Medical History Of Your Family

Christopher Friedrich, MD, PhD, associate professor of medical genetics at the University of Mississippi Medical Center in Jackson. He is also a member of the working group on family history at the Centers for Disease Control and Prevention Office of Genomics in Atlanta.

An accurate, up-to-date family medical history is one of the most important tools you have for safeguarding your health. It offers a road map to your own genetic strengths and weaknesses, pinpointing the ailments for which you need frequent screening tests and an aggressive prevention plan.

Dr. Christopher Friedrich tells what you need to know about your family medical history and what to do with this information...

■ *Your Health* ■

●**If I have a healthful lifestyle, do I still need to learn my family medical history?** Absolutely. Most diseases have an environmental *and* genetic component. For example, a high-fat diet and smoking may lead to coronary artery disease. But genetic factors help determine your vulnerability.

Likewise, your risk of developing lung cancer or emphysema depends on your smoking habits *and* on your genetic susceptibility to the effects of smoking.

Knowing your family medical history will allow you and your doctor to monitor for symptoms and alter your lifestyle so that you can drastically reduce your chances of developing these diseases.

Thousands of rare diseases, such as cystic fibrosis and hemophilia, are entirely hereditary. If one of these diseases runs in your family, you may want to consider genetic testing.

●**Isn't it my doctor's responsibility to ask about my family medical history?** Your doctor should ask about your family medical history during your first visit. However, completing this history is a cooperative effort, requiring your active input.

Your physician needs to know about any medical condition affecting your first-degree relatives—parents and siblings.

Tell your doctor if any first- or second-degree relative (grandparent, aunt or uncle) suffered from inherited diseases, such as sickle cell anemia…cystic fibrosis…hemophilia…Parkinson's disease…Marfan syndrome (a connective tissue disorder)…or muscular dystrophy.

Also tell your doctor if any of the following diseases are in your family: Alzheimer's, asthma/allergies, blood disorders, cancer, diabetes, epilepsy, eye conditions, heart disease, high blood pressure, kidney disease, mental illness, osteoporosis and stroke. And indicate if there has been any substance abuse or smoking in your family.

●**What other things do I need to know about the medical conditions that have affected my relatives?** The age when a disease first strikes can be *extremely* important, because this may indicate your family's level of genetic vulnerability. Heart attack, stroke, bypass surgery or angioplasty in a first-degree male relative under age 45 or in a female relative under age 55 may indicate strong genetic susceptibility.

The age when high blood pressure, diabetes or cancer strikes is also significant. The earlier these conditions show up, the more likely a genetic risk factor is involved.

●**Will my family medical history tell me anything other than possible lifestyle changes I should make?** Your family history can also indicate when early screening is warranted to detect diseases in their early stages when they're most treatable.

●If you have a first-degree relative with hypertension, you should get annual blood pressure checks starting at age 18.

●If you have a first-degree relative with heart disease or high cholesterol, you should start cholesterol testing in your mid-teens and continue on a schedule recommended by your doctor.

●If cancer of the breast, ovaries or colon has occurred in three or more relatives (or two relatives, including one under age 40), you should get mammograms (for breast cancer), CA-125 blood tests (for ovarian cancer) and colonoscopies (for colon cancer) beginning at age 40, or at the earliest age of diagnosis in the family, if under the age of 40.

●If you're male and your father, uncle or brother had prostate cancer, you should consider annual examinations and prostate-specific antigen (PSA) testing starting at age 45.

●**If my family history suggests a specific genetic vulnerability, should I undergo genetic testing?** Most genetic vulnerabilities have not yet been traced to specific gene mutations, so they can't be tested for. Even with diseases such as polycystic kidney disease and Marfan syndrome, which are linked to specific mutations, the case for testing isn't always clear.

In families with a history of breast cancer, which has been linked to two specific gene mutations (BRCA1 and BRCA2), testing is probably a good idea. If you turn out to have one or both mutations, then you can be extra vigilant with self-exams and mammograms.

One of the major advantages of genetic testing for cancer susceptibility is that it identifies those who may benefit from earlier and more frequent monitoring than is recommended for the general public. Testing will also identify those who did not inherit their family's mutation and do not need to undergo more intensive monitoring.

With inherited diseases, such as sickle cell anemia, it makes sense to test the extended family (aunts, uncles, cousins, nieces and nephews) as well as the immediate family to identify the carriers for the gene mutation (meaning they could pass the mutation to their own children).

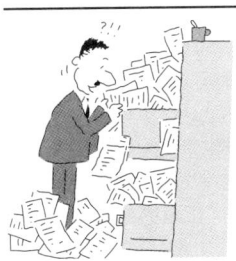

Do Your Own Medical Research

Carol Svec, a Raleigh, NC–based researcher, medical writer and patient advocate. She is the author of *After Any Diagnosis: How to Take Action Against Your Illness Using the Best and Most Current Medical Information Available* (Crown).

If you have always trusted your doctors to stay up to date on medical treatments, you are taking a big chance.

Every year, more than 3,000 biomedical journals are published. Every year, the Food and Drug Administration approves more than 500 new or updated drugs and more than 3,000 new medical devices. No doctor can keep up with all these innovations.

Patients must fill in the gaps by becoming experts on any medical condition from which they suffer. Studies show that informed patients spend fewer days in the hospital, lose fewer days of work, feel less depressed and report lower levels of pain.

EASIER SEARCHES

The Internet has made gathering medical information easier than ever before. There are nearly 10,000 Web sites on specific diseases and conditions.

To find reliable information, start with Web sites sponsored by government agencies (with URL addresses that end in *.gov*), educational institutions (with addresses ending in *.edu*) or nonprofit organizations (which end in *.org*).

Find one or two good Web sites and consult them periodically. For common disorders, such as diabetes, multiple sclerosis or asthma, checking back once a month is sufficient. For rare diseases, once every six months is plenty, because breakthroughs occur so infrequently.

Exception: For life-threatening diseases, check *every week* for updates and any new clinical trials.

Do not let the search become an obsession. Gathering information may help you feel "in control," but when the paper chase starts controlling you, it's time to scale back the search.

USING INFORMATION WISELY

Some physicians don't reveal all medical options to their patients—because they think patients will be confused by the choices or because the physicians specialize in a particular treatment.

For example, a surgical oncologist may be more inclined to recommend treating cancer with surgery, rather than with radiation or chemotherapy.

If you are well-informed, you'll be able to discuss all treatment options, make sound medical decisions and avoid health scams.

Work in partnership with your physician. Doctors know the medical facts, but patients know how they're feeling. *Some good ways to stay involved...*

•**Talk openly with your doctor about wanting to participate in your own care.** Most encourage their patients to become active information seekers. If your doctor objects, find a new one.

•**Keep your physician in the loop.** Don't try any new medication, supplement, herb or device without discussing it with your physician. Make sure it won't interfere with your current treatment.

•**Stay in touch *between* your appointments.** Questions often arise between office visits. Ask your doctor how he/she prefers to respond to these inquiries.

Good choices: Sending E-mail (if you're not worried about privacy), talking on the phone after office hours or consulting with a nurse or physician's assistant. If these strategies do not work, it may be necessary to book a separate appointment.

•Don't deluge your doctor with written material. Bring no more than three articles to your physician per visit. That's all a physician will be able to evaluate during the standard appointment.

•Track your progress. Request copies of all your medical reports (blood tests, X rays, etc.) and keep them in a file. Log all monitoring information, such as blood pressure or glucose levels. Note any changes since your last office visit, including new pain or other symptoms and steps you've taken to control them.

Take your file to each doctor's appointment. This information lets the doctor know what's happening between office visits, and it provides a quick reference in case you change doctors or require emergency care.

STOP SCARING YOURSELF

Health statistics can be confusing and frightening. When assessing these numbers, remember that they are based on the *average* outcome of research involving thousands of patients.

Example: If a disease is said to have a 50% death rate, the statistic is based on reports from a broad sample of people who have had the disease. This includes those people who have had extensive treatment as well as others who opted for no treatment.

Statistics are used for understanding the seriousness of a disease, but they should never be used to predict an individual's outcome. Do *not* let numbers alone make you lose hope. *Before you worry over a study reported in the news, find out…*

•Did the study involve humans? Animal studies are a valuable first step, but the same results are not always found in people.

•How many people participated in the study? The more subjects, the better. If a study uses fewer than 100 subjects, don't take it too seriously.

•Were the participants similar to you? Did they have the same disease? Were they of the same sex and of a similar age? Unless the subjects were people just like you, the study may not be relevant.

Beware of "Normal" Test Results

Leo Galland, MD, director, Foundation for Integrated Medicine, New York City, and author of *Power Healing: Use the New Integrated Medicine to Cure Yourself* (Random House).

Susan Leclair, PhD, professor of medical laboratory science at University of Massachusetts, Dartmouth.

Are you relieved when your doctor's office calls to say your lab test results are "normal"?

Counts that look okay do not necessarily mean you are okay. Nor do high or low counts always mean health problems.

Key: Patients should ask their doctors for copies of test results and to compare current and past results to see if anything has changed significantly. Your doctor should be doing this —but don't rely on it.

Among the counts that patients should be sure to ask about…

•Hemoglobin/hematocrit. High levels may signal dehydration…low levels, anemia.

•Mean corpuscular volume (MCV). Low levels usually mean an iron deficiency. High values often disappear with retesting. If not, they may indicate liver disease or a vitamin B12 deficiency, etc.

•White blood cells and platelets. Investigate high or low levels of either. Causes could range from an infection to bleeding disorders to leukemia.

•Albumin. Values under 4.0 may suggest liver problems or chronic inflammation.

•Blood glucose. A fasting level over 110 suggests a prediabetic condition…over 126, probably diabetes.

•Calcium. High counts usually disappear on repeat tests. If not, parathyroid glands may be malfunctioning.

•Cholesterol. High LDL ("bad") cholesterol counts are the most important. Total cholesterol is less significant.

There is no "one-size-fits-all" interpretation of results. Discuss them with your doctor in conjunction with symptoms and personal or family history of disease. That 10 minutes could add years to your life.

Female Doctors Have Better Bedside Manners Than Male Doctors

Women MDs spend an average of 23 minutes with patients, compared with 21 minutes for male doctors. Female physicians who talk more about lifestyle and social issues, such as the advantages of exercising with a friend or the challenges of raising teenagers, are more likely to engage in positive health-related discussions, including the patient's feelings about diet restrictions. Other studies have linked this communication style to patient satisfaction, compliance with medical recommendations and improvements in health.

Debra Roter, DrPH, professor of health policy and management, Johns Hopkins University, Baltimore.

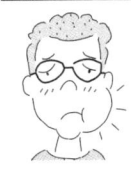

How to Relax at The Dentist

Many people feel apprehensive when going to the dentist. *To help alleviate stress, follow this advice...*

- **To feel more in control,** have the dentist explain the procedure.
- **Take an active role in decisions** about your treatment.
- **Communicate your fears to the dentist** so he/she can help you cope with them.
- **Agree on a signal,** such as raising your hand, to indicate that you need a short break during treatment.
- **Find a distraction**—many dentists now offer TV, headsets with music, etc.
- **Review pain-control options,** such as premedication with something to help you relax or local or general anesthesia.

D. Scott Navarro, DDS, national oral health adviser, Delta Dental Plans Association, Oak Brook, IL.

Doctors Making House Calls Again?

Doctors' house calls just might be making a comeback.

Reasons: Medicare pays physicians more for house calls than for office visits—perhaps up to 69% more in the most complicated cases—in order to compensate the doctor for his/her time and travel expenses. Many elderly patients may be frail or suffering from dementia and have difficulty getting to a doctor's office.

Centers for Medicare and Medicaid Services, Baltimore.

Important Presurgery Test

Before undergoing surgery, ask your doctor to check your albumin levels. A deficiency of this blood protein increases your chances of suffering postoperative bleeding or an infection by 50% or more. Few hospital patients are screened for low albumin prior to surgery. Albumin deficiency, which can be detected by an inexpensive blood test, may indicate malnutrition, and can generally be corrected with a more nutritious diet prescribed by a dietitian.

James Gibbs, PhD, research assistant professor, Institute for Health Services Research and Policy Studies, Northwestern University, Evanston, IL.

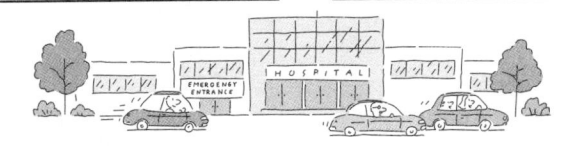

■ *Your Health* ■

Stop Herbs Before Surgery

Stop taking all herbs two weeks before surgery. *Ginseng* can increase heart rate and blood pressure—potentially dangerous for any patient undergoing anesthesia. *Ephedra* (ma huang) can raise blood pressure and heart rate to dangerous levels, and cause cerebral hemorrhage, stroke or heart attack. Be sure your doctor knows *everything* you take regularly—all medications, vitamins and herbal products.

Frederick W. Ernst, MD, anesthesiologist, Dothan, AL, and coauthor of *Now They Lay Me Down to Sleep* (available from the author, *www.fwernstmd.com*).

No Need for Lengthy Presurgery Fasting

More than 90% of patients surveyed had been told to ingest nothing after midnight the night before surgery. Fasting 12 hours or more may result in severe thirst, headaches and hypoglycemia. Since 1999, the American Society of Anesthesiologists has allowed preoperative patients to have clear liquids until two hours before surgery, a light breakfast six hours before and a heavier meal eight hours before.

Self-defense: Discuss guidelines with your doctor and anesthetist or anesthesiologist.

Jeannette Crenshaw, MSN, RN, family education coordinator, Presbyterian Hospital of Dallas, and leader of a study of 155 preoperative patients, reported in *The American Journal of Nursing*.

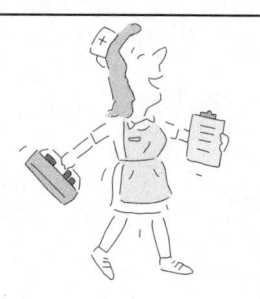

Safer Surgery

Bloodless surgery eliminates the risk of contracting hepatitis or other viral infections from someone else's blood. Also, many patients go home sooner and experience less fatigue. Collecting, filtering and reusing the patient's own blood during an operation carries only a slight risk of bacterial contamination.

The greatest blood loss occurs in cardiovascular, gynecologic and orthopedic surgeries. Patients considering such procedures should ask their surgeons what steps will be taken to minimize blood loss and reduce the need for a transfusion.

Patricia A. Ford, MD, medical director, The Center for Bloodless Medicine & Surgery, Pennsylvania Hospital, and assistant professor of medicine, University of Pennsylvania, both in Philadelphia.

Do You Need to See a Dietitian?

It's wise to see a dietitian when…you have a family history of an illness, such as heart disease, cancer or diabetes, and want to reduce your risk…you have trouble controlling snacking behavior…you feel low on energy, and a physical exam shows no reason…you are trying to lose weight, but the diet is not working …or you are a vegetarian trying to get all the nutrients you need.

Cost: $60 to $100 per hour. Check with your insurance company about coverage.

To find a qualified dietitian: Ask your doctor for a recommendation, or contact the American Dietetic Association (800-877-1600 or *www.eatright.org*).

Cynthia Sass, RD, dietitian in private practice, Tampa, and spokesperson, American Dietetic Association.

■ Your Health ■

3 Quick Fixes For Common Problems

How to Get to Sleep And Stay Asleep

An occasional night without sleep is an annoyance, but persistent insomnia—and the crushing fatigue that results—can threaten your health and the health of others.

The National Highway Traffic Safety Administration reports that insufficient sleep contributes to more than 100,000 traffic accidents each year. People with chronic insomnia often underperform at work...have family problems...and are four times more likely to suffer from depression than those who sleep soundly.

WHAT CAUSES INSOMNIA?

Some people are born with a neurological "hardwiring" that causes *hyperarousal*—the brain stays alert when it is time to sleep. Other causes...

•**Negative life experiences,** such as a stressful family life or childhood abuse. Stress and anxiety inhibit sleep by causing the brain to remain "on guard."

•**Medical problems,** such as restless legs syndrome, which causes leg pain or discomfort at night...and sleep apnea, a condition in which breathing periodically stops—sometimes hundreds of times each night.

Restless legs syndrome is usually treated with medication, vitamins and other preventive measures. Sleep apnea may require surgery, respiratory devices and/or exercise.

•**Menopause.** About one in four women experiencing menopause has insomnia. Hormonal changes and the resulting hot flashes and night sweats can disrupt sleep.

•**Disruptions of the body's internal clock.** Individuals with *advanced sleep phase syndrome* fall asleep very early in the evening and wake up very early in the morning. People with *delayed sleep phase syndrome* fall

---

Karl Doghramji, MD, director, Sleep Disorders Center, Thomas Jefferson University Hospital, and professor of psychiatry, Jefferson Medical College, both in Philadelphia, *www.jeffersonhospital.org/sleep.*

■ *Your Health* ■

asleep very late and wake up late the following day.

BEST TREATMENTS

Insomnia that is caused by a medical problem or hormonal change will generally clear up when the underlying condition is treated. Other cases usually require a combination of drug and behavioral treatments. Drugs will provide immediate relief. Behavioral therapy has long-term benefits that may make medication unnecessary. Psychotherapy may also be necessary to relieve anxiety.

Nearly everyone with insomnia sleeps better when they develop better lifestyle habits. *Some behavioral approaches...*

- **Relax an hour before bedtime.** Read, listen to music, take a hot bath. Or try yoga, meditation or deep breathing. Avoid activities that bring on anxiety, such as paying bills or watching the news.
- **After noon, avoid caffeine**—coffee, cola, black or green tea, chocolate and some pain medications, such as Excedrin. Even in small amounts, caffeine can disrupt sleep in vulnerable individuals. Foods containing *L-tryptophan*, such as milk and turkey, may promote sleep, but studies in this area are unclear.
- **Don't drink alcohol at night.** It makes sleep less restful.
- **Go to bed and get up at the same time every day,** even on weekends. Avoid naps, even short ones. They make it harder to fall asleep at night.
- **Exercise for at least 30 minutes daily.** Weight lifting, aerobic workouts and other exercise may promote sleep. Don't exercise within three hours of bedtime because it temporarily raises alertness. I recommend *outdoor* morning exercise—exposure to light helps regulate the body clock.
- **Listen to relaxation tapes.** Some people sleep better when they listen to recordings of whale songs or forest or ocean sounds before going to bed. When sleep is disturbed by traffic or other noise, sound generators that produce "white noise" can help, as can earplugs.

OTHER TECHNIQUES

For patients with more severe sleep problems, I sometimes suggest that they chart their sleep for about two weeks. They write down when they go to bed, wake in the night, get up in the morning, etc. so they can estimate how much time they actually spend sleeping. I then have them limit themselves to that amount of time in bed each night. This eliminates the frustration of tossing and turning.

Example: Suppose a patient normally spends eight hours in bed but sleeps for about five. I might suggest he/she go to bed at midnight and set the alarm for 5 am. If he is sleeping soundly, I might increase the time in bed by about 15 minutes every few days, as long as he continues to sleep soundly.

I also sometimes recommend light therapy. Patients sit in front of a light box for 30 minutes daily to reset their body clocks. They do this first thing in the morning if they have trouble falling asleep and in the afternoon or evening if they wake up too early. Middle-of-the-night awakenings usually aren't caused by body clock disturbances and aren't likely to respond to light therapy.

Light boxes and lamps that produce 10,000 lux—the recommended amount of light—are available from Light Therapy Products (800-486-6723 or *www.lighttherapyproducts.com*).

DRUGS

The most commonly prescribed drugs for insomnia, *zolpidem* (Ambien) and *zaleplon* (Sonata), are relatively safe and effective when taken under a physician's supervision. They provide rapid relief for many insomniacs. This can diminish the fear of further sleeplessness, which can be a strong force behind the perpetuation and escalation of insomnia.

Doctors generally advise these medications be used for short periods of time, usually two weeks. However, some chronic insomniacs need them for longer periods. Ambien, taken at bedtime, works for seven to eight hours. It helps people get to sleep and eliminates any middle-of-the-night awakenings. Sonata wears off in four hours. It can be taken at bedtime if you have trouble falling asleep or in the middle of the night if you wake up.

Long-acting *benzodiazepines* (Dalmane, Doral, Valium) are effective but may cause a daytime "hangover effect." The shorter-acting benzodiazepine, Halcion, causes less of a hangover effect, but a decrease in the drug's effectiveness over time can necessitate increasing the dose. It has also been linked to rebound insomnia, which can be even worse than the original insomnia.

Over-the-counter products that contain the antihistamine *diphenhydramine*—Benadryl, Tylenol PM, etc.—may work well for some individuals. But the effects of diphenhydramine are unpredictable. Some people don't get the necessary sedation to help them sleep. Others experience next-day drowsiness.

HERBS AND SUPPLEMENTS

The herb valerian, as a supplement or a tea, may help. Studies are needed before its use can be endorsed. There is little evidence that kava or melatonin supplements work—and they may be harmful. Melatonin supplements have been linked to infertility and heart damage. Kava may cause liver damage.

To find a doctor who specializes in sleep disorders, contact the American Academy of Sleep Medicine (708-492-0930 or *www.aasmnet.org*).

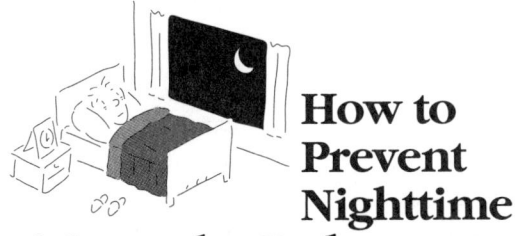

How to Prevent Nighttime Visits to the Bathroom

Put an end to nighttime bathroom visits by avoiding bladder irritants, such as citrus fruits, spicy foods and nicotine...and diuretic drinks, including anything containing caffeine or alcohol, for several hours before bedtime. Also, drink your last fluids of the day no later than three hours before bedtime. Most fluids will be in your bladder by the time you are ready for sleep, so you should be able to use the bathroom and then sleep through the night.

Gary Lemack, MD, assistant professor of urology, University of Texas Southwestern Medical Center, Dallas.

Nighttime Leg Cramp Relief

To alleviate a leg cramp at night, flex your foot up. Point toes at the ceiling and hold until cramping stops. Or stand up, bend your knee and place your weight on the affected leg for a few minutes—this stretches out the calf muscle. A heat pad or ice pack may provide some relief.

To prevent cramps: Drink six to eight glasses of water daily so you do not become dehydrated. Loosen bed covers so toes do not point downward while you sleep. Stretch calf muscles regularly during the day. Riding a stationary bike before bed and regular aquatic exercise may also help.

Mary McGrae McDermott, MD, assistant professor of medicine and preventive medicine at Feinberg School of Medicine, Northwestern University, Chicago.

A Simple Way to Avoid Infectious Diseases

David Gilbert, MD, past president of the Infectious Diseases Society of America, Alexandria, VA.

Each year, the bacteria and viruses that spread through hospitals infect two million Americans. About 90,000 of these people die as a result of these infections. Lax handwashing practices among health care workers are largely to blame.

The Centers for Disease Control and Prevention has issued new guidelines advising doctors and nurses to replace soap and water with fast-drying alcohol gels. Gels are much more convenient—and they kill more germs than soap and water. Regular use of alcohol gels could halve the rate of hospital-acquired infections, new studies indicate.

Outside the hospital setting, alcohol gels are a convenient way to "wash up" at restaurants, picnics, portable toilets and on airplanes. At home, the gels may be a good idea

■ *Your Health* ■

if someone in the family has a cold or has a severely compromised immune system, which makes him/her vulnerable to infections.

If everyone in the household is healthy, plain old soap and water suffices. Just be sure to wash your entire hand, including the back and between the fingers.

Exercise to Reduce Colds

Individuals who maintain an active lifestyle suffer 23% fewer colds than their less active counterparts. Extreme exercise, such as running a marathon, can suppress the immune system and increase the risk of getting a cold. But people who performed moderate exercise, such as walking or mowing the grass, reported getting fewer colds.

Theory: High activity levels increase immune defenses against viruses that cause colds.

Charles E. Matthews, PhD, assistant professor of medicine, Vanderbilt University, Nashville.

Feed a Cold, Starve a Fever

It really does make sense to feed a cold and starve a fever.

In what may be the first study to test the effectiveness of Mom's favorite adage, eating boosted the immune system's ability to fight rhinoviruses—the type that cause the common cold. And, fasting quadrupled the levels of *interleukin-4,* a chemical messenger involved in the immune response that helps ward off fevers. Ask your doctor for recommendations on your specific illness.

Gijs R. van den Brink, MD, researcher, laboratory for experimental internal medicine, Academic Medical Center, Amsterdam.

Natural Decongestant

To quickly unstuff your nose, sniff horseradish. It contains *allyl isothiocyanate,* a compound similar to the active ingredient in decongestants. Take a sniff two or three times daily. Keep your nose six inches from the jar, and don't spread your germs by breathing directly onto it. Better yet, keep a separate jar for decongestant purposes.

Caution: If congestion lasts for more than a week, or is accompanied by green mucus, postnasal drip, pain or toothache, be sure to see your doctor.

Sanford M. Archer, MD, associate professor of otolaryngology, University of Kentucky Medical Center in Lexington.

Drug-Free Relief For Hay Fever

Nose filters could provide a drug-free alternative for hay fever sufferers. The filters trap up to 97% of ryegrass and ragweed pollen without interfering with normal breathing.

The filters, which should be on the market in a few years, are expected to be a boon for people who cannot tolerate nasal steroids or antihistamines.

New Scientist, Reed Business Information Limited, 151 Wardour St., London.

Natural Way to Treat Constipation

Corn syrup, long used as a folk remedy, will draw water into the bowels to soften stools, making them easier to pass.

Recipe: Drink one tablespoon of corn syrup stirred into a glass of warm water twice a day for one or two days.

Caution: Don't use this remedy if you're diabetic, dehydrated or taking diuretic medication, such as *furosemide* (Lasix) or *triamterene* and *hydrochlorothiazide* (Maxzide).

Victor S. Sierpina, MD, associate professor of family medicine, University of Texas Medical Branch, Galveston.

Better Treatment for Carpal Tunnel Syndrome

Exercise and yoga may work better than splints for treatment of carpal tunnel syndrome (CTS).

In one recent study, a structured program of aerobic exercise, including walking, rowing or cycling, relieved pain by 33%. In another, doing Iyengar yoga for eight weeks improved grip strength and decreased pain more than wearing splints did.

Marian Garfinkel, EdD, Philadelphia-based leader of the yoga study, reported in *The Journal of the American Medical Association*.

Peter Nathan, MD, orthopedic surgeon in private practice, Portland, OR, and leader of the exercise study, published in the *Journal of Occupational and Environmental Medicine*.

Acupressure Cure For Hiccups

To put an end to persistent hiccups, simply place both your index and middle fingers behind your jawbone on the soft area under each earlobe. Press inward with your fingers until the spots feel sore, then hold for two minutes while breathing deeply. This should stop the involuntary diaphragm contractions that cause hiccups.

Michael Reed Gach, PhD, director, Acupressure Institute of America, Berkeley, CA, and author of *Acupressure's Potent Points* (Bantam Doubleday Dell).

What to Do If You Feel Faint

Feeling light headed or seeing black spots? You can temporarily prevent yourself from passing out by crossing your legs at the ankles and contracting the muscles in your legs, abdomen and buttocks.

People prone to fainting who practiced this technique either avoided fainting altogether or delayed it for an average of two-and-a-half minutes, which is often enough time to find a safe place to sit or lie down. If you still feel yourself losing consciousness, lower yourself to the ground to reduce the chances of injuring yourself when you fall.

Fainting can be triggered by blood pooling in the legs and abdomen, which causes a drop in blood pressure.

C.T. Paul Krediet, researcher, department of internal medicine, Academic Medical Center, Amsterdam.

No Stitches Necessary

A new study shows that simply washing and bandaging a cut promotes healing just as quickly and completely as stitches—and this method requires less time in the emergency room and costs much less.

You should get stitches when: A cut is longer than one inch...you cannot stop the bleeding...there is numbness or it hurts to move the injured area, which indicates possible nerve or tendon damage.

James Quinn, MD, associate clinical professor of medicine, University of California, San Francisco, and leader of a study of 91 patients with hand lacerations, published in the *British Medical Journal*.

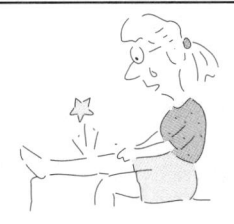

■ *Your Health* ■

Should You Ice an Injury Or Use Heat?

When to use ice or heat depends on how long ago an injury occurred.

Use ice for the first 48 hours after an injury. Apply for 20 minutes, remove for 20 minutes, then repeat. Do not apply directly to skin—put a thin towel over skin for protection, or freeze a paper cup full of water, tear off the top rim and move the ice over the injury.

Use heat 20 minutes at a time at least 24 hours after a minor injury or 48 hours after a more serious one. Place a heat pack directly on the injured area—do not add pressure. Do not apply to broken skin.

Carl W. Nissen, MD, assistant professor of orthopedic surgery at the University of Connecticut Health Center in Farmington.

Folk Remedies for Summer Ills

Joan Wilen and Lydia Wilen, of New York City. The sisters are authors of Chicken Soup & Other Folk Remedies *(Ballantine) and* Folk Remedies That Work *(Harper Perennial). Growing up in Brooklyn, their mother and grandmother had folk remedies for almost everything.*

Try these home remedies for hot-weather health challenges. They work wonders, even if we don't always know why.

MOTION SICKNESS

• **Mix eight ounces of warm water with one-half teaspoon of ground ginger powder.** Drink this 20 minutes before traveling. It is more effective than popular motion sickness medications. Taking two ginger pills, available at health food stores, also does the trick.

• **Suck on a lemon wedge** if you feel queasy while en route.

• **Inhale the smell of newsprint.** Make sure the newspaper was printed in the traditional method. To be effective, the ink should have a distinct smell and come off on your fingers.

SUNBURN

Always apply sunscreen. *But if you do get a sunburn...*

• **Take a cool shower as soon as possible.**

• **Steep six regular tea bags in one quart of hot water.** When the tea is strong and cool, drench washcloths in it and apply them to the sunburned area. Repeat until you feel relief.

• **Burned your feet from walking on hot sand?** Apply tomato slices to the soles of your feet, and secure them in place with elastic bandages or handkerchiefs. Elevate your feet for 20 minutes.

ALLERGIES

• **Use honeycomb to quell the wheezing,** itchy eyes and runny nose of an allergy attack. Cut off a one-inch square of fresh honeycomb (available at most health food stores), suck out the honey and chew the wax for five minutes. Then spit the wax out. You may even be able to immunize yourself against future attacks if you do this daily.

Caution: Diabetics and those allergic to honey should not try this. Never give honey to a child younger than one year old.

• **If your allergies start acting up in an air-conditioned car,** it may be due to the chemicals and/or mold in the air-conditioning unit. Turn off the air conditioning, and open the windows instead.

LEG CRAMPS WHILE SWIMMING

• **To relax the leg muscle,** paddle in place while forcing the toes of the cramped leg up, toward the knee.

• **Pinch your philtrum,** the skin between your nose and lip. Place your thumb below one nostril, your forefinger below the other, and then gently squeeze the skin between for 20 seconds.

SWIMMER'S EAR

• **To prevent swimmer's ear,** blow up a balloon three times after swimming. This dislodges trapped water that causes infection.

MOSQUITO BITES

To ward off mosquitoes...

• **Avoid consuming sugar or alcohol.**

• **Rub fresh aloe vera or parsley on skin.**

If you get bitten: Apply wet soap or a mixture of equal parts vinegar and lemon.

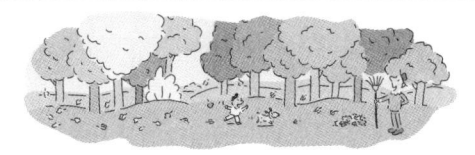

Quick Action Helps Stop Outbreaks of Poison Ivy

To prevent an outbreak *after* exposure to poison ivy...

•**Immediately cleanse exposed skin** with rubbing alcohol and rinse with water.

•**As soon as possible,** shower with soap and water.

The allergy-causing resin *urushiol* can be removed from clothes, shoes, tools, etc. by cleaning them with a mixture of alcohol and water. Be sure to wear rubber gloves.

A climbing plant, poison ivy grows in three-leaf groupings. The leaves are green during the summer and red in the fall.

William L. Epstein, MD, professor of dermatology, University of California, San Francisco.

Stress-Busters to Go

Mina Hamilton, author of Serenity to Go: Calming Techniques for Your Hectic Life *(New Harbinger). She has taught yoga and stress reduction for 12 years in New York City.*

A hot bath is a proven stress reliever. So is a soothing massage. But sometimes you need to relax *right now*—while you're stuck in traffic or trapped at the end of a slow checkout line.

After years of teaching yoga and stress reduction, I have discovered how to integrate relaxation techniques into the rough and tumble of daily life. Remember—no matter what situation you're in, you can always choose how to respond.

Here are four real-life situations that allow you to put simple stress-busting techniques into action...

PLACED ON HOLD

Next time you're on hold with a customer-service line, use your nondominant hand to hold the receiver a few inches from your ear (far enough to soften the canned music, but close enough to hear when a human being answers). Loosen your grip on the receiver. If you're slouching, lengthen your spine. You may keep your eyes open or gently close them.

Mentally scan your body, from your head to your toes. Relax tense muscles, and breathe deeply and slowly from the gut.

While the music drones on in the background, use your second and third fingers to massage your forehead. Place the fingertips between your eyebrows, and press down gently for two seconds. Then move the fingers toward your hairline in a single, slow motion.

Once you reach the hairline, lift the fingers off the skin and bring them back to the spot between your eyebrows. Imagine your forehead becoming as placid as a mountain lake.

Move on to your cheeks. Place the second and third fingers on the skin, and make small circular motions. Massage one cheek at a time.

Now focus on your jaw muscle. Massage it along the jawline in a circular motion. Let your mouth fall slightly open as you perform these mini-massages. When someone finally answers the phone, you may feel disappointed!

TRAPPED IN TRAFFIC

It's only too easy to develop hostile attitudes toward other drivers. We think of them as anonymous faces inside massive chunks of metal. We forget what we have in common with our fellow human beings.

Take a look at the people around you. *What kind of lives do they lead? Where is that white-haired man going? Was that young businesswoman up all night with a sick child?*

Instead of thinking of rude drivers as jerks, think about how much you share with them. Everybody trapped in this jam wants a loving spouse, a good job, the best education for their kids—just like you do.

STUCK AT YOUR COMPUTER

Those of us stuck at a desk, staring at a computer screen for hours, need to rest our eyes for at least two minutes every hour.

■ *Your Health* ■

To do this, turn your chair away from the computer. If you wear glasses, take them off. Focus on an object 10 feet away from your desk for a moment. Next, shift your eyes to look at something close, such as a plant or a nearby desk. Without straining, shift your eyes back and forth between these two places. Take long easy breaths as you do this.

NO PLACE TO SIT

So you couldn't get a seat on the bus. If you've been sitting in a chair all day long, here's a chance to lengthen and stretch your spine.

Stand straight, with your knees gently bent and your feet slightly separated. Relax your neck and jaw. Allow your shoulders to drop. Elongate your spine by imagining that it is growing taller as you feel the muscles in your back stretching upward. Breathe deeply. Now slowly turn your torso, shoulders and head to the left. Then slowly turn to the right. You will feel better and calmer.

Quick Stress Reduction

Intense relaxation not only reduces stress, it may also improve immune function.

Good news: It takes as little as *five minutes*.

What to do: Lie on your back with your legs placed at a 90-degree angle against a wall...close your eyes and place a soft cloth or towel over them. Slowly relax all your muscles, letting your body weight sink into the floor...take three deep abdominal breaths, inhaling through your nose. Continue to focus on your breathing. Perform this exercise for five to 10 minutes daily.

Judith Hanson Lasater, PhD, physical therapist and yoga instructor in San Francisco. She is author of *Relax and Renew: Restful Yoga for Stressful Times* (Rodmell).

Easy Way to Swallow Pills

If you have trouble swallowing pills, try the following tactics...

•**Take a gulp of water *before* putting the pill in your mouth.** This lubricates your throat and makes the pill easier to swallow.

•**Put the pill as far back on your tongue as possible.**

•**Ask your doctor or pharmacist if your pill can be crushed**—or capsule opened—and dissolved in liquid.

Susan Proulx, PharmD, president, MedERRS (Medication Error Recognition and Revision Strategies), a subsidiary of the Institute for Safe Medication Practices, Huntingdon Valley, PA.

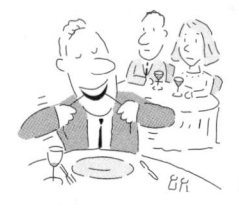

Simple Ways to Stay Healthy

There are a variety of simple things you can do to greatly improve your health...

•**Always wash your hands** after using the restroom. One-third of people don't have this disease-fighting habit.

•**Never use a cell phone while driving.**

•**Floss regularly**—flossing protects against gum disease, heart disease and stroke.

•**Avoid watching the nighttime news.** Its steady diet of troubles can make it hard for you to sleep restfully.

•**Do not procrastinate.** Putting things off is stressful.

Shape, 21100 Erwin St., Woodland Hills, CA 91367.

Your Health

4

Fitness Made Simple

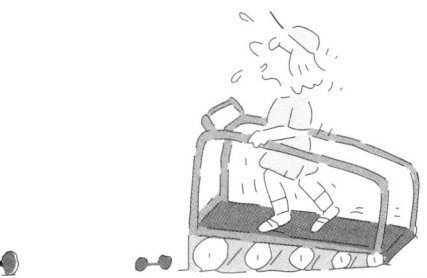

Outsmart These Fat Triggers to Lose Weight and Keep It Off

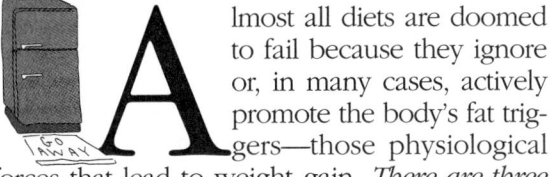

Almost all diets are doomed to fail because they ignore or, in many cases, actively promote the body's fat triggers—those physiological forces that lead to weight gain. *There are three ways that misguided dietary patterns, food choices and lifestyle habits promote weight gain...*

- **They slow the rate at which your body burns calories**—the opposite of what you want to do.

- **They disturb the normal metabolic process that converts glucose into energy,** producing sharp spikes of insulin and wildly fluctuating levels of blood sugar, which can trigger bingeing.

- **They make it almost impossible to eat sensibly** by generating appetite surges and uncontrollable food cravings.

Some triggers kick in immediately. Others will work over time, which is why some diets seem to work for weeks, even months, before weight is regained.

I have identified 43 fat triggers. *Here are the most common...*

UNDEREATING

Most people are surprised to hear that the biggest fat trigger is too few calories. Certainly the basic principle of weight loss is to take in fewer calories than you burn—but there's a point of diminishing returns. Fall below that level, and your metabolism goes into conservation mode. Within days, you're burning calories more slowly and finding it harder to lose weight.

The weight that does come off when you cut calories too drastically is lean tissue, like muscle —the energy-burning furnace of your body. This slows metabolism even further.

Stephanie Dalvit-McPhillips, PhD, nutritional biochemist in Willoughby, OH. She counsels people with weight disorders and is author of *The Right Bite: Outsmart 43 Scientifically Proven Fat Triggers and Beat the Dieter's Curse* (Fair Winds).

43

■ *Your Health* ■

Two other effects of overenthusiastic calorie reduction torpedo weight-loss efforts as well. Your body, feeling starved and looking for efficient ways to put on weight, increases production of the enzyme *lipoprotein lipase*, which metabolizes food into fat. At the same time, too little food leads to sharp drops in blood sugar. The resulting extreme hunger can drive you to binge eating.

The consequence of the starve/binge cycle is to replace muscle with fat.

How many calories are enough? It depends on your weight, metabolic rate and other factors. For most women, 1,400 to 1,500 calories daily leads to efficient weight loss...for men, 1,800 to 2,000.

Related fat triggers...

●**Skipping meals.** Even brief visits to the fasting state will lower metabolism and blood sugar, which can lead to bingeing. If you pack your daily calorie consumption into two large meals, a higher proportion is deposited as fat.

Small, frequent meals increase your metabolism. Try to eat every two to four hours. Consume a carbohydrate with some protein, such as one-half cup of strawberries with one-half cup of low-fat cottage cheese. The carbohydrate supplies energy, while the protein keeps blood sugar levels stable.

●**Too little fat.** The body needs essential fatty acids to repair cells, produce hormones and start the chemical reaction to burn fat. A diet in which fat has been ruthlessly removed can lead to strong cravings and fatty-food binges.

Be sure to include in your diet heart-healthy fat sources—especially olive or canola oil and two or three servings of fish a week.

●**Too little fiber.** It's the volume of food that fills you up and makes you feel satisfied. Fiber has more volume. It also speeds the passage of food through the intestine, so you absorb fewer calories.

Eat 25 to 35 grams of high-fiber foods—whole grains, fruits, legumes and vegetables—every day.

●**Too little water.** Thirst is easily mistaken for hunger. We often reach for a snack when water is what we really need. Drink at least eight eight-ounce glasses of water daily.

Fruit juices have some nutritional value, but they are high in calories and lack the filling fiber of fruits themselves. Get your vitamin C from oranges, not orange juice.

THINGS TO AVOID

●**Alcohol.** It has seven calories per gram—nearly as much as fat, which has nine calories—and no nutritional value. Just one or two drinks can lower blood sugar within two to four hours, generating powerful hunger. When alcohol is combined with sugar, as it is in many mixed drinks, it triggers a strong release of insulin. This makes blood sugar plummet, creating a ravenous appetite.

●**Nicotine.** It causes a temporary rise in blood sugar and then a sharp drop. If you're particularly sensitive, even secondhand smoke can stoke your appetite.

Why do some people gain weight when they quit smoking? Research has shown that quitters who gained weight had poor eating and exercise habits. Those whose weight remained stable were eating and exercising sensibly.

●**Caffeine.** For people sensitive to it, caffeine temporarily raises blood sugar by mobilizing carbohydrates from the liver. This camouflages hunger for a short time. When your blood sugar finally drops, you realize that you are starved—and binge.

●**Artificial sweeteners.** In some sensitive individuals, sugar-free gum and diet soda can trick the body into releasing insulin, which will drive blood sugar down and appetite up.

EXERCISE ERRORS

Exercise is an essential ingredient of any weight-loss program. If performed properly, it burns calories and takes the edge off hunger. But too much too soon is counterproductive. If you're out of shape and embark on a rigorous exercise regimen, your body burns glucose, not fat. This lowers blood sugar levels, making you feel hungrier. This effect is particularly striking with anaerobic exercise, such as weight lifting.

Start exercising gradually—walk briskly for 10 minutes at a time every other day, then 20 minutes, then more, and increase your frequency to daily. Aim for 30 minutes of exercise

Fitness Made Simple

a day. After four weeks of eating healthfully and exercising aerobically, add weight training.

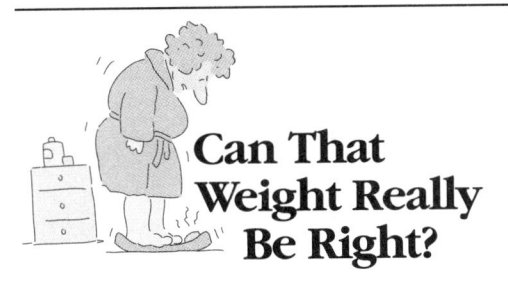

Can That Weight Really Be Right?

Scales found in weight-loss and fitness centers are often off by up to five pounds. And half of all scales found in doctors' offices are off by at least 1.5 pounds.

Self-defense: Ask if the scale has been calibrated in the past year...use scales that appear to be in good condition and are placed on a carpeted floor. Carpet acts as a shock absorber, which helps the scale maintain calibration.

Risa J. Stein, PhD, assistant professor of psychology, Rockhurst University, Kansas City, MO. Her study was published in *Obesity Research*.

Turn Off Hunger

Researchers have discovered that a certain hormone produced in the intestine after meals shuts off the appetite switch in the brain. Studies found that volunteers injected with the hormone, *peptide YY3-36,* took one-third less food from a buffet table than those who weren't injected. This finding could lead to new treatments for obesity.

The Lancet, 32 Jamestown Rd., London.

Most People Don't Realize When They're Full

People who wore blindfolds ate 22% less food than those who could see their plates.

Reason: Most of us rely on external cues—an empty plate or the bottom of a bag—to tell us when we're full. Blindfolded subjects rely instead on signals from their stomach.

If you are trying to lose weight: Try using a blindfold once to become more aware of your satiety cues.

Yvonne Linne, MD, PhD, researcher, obesity unit, Huddinge University Hospital, Stockholm.

Stop Food Cravings And Lose Weight

Elizabeth Somer, RD, nutritionist in Salem, OR. She appears regularly on NBC's *Today* show and is a contributing editor to *Shape* magazine. She is author of *Food & Mood* and *The Origin Diet* (both from Owl Books).

If you're berating yourself because you simply can't seem to cut back on potato chips, ice cream or some other tempting food—stop. Your problem may *not* come from a lack of willpower.

Food cravings are linked to low levels of critical nutrients and/or an imbalance of brain chemicals that affect appetite as well as mood.

Example: Low levels of *serotonin,* a "feel good" neurotransmitter, trigger cravings for carbohydrate-rich foods, including cookies, pasta and candy. Such foods elevate levels of *tryptophan,* an amino acid that is converted into serotonin in the brain.

Cravings can often be reduced by eating a healthful breakfast and a nutritional meal or snack every four hours throughout the day... and getting at least 30 minutes of exercise five days a week.

Other helpful solutions for common problem foods...

FAT

The craving for fat is driven, in part, by a brain chemical called *galanin*. Galanin levels are lowest in the morning, rise during the day and peak in the afternoon. Eating fatty food keeps galanin circulating in the body, which stimulates a strong craving for *more* fat later in the day.

45

■ *Your Health* ■

This physiological response makes sense in evolutionary terms. Fat was once scarce, so people had to eat as much as possible whenever it was available in order to survive.

Today, with rich food all around, fat cravings can lead to obesity, diabetes and heart disease. *Much better for you...*

●**Eat half a small avocado or one ounce of nuts daily.** These foods usually satisfy fat cravings because they contain monounsaturated and polyunsaturated fats, which are more healthful than the saturated fat found in meat and rich desserts.

●**Satisfy cravings with fat-free creamy foods,** such as fruit-and-yogurt smoothies or puréed squash soup. Their creamy textures help reduce cravings.

CARBOHYDRATES

Carbohydrates, such as candy, pie, doughnuts and cake, provide a temporary serotonin boost. But the cravings return as soon as serotonin levels wane. *Better approach...*

●**Eat complex carbohydrates.** Whole wheat toast...a whole wheat bagel...a bowl of air-popped popcorn are all low in fat and calories, but raise serotonin levels.

●**Stock up on healthful snacks** so you will be prepared if you tend to crave carbohydrates in the afternoon.

Good choices: Low-fat bran muffin, English muffin, baked tortilla chips and salsa, or lemon sorbet with fruit.

●**Use artificial sweeteners,** such as *aspartame* (NutraSweet), *sucralose* (Splenda) or *acesulfame-K* (Sunett). Consumed in moderation, these products satisfy your sweet tooth but spare you the calories found in sugary snacks.

SALT

The human body needs only about 500 milligrams (mg) of sodium daily, or about one-quarter teaspoon. Most Americans consume *10 times* that amount. Salty foods increase blood pressure in people who are sensitive to salt. These foods also contribute to weight gain because they are typically high in fat.

Salt cravings usually result from eating habits that are surprisingly easy to unlearn. *Here's how...*

●**Snack on crunchy foods,** such as baby carrots or celery. Foods with a crunchy texture help satisfy the craving for salty snacks, such as potato chips.

●**Use seasonings.** Lemon juice, fresh ginger, cilantro, red pepper flakes and other spices enhance the flavor of unsalted foods.

CHOCOLATE

Chocolate boosts levels of serotonin and the morphine-like neurotransmitters called *endorphins*. It also contains caffeine and *theobromine,* a caffeine-like compound that provides a mental lift...*phenylethylamine,* the so-called "love" chemical that increases heart rate and blood pressure...and *anandamide,* a brain chemical that mimics the mood-lifting effects of marijuana.

It's no wonder chocolate is the most commonly craved food. Those who crave it find it is almost impossible to give up. *Instead...*

●**Eat very *small* amounts.** Just two small pieces of chocolate, one cup of sugar-free hot chocolate or one small cookie will often correct your brain chemistry without providing too many calories or fat.

●**Eat chocolate only *after* meals.** You will enjoy the taste treat and the boost in brain chemicals, but you'll be less likely to overindulge than if you eat chocolate between meals when you are hungry.

●**Substitute fat-free chocolate syrup for regular chocolate.** It provides the same pleasurable effects but only a fraction of the calories. I often advise clients to use one-quarter cup of chocolate syrup as a dip for fresh fruit.

Reduced-Fat Foods Could Cause Weight Gain

Low- or reduced-fat foods actually may cause weight gain. That's because many people eat more of these foods in the mistaken belief that they are also low in calories. No scientific evidence exists to support the use of low- or reduced-fat foods as a weight-loss tool.

Fitness Made Simple

Better: Eat at least five servings of fruits and vegetables daily. They are naturally low in fat and calories and are filling.

Judith Wylie-Rosett, EdD, RD, professor and head of the division of health, behavior and nutrition, department of epidemiology and social medicine, Albert Einstein College of Medicine, Bronx, NY.

Healthier Peanut Butter

Regular peanut butter is healthier for you than reduced-fat peanut butter. Reduced-fat versions contain less monounsaturated fat, the kind that is good for the heart. To replace fat, manufacturers add sugar—so you end up with as many calories in reduced-fat peanut butter as in the regular type.

Holly McCord, RD, author of *Prevention's The Peanut Butter Diet* (St. Martin's) and nutrition editor, *Prevention*, Emmaus, PA 18098.

Weight-Loss Secrets That Really Work

Lawrence J. Cheskin, MD, director of the Johns Hopkins Weight Management Center and associate professor of human nutrition at Johns Hopkins Bloomberg School of Public Health, both in Baltimore. He is author of *New Hope for People with Weight Problems* (Prima).

Consume fewer calories. Exercise daily. Reduce fat intake. Everyone knows the standard advice for losing weight. Unfortunately, up to 90% of those who initially lose weight gain it back within one year.

HIDDEN CAUSES OF WEIGHT GAIN

Only 2% of people who cannot lose weight have physical reasons for gaining the weight, including a slow metabolism or inefficient fat-storing mechanisms. The adrenal gland disorder Cushing's syndrome and an underactive thyroid (hypothyroidism) can also lead to weight gain.

More often, people put on weight because they eat too much and/or do not get enough exercise. Sadly, our sedentary lifestyle makes it difficult for us to maintain a healthful weight. Many people also eat to relieve stress or boredom. They fail to lose weight because they don't recognize the cues that cause them to eat inappropriately.

Helpful: Wear your watch upside down for a few weeks. Most people look at their watches when they're thinking about eating. When you see it's upside down, ask yourself *why* you're eating. If you're truly hungry, eat—but resist the urge if you're merely doing it out of habit. Instead, go for a walk...read the newspaper... or call a friend.

When buying food, it's not enough to check the labels for fat and calories. You must also check serving sizes. Many packaged foods that appear to contain one serving actually contain two or more. This means you might be consuming more fat and calories than you think.

Example: Bottled cranberry juice has approximately 120 calories per eight-ounce serving. But a 20-ounce bottle contains two and a half servings. If you drink the whole bottle, you're really getting 300 calories.

Surprisingly, gyms can also be a problem for dieters. They are often inconvenient, and people are sometimes too self-conscious to go. I favor home and neighborhood workouts —riding an exercise bike or walking around the block.

Many people fail to realize that medication can cause unintended weight gain, too. These drugs include hormones...steroids...and antidepressants, such as *amitriptyline* (Elavil) and *imipramine* (Norfranil). If you've gained more than a few pounds within one month of starting a drug, ask your doctor or pharmacist to review your medications. There may be effective alternatives.

For people who *still* can't lose weight, the best approaches...

WEIGHT-LOSS PROGRAMS

If you are too busy or self-conscious to participate in a group weight-loss program, such as Weight Watchers (800-651-6000 or *www.weightwatchers.com*)...or Take Off Pounds Sensibly (800-932-8677 or *www.tops.org*), the interactive, Internet-based weight-loss programs can be an effective alternative.

■ *Your Health* ■

A recent study in *The Journal of the American Medical Association* found that people who participated in an Internet-based program lost an average of 10 pounds in six months.

Good weight-loss information on the Web: *www.ediets.com.*

Cost: $65* for a thirteen-week program.

WEIGHT-LOSS DRUGS

People who combine drugs with diet and exercise may lose an additional 5% of their weight over six months. But all drugs have side effects, so I recommend them only for people who are at least 40 pounds over their ideal weight.**

Leading weight-loss drugs...

•**Fat-blockers.** *Orlistat* (Xenical) attaches to enzymes that digest fats. Fats pass out of the body in the stool instead of entering the bloodstream.

•**Appetite suppressants.** *Phentermine* (Fastin), *sibutramine* (Meridia) and the other appetite suppressants alter brain chemistry to make you feel satisfied with eating smaller amounts of food.

Warning: Do *not* take over-the-counter weight-loss drugs. They often contain such ingredients as caffeine and ephedrine, which may cause heart irregularities.

KETOGENIC DIETS

Seriously obese patients can benefit from so-called *ketogenic diets*.

How they work: A high-protein diet, in which 60% to 80% of calories come from protein, curbs appetite and helps maintain muscle mass during weight loss. Restricting carbohydrate intake results in *ketogenesis*—a process in which the production and breakdown of fat by-products curbs appetite and increases the burning of fat tissue.

However, this approach may cause heart and kidney damage. To prevent this, I recommend a *modified* ketogenic diet that consists of 20% to 30% carbohydrates...10% to 20% fat ...and the rest protein.

*Price subject to change.

**Use of weight-loss drugs and the diets described here require a doctor's supervision.

VERY LOW-CALORIE DIET

People who are 100 pounds or more over their ideal weight often get good results from a very low-calorie diet—defined as less than 800 calories daily. This approach can cause weight loss of up to three pounds per week.

SURGERY

People with a body-mass index of 40 or higher† are candidates for a new surgical procedure that uses a *laparoscopically adjustable gastric band,* FDA approved in June 2001.

How it works: A plastic band is tightened around the stomach to reduce the amount of food it can hold. To perform this procedure, a bariatric surgeon inserts flexible instruments through keyhole incisions in the abdomen.

To locate a bariatric surgeon in your area: Contact the American Society for Bariatric Surgery (352-331-4900 or *www.asbs.org*).

†To calculate your body-mass index, go to the National Heart, Lung and Blood Institute Web site at *www.nhlbisupport.com/bmi*.

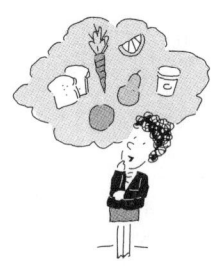

A Harvard MD Weighs in On the Eating Debate

George L. Blackburn, MD, PhD, associate professor, surgery and nutrition, and associate director, division of nutrition, Harvard Medical School, Boston. He is chief of the Nutritional/Metabolism Laboratory and director of the Center for the Study of Nutrition Medicine, both at Beth Israel Deaconess Medical Center, Boston.

For years, we've been told that a low-fat, high-carbohydrate diet is the best way to lose weight and reduce the risk of heart disease. It is the basis of the federal government's Food Pyramid for healthful eating.

Recently, though, some reputable researchers have suggested that a high-protein, high-fat, low-carb diet is actually more healthful and effective. The premise behind this diet—often called the Atkins diet because it was first popularized by the late Robert Atkins, MD, over 30 years ago—is that it is carbohydrates, not fat, that make us gain weight. If we consume fewer carbohydrates, we will lose weight—and live much longer.*

Distinguished expert in the field of nutrition and obesity, Harvard's George L. Blackburn, MD, PhD, helps sort fact from fiction...

•**When trying to lose weight, is what you eat more important than the number of calories?** Probably not. The bottom line is always total calories taken in minus total calories expended. If you burn more calories than you consume, regardless of the source, you will lose weight. If you consume more calories than you burn, you will gain weight.

•**But people lose weight on the Atkins diet, which can be high in calories. Why?** Like almost all fad diets, a high-protein, high-fat diet cuts down on variety, which reduces interest in food and thus limits intake. Also, protein—especially animal protein—seems to induce the feeling of being satisfied.

Some proponents claim that the Atkins diet burns fat by controlling insulin production. Another theory is that *ketones*—chemicals produced when carbohydrate intake is very low—play a role. But these are just hypotheses.

Whatever the mechanism, obese people will generally lose 20 to 30 pounds over a three- to six-month period.

•**What happens long term?** There are no scientific control studies that prove weight loss continues past that point or that the weight stays off.

•**Is the Atkins diet better than other diets for losing weight?** The jury is still out on that one. There have been no head-to-head trials in which a control group was following a different weight-loss regimen. It's an area that deserves serious study.

•**The Atkins diet encourages fat consumption. Is that healthful?** High LDL (bad) cholesterol remains the number one risk factor for coronary heart disease, and saturated fat is known to increase it. But it appears that you can take in substantial amounts of fat without increasing cholesterol—*while your weight is decreasing*. As long as you burn all the fat you consume, it doesn't end up in your arteries.

Once you stop losing weight, it's another story. We don't know if you can exceed the recommended levels of dietary fat and still stay healthy.

There are other health problems as well. Low-carbohydrate, high-protein diets, such as Atkins, raise blood acid levels, which can increase the risk of osteoporosis and promote the formation of kidney stones in vulnerable individuals. You shouldn't start the Atkins diet or change your eating habits in any radical way without talking to your doctor.

•**How about the high-carbohydrate, low-fat diet promoted in the Food Pyramid? Some people now say it *causes* obesity.** There is no evidence of this. It is true that the rate of obesity in this country has gone up markedly over the last 20 years. But that's probably because people are dining out more—and eating larger portions than they would at home. Also, people are exercising less.

As for carbohydrates themselves, it is important to distinguish among different kinds. The Food Pyramid calls for fiber-rich whole-grain foods, vegetables and fruits. No one is advocating unlimited white bread, white rice and sugar.

Some people do need to be cautious about consuming too many carbohydrates. They have *Syndrome X*—high triglyceride levels, low HDL (good) cholesterol and an increased risk of heart disease and diabetes—which could be aggravated by any simple sugars and refined starches. This is another reason to discuss diet plans with your doctor.

•**Overall, what is a sensible plan for losing weight?** It doesn't matter what you do for a few days, weeks or even months. You need a diet *for the rest of your life*. The idea is to find one that is flexible and satisfying.

One thing people tend to overlook even though it makes a real difference in weight control is water. Volume makes you feel satisfied, and water, especially when it's in food, has a lot to do with that. Eat lots of fruits and vegetables—they have a high water content and are rich in dietary fiber, which also fills you up. Soup is also a good diet food.

*For more information on the Atkins diet, go to *http://atkins.com*.

■ *Your Health* ■

It takes some time and practice to change the way you eat. Most people eat 21 meals a week. In at least 10 of them, try to include whole grains, vegetables and fruits, moderate amounts of protein and limited fats. This may mean brown-bagging some lunches.

For the other meals, concentrate on controlling portions and eating slowly. Take at least 20 minutes between the first and last bites of the meal.

Guidance from a dietitian or other health professional can be worthwhile. It is also helpful to have family members and others with whom you eat regularly eating healthfully, too. Healthful eating should be a communal effort.

Always Have Breakfast

Breakfast eaters tend to stay thinner than skippers, because breakfast speeds metabolism and diminishes midday food cravings. Breakfast also helps boost mood and sharpen memory. If you really dislike eating early in the day, pack a simple breakfast and eat it later in the morning.

Examples: Half a mini whole wheat pita topped with part-skim ricotta cheese and a few chopped nuts...five fat-free bagel chips with one-third cup of shredded reduced-fat cheese melted on top.

Good Housekeeping, 959 Eighth Ave., New York City 10019.

Beware of Unintended Weight Loss

Unintended weight loss is linked with increased risk for death in older adults. Dramatic weight loss has long been recognized as a sign of potential health problems, including cancer and chronic infection. But according to a new study, even losing as little as 5% of total body weight over a three-year period more than doubled the likelihood of dying during the following three years. Gradual, unintended weight loss may also signal health problems that need treatment.

If you experience unintended weight loss: See your doctor.

Anne B. Newman, MD, MPH, associate professor of medicine and epidemiology, University of Pittsburgh School of Medicine.

Easy Way to Increase Fat Burning

Caffeine before a workout can accelerate fat burning. It works best when it's taken on an empty stomach. For maximum absorption, drink one cup of coffee or tea without sugar and with a little milk. If you are sensitive to coffee or dislike black tea, try *guarana tea,* a natural caffeine source that is often sold in health food stores.

Ori Hofmekler, New York City–based fitness expert and author of *The Warrior Diet* (Dragon Door), www.warriordiet.com.

Two Big Benefits of Magnesium

Magnesium reduces fatigue and promotes weight loss by helping the body convert food into energy.

Recent finding: Women used 15% more oxygen while riding a stationary bicycle when they ate a diet that was low in magnesium than when they ate sufficient amounts of the mineral. Increased oxygen consumption during physical activity indicates exercise inefficiency.

Implication: People who fail to consume the recommended daily intake of magnesium —320 milligrams (mg) for women and 420 mg for men—are more likely to experience fatigue. That means they're unlikely to have the energy they need to exercise regularly for effective weight control.

Good sources of magnesium: The green vegetables, legumes, nuts and unprocessed grains. Except for bananas, fruits contain little magnesium.

Henry Lukaski, PhD, research leader for mineral nutrient functions, Human Nutrition Research Center, US Department of Agriculture, Grand Forks, ND.

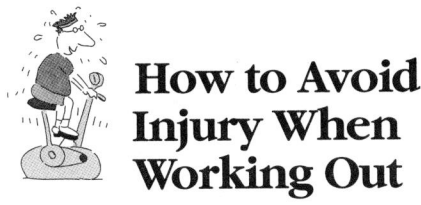

How to Avoid Injury When Working Out

Jolie Bookspan, PhD, sports medicine specialist and physiologist in private practice in Philadelphia. She is author of six books, including *Health & Fitness in Plain English* (Healthy Learning).

Fitness enthusiasts often assume that they won't get injured as long as they work out frequently. Unfortunately, that's not true. Even people who exercise several days a week are at risk for injury if they spend most of their time sitting, slouching and/or bending or walking incorrectly.

THE WARM-UP

For years, we've been told to stretch before working out. But warming up is key to avoiding exercise injury. In fact, stretching itself can *cause* injury if it's attempted before warming up.

To warm up, you must perform enough physical activity to raise your body temperature.

Helpful: For 10 minutes—or until you break a sweat—move around. For example, walk, jog slowly or bike.

After warming up, slowly ease into your stretch and hold the position. Don't bounce while stretching—it can cause muscle and joint pulls and tears. *Never* stretch to the point of pain.

AVOIDING INJURIES

Here are some surprisingly simple ways to avoid five common exercise injuries...

• **Strain of the Achilles tendon.** A sedentary lifestyle, walking with your toes pointing out (i.e., duck-footed) and wearing shoes with heels can shorten the Achilles tendons. Short, tight tendons are subject to strain during almost any activity. When this occurs, pain is felt anywhere from the heel to the calf.

Self-defense: Stretch your Achilles tendons with a simple wall exercise. Stand facing a wall. Place the ball of your right foot against the wall with your heel resting on the floor. Lean forward, pressing your right hip toward the wall. Stretch the whole foot for a few seconds. Repeat with left foot. Perform this exercise a few times each day.

If you have Achilles tendon pain: Have your cholesterol checked. High cholesterol levels can stiffen blood vessels in the tendon and predispose it to injury.

• **Ankle sprain.** People with loose ligaments and stretched muscles on the sides of the ankles, weak leg muscles, prior ankle sprains that were incompletely rehabilitated and bad balance are especially prone to ankle sprain. This is because their ankles tend to roll outward, either overstretching or tearing the ligaments.

Self-defense: Forget high-top shoes and elastic bandages. Prevent ankle sprain with strengthening and balancing exercises.

To strengthen your *evertor* muscles (those that lift the outside edge of your foot), loop a bungee cord (without the hook), any stretchy tubing or band or a pair of pantyhose around both feet while sitting or standing. Roll the outside edges of your feet upward. Hold for a few seconds. Repeat. Gradually increase to 10 repetitions. Do this exercise at least once daily.

Helpful: Balance exercises are crucial to preventing recurrence of ankle sprain. While talking on the phone or waiting in line, stand on one foot for as long as you can. Repeat with other leg.

• **Anterior cruciate ligament (ACL) tear.** When you stop short while lunging for a ball during tennis or hit a mogul too hard while skiing—but do not have the muscular strength to compensate—you can overstress or tear a

■ *Your Health* ■

ligament inside your knee (ACL). This causes pain and swelling.

Self-defense: Strengthen your leg muscles, including the quadriceps (the muscles in your front thighs) and hamstrings (the muscles in your back thighs).

Running, biking and stair climbing are the most effective ways to build these muscles. For best results, combine with squats and lunges.

Helpful: When lifting things, hold your torso upright, use your leg muscles and bend with your knees.

•**Rotator cuff strain.** Also known as swimmer's, tennis or pitcher's shoulder, rotator cuff strain often comes from bad head and arm posture during activities that require you to lift the arm. This can even include movements that do not lift the arm completely overhead.

If you hold your head forward in a "craned" posture, it can impinge on any of the four muscles and tendons that make up the rotator cuff. This can lead to pain anywhere from the shoulder to the middle of the arm. People who do not use the muscles of the torso when moving their arms also experience stress on the shoulder.

Self-defense: Begin by always practicing good posture.

To strengthen the rotator cuff, tie a strip of rubber tubing (found in most medical supply and sporting-goods stores) around a pipe, pole or anything that will hold it securely, at shoulder height.

While gripping the rubber tubing with your right hand, turn sideways and bend your right elbow. Pull the tubing across your torso, keeping your posture straight by using your leg, back and abdominal muscles.

Return the tubing to the starting position while continuing to use your muscles. Don't let the band pull your elbow back. Repeat with your left arm. Work up to 10 repetitions daily with each arm.

•**Shin splints.** Weak shin muscles, poor shock absorption when you land from walking, running or jumping, and running on your toes can all contribute to shin splints.

Self-defense: While sitting or standing, place your feet flat on the floor, with your toes under anything that provides resistance, such as the bottom of your desk. Lift your toes, and hold for two seconds.

You can do this exercise either one foot at a time or with both feet at once. If there's no object nearby to create resistance, you can even use the toes of one foot to hold down those of the other foot.

Repeat 10 times on each foot, working up to at least a few sets of 10 each day.

Helpful: Walk and run lightly, coming down heel first, then with the rest of the foot.

When you jump, land toes first, then allow your heels to come down, bending your knees and using your leg muscles to ensure a soft landing on your feet.

Short Bursts of Exercise For Bigger Benefits

Short bursts of exercise are just as effective as—and in some ways even better than—long workouts. Women who exercised for either 10 or 15 minutes at a time for a total of 30 minutes a day for three months improved their cardiovascular fitness just as much as women who worked out in 30-minute blocks. And the once-a-day group lost six pounds on average. The twice-a-day group lost 6.5 pounds. Women who exercised three times a day lost an average of 9.5 pounds.

W. Daniel Schmidt, PhD, department chair and associate professor, department of physical education and health promotion, University of Wisconsin, Oshkosh.

Take the Stairs

Stair climbing is a "weight-bearing" exercise that builds bone mass and helps prevent the onset of osteoporosis.

Key: Like muscle, bone just gets denser and stronger as a result of being put to work.

The bone-building exercises include jogging, walking, dancing and racquet sports. Resistance training with weights and machines is excellent because it builds both bone and muscle mass.

Contrast: Biking and swimming aren't good bone-building exercises.

Lynn Chard-Petrinjak, communications manager for the National Osteoporosis Foundation, Washington, DC, *www.nof.org*.

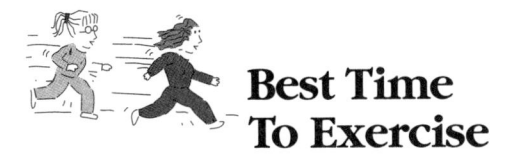

Best Time To Exercise

Although some people enjoy waking themselves up with an early morning jog, a recent study suggests that morning exercise can suppress the immune system.

Reason: Levels of *Immunoglobulin A,* a class of antibodies that protect the body against infection, are markedly lower early in the day. Exercising when the immune system is most vulnerable can increase risk of infection.

However: Recreational athletes should exercise whenever they can, whatever the time of day. The benefits of exercise will most likely outweigh the risks.

Craig Sharp, DSc, professor of sports science, Brunel University, Middlesex, England.

The No-Exercise Workout

Connie Tyne, director of The Cooper Wellness Program in Dallas.

The Institute of Medicine, *www.iom.edu*, which advises Congress on health matters, recently said that we need to exercise for a full hour daily for optimum health. But with numerous family and work responsibilities, it won't be easy to fit this in.

I am a true multitasker, so I do toe raises while on the telephone…squats while brushing my teeth…and leg curls while drying my hair. These microsessions are like tossing loose change into a jar.

Also, take advantage of TV time. One half-hour TV show includes eight minutes of commercials. Watch TV while on a treadmill or an exercycle—go faster during commercials to burn more calories and slow down during the actual program.

Other ways you can accumulate exercise time: Walk the dog…run around with your kids …pace while on the telephone…dance with a child, your spouse or even by yourself. Any activity that gets the heart and muscles going counts—housework, pushing a lawn mower, shoveling snow.

Exercise is cumulative, so three 10-minute bouts are just as good as one 30-minute session.

You might want to try a pedometer to see how much exercise you're getting doing everyday activities. You may be surprised. With your doctor's okay, aim for at least 8,000 steps a day. Boost your count gradually, adding another 100 to 200 steps per week.

What else could *you* be doing while reading this?

Heartburn from Exercise

Exercise-induced heartburn will be a burning sensation in the chest or a bitter taste in the mouth. Do not exercise on a full stomach or eat protein-rich or fatty foods for two hours before exercising. Also avoid citrus, chocolate, onions, peppermint, spearmint, spicy foods and caffeinated or carbonated drinks. If you like sports drinks, use ones that contain about 5% carbohydrate, and dilute those that have higher concentrations. Drink five to 12 ounces of fluid every 15 minutes while exercising.

Robert Robergs, PhD, director, exercise physiology laboratories, University of New Mexico, Albuquerque.

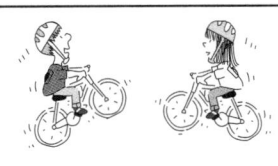

■ *Your Health* ■

Exercise in a Pill?

Scientists at Duke University School of Medicine are working on a drug that stimulates a muscle-building protein called *calcium/calmodulin-dependent protein kinase* (CaMK). It has the same effects on muscle cells as vigorous exercise—and could allow sedentary people with health problems to increase muscle strength.

CNN.com, on-line news from the Cable News Network.

New Exercise Guidelines

Be physically active for an hour a day to maintain health and normal body weight. The previous recommendations of 30 minutes of daily or almost-daily physical activity were not enough. Daily physical activities should be moderately intense, such as cycling, swimming or brisk walking.

Joanne Lupton, PhD, professor of nutrition at Texas A&M University, College Station, and chairperson of the Institute of Medicine panel making the recent exercise recommendation.

Better Fitness Walking

To get much more out of your fitness walking routine…

•**Stand tall** and don't lean forward.

•**Land on your heel** and roll to your toes for liftoff at each step.

•**To speed up, take smaller but quicker steps** and swing your arms, keeping them close to your body and your forearms parallel to the ground.

•**Maintain posture** by keeping your ears directly above your shoulders, hips, knees and feet, and tipping your chin up a half inch.

Suzanne Nottingham, spokesperson for the American Council on Exercise, Mammoth Lakes, CA.

Exercising with Asthma

Exercisers with asthma should take special precautions before each session…

•**Take two puffs on an inhaler 10 to 15 minutes before the activity.**

•**Notice the temperature and humidity of the exercise area**—heat and water loss can exacerbate symptoms.

•**In cold, dry weather,** put a scarf around your face to hold in heat and moisture.

•**Do not exercise in very cold weather.**

•**Consider air quality,** and take appropriate medicines if necessary.

Eric Small, MD, founder and director, Sports Medicine Center for Young Athletes, New York City, and author of *Kids & Sports* (Newmarket).

Painless Ways to Build Exercise into Your Daily Routine

Steven N. Blair, physical education doctor (PED), president and CEO, The Cooper Institute, Dallas, *www.cooperinst.org*. Formerly senior scientific editor of the Surgeon General's *Report on Physical Activity and Health,* he is coauthor of *Active Living Every Day: 20 Weeks to Lifelong Vitality* (Human Kinetics).

Improving your physical fitness need not require an arduous exercise regimen. And you certainly do not have to go to a gym, wear special clothes and sweat a lot.

But if you want to improve your health and fitness, you must increase your physical activity. This can be done gradually, at home or at work or with the help of a professional program. Your goal should be to change your behavior, not wear yourself out.

Burning 200 to 300 more calories per day through moderate-intensity exercise lowers the risk of heart disease, stroke, diabetes, some cancers and other conditions related to stress or being overweight. You'll also increase fitness, which will give you more energy and lead to greater enjoyment of life.

ACTIVITIES FOR HEALTH

Some of the most effective ways to boost physical activity are often overlooked...

•**Increase the number of steps you take each day.** That by itself will go a long way toward burning calories and exercising muscles.

Helpful: Use a pedometer to record the number of steps you take every day. My favorite is the DIGI-WALKER, which accurately documents steps you take. It is sold at sporting-goods stores and is also available directly from New Lifestyles (888-748-5377 or *www.new-lifestyles.com*).

Cost: Starting at $26.95* plus shipping and handling.

Most people over age 50 who work in sedentary jobs and do not exercise regularly take about 2,000 to 4,000 steps a day. It's easy to increase this.

When you go to the mall, for instance, don't drive around until you find a parking place next to the door. Park in the first available space and walk to the entrance. You'll increase the number of steps you take and often save time in the long run.

Before taking the car out for a short errand, think about walking. You'll often be delighted at how much you see in the neighborhood. If you take public transportation, getting off one stop early can be similarly enjoyable and will add exercise to your trip as well.

•**Stand instead of sit.** Standing burns more calories than sitting, which is what many people do for 12 hours a day.

When you talk on the phone, get in the habit of standing. And at least sit up when you watch television instead of stretching out on a sofa. Sitting burns more calories than lying down.

•**Move around.** Even slow walking burns twice as many calories per minute as sitting. If you have a mobile phone or a phone with a long cord, don't merely stand each time you have a conversation. Instead, walk around as you talk.

•**Do household chores.** Catch up on your gardening. Or repaint a wall, repair the kitchen cabinet, hang some new pictures or rearrange the furniture.

*Price subject to change.

•**Take up a sport or physical activity.** Try one that always interested you or one you once enjoyed but gave up as your responsibilities grew.

Examples: Bicycling, tennis, swimming, bowling, golf, running.

Call local clubs in your area. You may be surprised to find out how many people are resuming a sport after many years or taking it up for the first time.

KEEP ON TRACK

Increasing your physical activity, even gradually, isn't always easy. The big problem is reversing the long-established behavior of avoiding unnecessary exertion. *Helpful...*

•**Set goals.** Aim low at first. When you reach your first objective, set the next goal slightly higher. The satisfaction of reaching a goal will inspire you to go on to the next.

On the other hand, nothing is more discouraging than setting a high goal and then failing to meet it. *Examples of reasonable goals...*

•If a pedometer shows that you take about 3,000 steps a day, set a goal for increasing the number by 500 a week until your daily rate is in the 8,000 to 10,000 range.

•If your goal is to lose 30 pounds, set a goal of five pounds a month.

•**Monitor your progress.** Recording your physical activities in a diary can help develop momentum for reaching your goals. Keep the entries short so the diary itself doesn't become a chore. Simply record each day's physical activity, and make a note of whether you met your goals.

If you use a pedometer, record the number of steps you take each day. It also helps to estimate how many hours a day you sit and how many you spend moving around. Over a period of several weeks, the log should show a decrease in the amount of time spent sitting and an increase in moving around.

•**Join a group.** Although you can easily increase your physical activity without joining a health or fitness club, being a member of a group offers two major advantages—you'll have access to a professional trainer and the support of fellow members.

■ *Your Health* ■

Look for a group that helps its members to achieve a modest, but steady, increase in their physical activity.

Human Kinetics, a publisher with which I'm affiliated, is in the process of establishing Active Living fitness centers at health clubs, hospitals, work locations and Ys throughout the country. These centers teach changes in lifestyle, encourage goal-setting and establish support systems to help people stay physically active. Those are the qualities to look for in any activity group.

Information: 217-351-5076 or *www.active living.info.*

•**Gather support.** Research on physical activity shows that people with support from friends or family members are far more likely to succeed than those who try to do it on their own. Support can be especially critical during the early stages of a fitness program. *Recommended…*

•When you decide to increase your physical activity, tell two or three friends about your goals, and ask them to help you. Choose these people on the basis of how supportive they've been in the past—those who will phone you periodically to check on your progress or to encourage you to reach difficult goals…or better still, those who will go for a walk with you at lunchtime.

•If someone you hoped would support you doesn't follow through, immediately enlist the support of someone else.

•When you evaluate fitness programs, ask what type of support they offer. The best programs encourage participants to support one another after class and to find support among other friends.

Safety: All the moderate-intensity lifestyle activities discussed here are safe. You are just doing more of what you normally do. If you have a history of heart problems, osteoporosis or other conditions that could interfere with physical activity, check with your doctor. If you experience worrisome symptoms during exercise, such as pressure in your chest or extreme breathlessness with mild exertion, stop your exercise and check with your doctor.

Information: Visit *www.americanheart.org*.

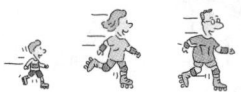

More from Steven Blair…

Can Fat Be Fit?

A growing number of experts are challenging the standard belief that being overweight indicates one is unfit and subject to serious health risks. They say that being unfit and sedentary may contribute to weight gain—but it is the lack of fitness that creates health risks associated with high body weight, not the weight itself.

In fact, people who are "fat but fit" face fewer health risks than those who are thin and unfit.

Example: Long-term studies done at The Cooper Institute in Dallas have found that death rates for both women and men who are thin but unfit are at least twice as high as for their counterparts who are obese but fit.

Being fit in these studies means merely engaging in a cumulative 30 minutes of moderate intensity activity, such as walking, daily.

Key: The greatest health benefits come from taking the first steps toward fitness—study data show about 50% lower mortality in the moderately fit as compared with the low fit…while highly fit individuals lower their mortality risk by only another 10% to 15%.

Recommended: Be physically active. This will greatly reduce health risks regardless of your weight.

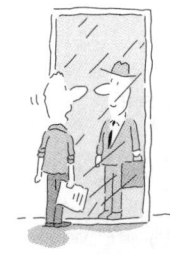

Enjoy a Better Body Image At Any Age

Thomas F. Cash, PhD, professor of psychology at Old Dominion University in Norfolk, VA, and psychologist in Virginia Beach. He is author of several books on body image, including *The Body Image Workbook: An 8-Step Program for Learning to Like Your Looks* (New Harbinger).

The physical changes that accompany aging don't have to make you feel bad about your looks—but often they do.

Negative feelings about your body can lower your self-esteem, causing you to experience social anxiety and, as a result of your feeling unattractive, jeopardize sexual fulfillment.

The good news: It's never too late to transform the relationship you have with your body from a self-defeating, time-consuming struggle to self-acceptance and even enjoyment. *Here's how to do it...*

- **Assess how you currently see yourself.** Set goals for changing the way you feel about your looks. *Ask yourself...*

  - *How satisfied am I with my face, torso, hair, muscle tone and other aspects of my body?*

  - *What is my ideal vision of myself? How close am I now to that vision?*

  - *How often do I have negative feelings about my appearance? Negative thoughts?*

  - *To what extent do these feelings and thoughts limit my life? Social opportunities?*

- **Understand the causes of your negative body image.** Being good-looking doesn't guarantee a positive body image, just as being obese or homely doesn't guarantee self-loathing.

Body image is a state of mind. It is shaped over time in response to cultural influences, experiences with family and friends, and your own physical development.

Helpful exercise: Identify your body image ABCs...

  - *Activators* are the specific events and situations that trigger your thoughts and feelings about your body.

  - *Beliefs* include the thoughts, perceptions and interpretations that typically occur in your mind in response to the activators.

  - *Consequences* are how you tend to react emotionally as well as behaviorally.

Also helpful: Keep a body-image diary to record present-day ABC episodes that perpetuate your negative body image. By recording these episodes, you'll gain insight that will help you change the way you think about your body.

- **Manage body image through relaxation exercises.** Any negative thoughts and feelings about your appearance can lead to anxiety and stress. But, if you practice your relaxation and deep-breathing exercises every day, you will soon be able to relax before anxiety takes hold.

Helpful: Audiotapes can guide you through muscular relaxation and deep-breathing exercises. You can find suitable tapes at music and some natural foods stores.

- **Challenge your assumptions about appearance.** We all have these "appearance assumptions."

Example: *The only way I could ever like the way I look is if I change it.*

Record the appearance assumptions you hold to be true and ask yourself: *What's wrong with this belief? What facts contradict my assumptions?*

Consider the assumption that physically attractive people have it all. Remind yourself of the following realities—beauty can breed envy and jealousy...it raises people's expectations about a person, and those expectations aren't always met...it is a weak foundation for self-esteem.

- **Correct your private "body talk."** Discover, dissect and dispute the negative messages your inner voice repeats about your body.

Examples: *Elizabeth Taylor and I were born the same year, yet she's aging gracefully and I'm not.* Or, *I wasn't asked to see my grandchild's school play because he's ashamed of my weight.*

Talk back to that voice with a new, more positive message...

  - Remind yourself that not seeing yourself as a "10" on a 10-point scale of attractiveness doesn't necessarily make you a "1."

  - Consider how you think about other people's looks. Is it fair to compare yourself to them?

  - Replace the emotionally charged language of your thoughts with more objective descriptions. Instead of referring to yourself as having *hippo hips,* see yourself with rounded hips... instead of *chrome dome,* see yourself as having experienced hair loss.

- **Don't overscrutinize your appearance.** *Appearance-preoccupied rituals are often time-consuming and reinforce discontent with your body image, so work on changing them...*

  - Obstruct them. If you repeatedly pull a mirror out of your purse or pocket to check on

■ *Your Health* ■

your appearance, leave the mirror at home until you feel you have broken the habit.

• Delay them. Whenever you feel the urge to fix your hair or makeup, put off acting on it for a while—and make it a little longer each time. Soon, it will no longer be an urge, but instead a normal activity you engage in a few times a day.

• Restrict them. Allow yourself to perform the ritual one or two times a day, or allow yourself to perform it only at certain times of the day —morning and evening, for instance.

• **Treat your body right.** Think of your body as your friend. Nurture it by keeping it fit and eating healthful foods. The better you feel, the better your body image will be. *Other ways to befriend your body...*

• Write a letter in which you apologize to your body for prior mistreatment. Assure it you want to change the relationship, and thank your body for the good things it has given you.

• Accept compliments on your appearance graciously and without negative self-talk.

• Offer compliments to your reflection in a mirror at least once a day. Notice your smile, your energetic stance, the sparkle in your eyes.

• Remind yourself daily that you are in the process of developing a satisfying body image and living a fuller, more satisfying life.

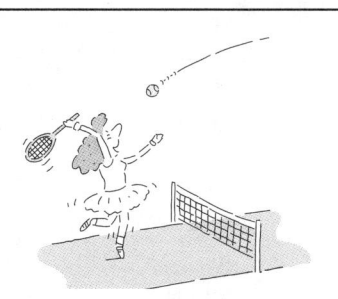

Choosing a Gym Doesn't Have to Be a Workout

Michael F. Roizen, MD, professor of anesthesiology and medicine, Upstate Medical University of the State University of New York, Syracuse, and author of *RealAge: Are You as Young as You Can Be?* (HarperResource).

Joining a health club can be a great investment—or a boondoggle. Only one-third of people who join a gym work out more than 100 days a year. *Here's what you need to do before you join...*

• **Try it out.** Most clubs will let you work out free at least once before joining. Use the free session to test the equipment as well as the atmosphere.

• **Determine your workout needs.** Some people like being pampered in an upscale gym. Others are happy in a concrete room with just a treadmill and free weights.

• **Ask about classes.** Does the schedule work with yours? Is there an extra charge, or are the classes included with membership?

• **Make sure someone will be there to answer questions.** Good gyms have trainers available who will teach you to use the equipment properly. There should be no charge for this service.

• **Find a place that's close.** Most people will continue with their workouts only if the club is within 12 miles of their home or office.

5

The Best in Natural Healing

Should You Forgo Surgery?

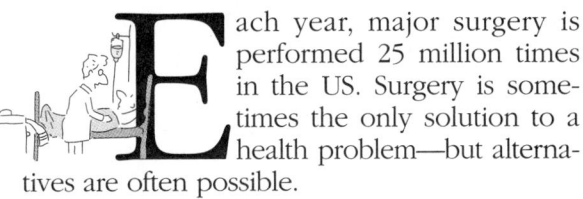

Each year, major surgery is performed 25 million times in the US. Surgery is sometimes the only solution to a health problem—but alternatives are often possible.

In some cases, diet, herbal treatment, acupuncture, yoga and other alternative treatments can eliminate the need for an operation.

Here are some common surgeries for which an alternative is often possible*...

CATARACT REMOVAL

A cataract is cloudiness in the eye's lens. By age 70, up to 70% of Americans suffer from decreased vision because of this condition.

Until recently, alternative medicine has primarily focused on measures to prevent cataracts or to slow their growth. But now, the evidence shows that these same measures may actually reverse cataracts, eliminating the need for surgery altogether.

Nonsurgical program for cataracts...

•**Eat a low-fat, high-fiber diet.** Avoid refined sugar and flour. These foods elevate blood sugar levels, which increases risk for cataracts and accelerates their growth.

•**Take daily vitamin and mineral supplements.** This should include 25,000 international units (IU) of beta-carotene...400 IU of vitamin E (mixed tocopherols)...200 micrograms (mcg) of selenium...50 milligrams (mg) of zinc...and 1,000 mg, three times daily, of vitamin C.

•**Make lifestyle changes.** Wear sunglasses outdoors (if you're often exposed to bright fluorescent light, try lightly tinted glasses indoors)...maintain a healthy weight...avoid tobacco smoke. Sunlight and tobacco smoke

---

*Check with your doctor before trying any of these regimens.

Sandra A. McLanahan, MD, executive medical director of the Integral Health Center in Buckingham, VA. She is coauthor of *Surgery and Its Alternatives: How to Make the Right Choices for Your Health* (Kensington).

Your Health

can damage eye tissues. Excess body weight increases levels of the stress hormone *cortisol,* which accelerates cataract growth.

• **Try herbs.** Da Wei Di Huang Wan (also known as Eight Flavor Rehmannia) is a combination of eight Chinese herbs. It has been reported in the *Journal of the Society for Oriental Medicine* in Japan to be effective in reversing early cataracts. Double-blind studies are still needed to confirm these findings.

This regimen should begin to improve cataracts within six weeks.

CORONARY BYPASS

Coronary heart disease (CHD) blocks blood flow through the arteries that feed the heart. This can cause chest pain (angina), which is frequently severe. But the bigger danger is heart attack.

When CHD is sufficiently advanced (based on the location and severity of blockage), surgery may be recommended to "bypass" the blocked arteries with grafts of blood vessels from elsewhere in the body. However, studies pioneered by renowned heart specialist Dean Ornish, MD, have shown that simple lifestyle changes are 90% effective at reversing coronary artery blockage.

Important: If your heart disease is unstable or has suddenly worsened or if the risk for heart attack is high, surgery may be your only option.

Consider this nonsurgical treatment for coronary heart disease...

• **Cut dietary fat.** Fats in your diet should constitute no more than 10% of daily caloric intake. Consume monounsaturated, rather than saturated, fat. Eating less fat reduces the risk for fatty plaque buildup in the arteries (atherosclerosis) and helps prevent clots from forming.

Limit cholesterol intake to 5 grams per day. Avoid refined sugar and salt.

• **Take vitamin supplements every day.** The most effective supplements include folate (400 mcg) and vitamin B-6 (3 mg). These vitamins improve circulation and reduce levels of homocysteine, an amino acid that appears to promote atherosclerosis.

• **Exercise for one full hour,** at least three times weekly. Choose aerobic activities, such as vigorous walking, swimming or biking. Exercise will reduce blood pressure and improve circulation.

• **Practice meditation,** deep breathing and/or yoga. Stress-reduction techniques work to lower blood pressure and balance out stress hormone levels, enabling the heart to repair damaged tissues.

• **Socialize more often.** Membership in religious groups, support groups and even in bowling leagues has been shown to reduce heart attack risk.

• **Get treatment for related health conditions.** If you have high blood pressure or diabetes, be sure they are being treated effectively. Both conditions promote atherosclerosis.

This type of regimen should help coronary heart disease within a few weeks. Significant changes can be seen within a few months.

HIP REPLACEMENT

Proper diet and exercise can often prevent or arrest hip problems.

Try this nonsurgical program for hip pain and disability...

• **Avoid red meat,** dairy products, refined sugar, salt and caffeine. Eliminating vegetables in the nightshade family (tomatoes, potatoes, eggplant and peppers) may also be helpful. These foods promote inflammation, which can contribute to arthritis.

• **Take daily vitamin and mineral supplements.** To help relieve pain and inflammation, take 1,000 mg of calcium...500 mg of magnesium...and 400 IU of vitamin E (mixed tocopherols). To promote cartilage repair, take 1,000 mg of vitamin C.

• **Try glucosamine sulfate.** This dietary supplement helps maintain and rebuild the cartilage that lines the joint.

Typical dosage: 500 mg, three times daily.

• **Take evening primrose oil.** This herb reduces inflammation and improves circulation.

Typical dosage: 500 mg, three times daily.

• **Lose weight.** This reduces the load borne by the joints.

• **Practice yoga.** This improves circulation and promotes healing.

The Best in Natural Healing

- **Consider acupuncture,** massage or chiropractic treatment. These therapies reduce pain by increasing the body's natural pain-killing endorphins.

This regimen should alleviate hip pain and disability within three months.

For a referral to a physician who is familiar with alternatives to surgery, contact the American Association of Naturopathic Physicians (866-538-2267 or *www.naturopathic.org*).

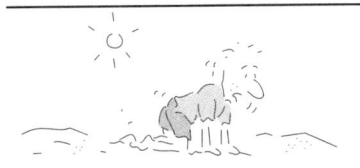

How to Survive a Medical Emergency Without a Doctor

William W. Forgey, MD, secretary and past president of the Wilderness Medical Society in Colorado Springs, *www.wms.org*. He is the author of *Wilderness Medicine: Beyond First Aid* (Globe Pequot) and *The Basic Essentials of First Aid for the Outdoors* (ICS). Dr. Forgey is in private practice in Merrillville, IN. For more information on medical treatment in the outdoors, visit *www.docforgey.com*.

When an emergency strikes, our first response is to call 911. But if you're camped on an isolated mountainside or exploring a remote island, you won't have that option.

Here's how to treat common medical emergencies when they occur in a remote area...

SEVERE CUT

Applying direct pressure with the heel of your hand should stop the bleeding. To avoid contact with the victim's blood, use a plastic bag as a barrier.

To clean the wound, fashion your own irrigation device. To do this, fill a plastic resealable bag with clean water from your canteen. Zip the top shut, punch a tiny hole (the size of a pencil tip) in one corner, and squeeze the bag to force the water out of the hole.

If you don't have a bandage, plastic food wrappers make an effective wound covering. Affix with tape. If tape is not available, rip clothes into strips and tie around the area to hold the covering in place.

If the wound becomes red, swollen or pus-filled, apply granulated sugar. It helps to kill off bacteria.

SPRAIN

Wrap the limb to provide support. T-shirts are a good source of stretchy cloth. If you need a cane, fashion one from a tree branch.

BROKEN BONE

To determine if a bone is broken, use three fingers to press along the length of the bone. If the bone hurts at any spot, it could be broken. Stabilize the limb with splints made from the stays of a backpack frame or strips of a foam sleeping pad. Affix the splint with tape or torn cloth.

A crooked (angulated) fracture can compress arteries, stopping blood flow. To straighten it before applying a splint, grasp both sides of the fracture and gently pull in opposite directions.

POISON IVY

Soothe the rash by applying a cloth soaked in a concentrated salt/water solution.

HYPOTHERMIA

Even during the summer months, a person can experience acute hypothermia if they are immersed in water that is less than 50°F for more than 20 minutes.

If this occurs, the victim should be kept still. Physical activity increases blood flow to the skin. Since the skin is already very cold, moving the victim further reduces core body temperature. Place the victim inside a warm area, such as a tent. If no shelter is available, build a roaring fire to warm the victim.

HEATSTROKE

A person whose skin is hot, flushed and dry and who feels fatigued and/or disoriented should be immersed in cool water.

If no lake or stream is nearby, move the victim into shade. Cool with ice, if available, or spray with water or any cold fluid while vigorously fanning the person.

Also, massage his/her limbs. That helps to move blood from the extremities to the core circulation more readily.

HEART ATTACK

If a person experiences chest heaviness or pain with exertion...pain in the neck or arms...

■ *Your Health* ■

sweating, clammy appearance...and/or extreme shortness of breath, have him lie down to lessen oxygen demand.

Position him so that his head is elevated at a 45° angle. If you have aspirin, give him one regular-strength tablet or two baby aspirin. If he is carrying any prescription heart medication, such as *nitroglycerin,* give him a dose.

EMERGENCY PREPAREDNESS

The *best* way to protect yourself in remote areas is to be prepared...

•**Dress to survive.** If you're going for a jog, walk or hike in the woods, carry emergency supplies. *In addition to bottled water, a hat, sunglasses and insect repellent, your pack should include...*

•A rain poncho or large garbage bag to make into a poncho. It can also be used as a makeshift shelter.

•An extra set of dry clothing in case you need to spend the night outside.

•A signal mirror.

•**Bring a medical kit.** Carry a medical kit that contains sterile gauze...scissors...adhesive and elastic bandages...waterproof tape...splint ...antibiotic ointment...eye drops...latex examination gloves...irrigation syringe...over-the-counter pain reliever, antihistamine, diarrhea and heartburn medications.

Such kits can be purchased at outdoor and sporting-goods stores for about $30 and up.

•**Make sure you use outdoor equipment safely.** Most serious burns in the wilderness happen when boiling water is spilled from a pot that's perched on a rock or when a cooking stove is used incorrectly.

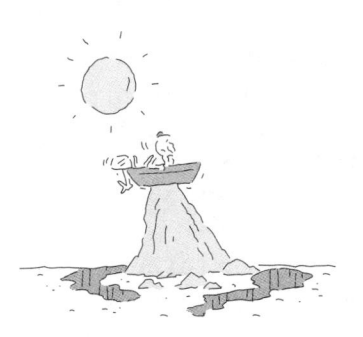

The Ultimate Disease-Fighting Diet

Bradley J. Willcox, MD, principal investigator of geriatrics, Pacific Health Institute, Honolulu, HI, and assistant professor of geriatrics, University of Hawaii. He is coauthor of *The Okinawa Program: How The World's Longest-Lived People Achieve Everlasting Health—and How You Can Too* (Three Rivers).

For years, US government scientists have been urging Americans to consume at least *five* daily servings of fruits and vegetables. But that's not nearly enough, according to new research.

For maximum longevity, look to the fruit- and vegetable-rich diet of the world's longest-lived people—the men and women living in Okinawa, Japan.

During 25 years of study, researchers have found that Okinawans have healthier arteries ...lower risk for hormone-dependent malignancies, such as breast and prostate cancer... stronger bones...sharper minds...lean, fit bodies...and excellent emotional health.

Okinawans eat mainly high-carbohydrate, low-calorie, plant-based foods—the same diet deemed optimal for long-term health by more than 2,000 scientific studies.

At first glance, the Okinawa diet seems like a lot of food to eat each day. The trick is to remember that a daily serving, as defined by the US Department of Agriculture (USDA), is quite small.

Example: For raw, leafy vegetables, a serving is one cup. For whole grains, a serving is one-half cup of cooked cereal, one slice of bread or half a bagel.

If you adhere to the Okinawa program, in which plant-based foods comprise two-thirds of the diet, you will exceed the USDA dietary recommendations.

Here is how scientists have adapted the Okinawa diet for Americans...

•**Eat until you are 80% full.** Okinawans say, *hara hachi bu,* "Eat until you are eight parts full (out of 10)."

Restricting calories is a proven way to prolong life and vitality. Fewer calories will mean fewer free radicals, the molecules responsible for the biochemical damage that causes aging.

This doesn't mean Okinawans eat less. In fact, they eat more food by weight than North Americans. But they eat small amounts of fat and sugar, which are calorie-dense.

To eliminate excess calories...

• Flavor meals with spices instead of fat.

• When cooking, spray the oil instead of pouring—two seconds of spraying equals one-half teaspoon of oil.

• Use heart-healthy canola oil.

• Start your lunch with a chunky, low-fat soup. If you do, you'll eat 20% fewer calories.

• When dining out, order lean fish instead of steak...ask for fatty sauces and dressings to be served on the side...and share desserts.

•**Eat nine to 17 servings of vegetables and fruits daily.** A diet rich in fruits and vegetables decreases your risk for heart disease, cancer, stroke, high blood pressure and obesity.

Fruits and vegetables are full of healthful nutrients—but low in calories. They also contain antioxidants, which help to protect you against free radicals.

To increase your consumption of fruits and vegetables...

• At breakfast, eat a fruit salad with cantaloupe, strawberries, blueberries and apples.

• At lunch, include vegetables like tomato, broccoli and celery in a salad.

• At dinner, make a vegetable soup with onions, zucchini and carrots.

•**Eat seven to 13 servings of whole-grain foods daily.** Whole grains are rich in nutrients, antioxidants and fiber. These constituents decrease your risk for heart disease, stroke, diabetes and cancer.

Many different types of whole grains—from amaranth, barley and bulgur to rice, triticale (a high-protein hybrid of wheat and rye) and wheat—are in cereals, breads and pastas.

For maximum benefit: Choose breakfast cereals that contain at least 7 grams of fiber per serving.

•**Eat two to four servings of calcium foods daily.** Calcium fights osteoporosis and may help to prevent colon cancer, high blood pressure and premenstrual syndrome. Good plant sources of calcium include green, leafy vegetables...calcium-fortified soy products, like tofu and soy milk...and calcium-fortified orange juice.

Important: Low-fat dairy products may not be the best source of calcium. The protein in dairy products may leach the calcium from your bones.

•**Eat two to four servings of flavonoid-rich foods daily.** Blood levels of flavonoids —beneficial compounds found in all plants— are up to 50 times higher in the Japanese than in white Americans, according to a recent study. A high-flavonoid diet may help prevent heart disease as well as breast, prostate and colon cancers.

Isoflavone-rich soy products contain flavonoid levels that are up to 1,000 times greater than those found in other foods.

Flaxseed contains high levels of lignans, which are similar compounds. And, beans are another good source, followed by tea, onions and apples.

To increase your intake of the flavonoids and lignans...

• Eat soy products twice a day. Choices include tofu, miso (a salty paste often used as a flavoring), soy milk, soy nuts and soy burgers.

• Take one tablespoon of flaxseed oil daily, or use it instead of butter or as a salad dressing.

• Drink three cups of tea daily.

• Emphasize flavonoid-rich fruits and vegetables, such as broccoli, kale, celery, onions, snow peas, turnip greens, apples, strawberries, grapes and apricots.

•**Eat one to three servings of omega-3 foods every day.** Most Americans do not consume enough of the omega-3 fatty acids. These dietary constituents protect your brain, arteries and immune system.

To boost your intake of omega-3 foods...

• Eat fatty fish (salmon, tuna and mackerel) three times a week.

• Add flaxseed to your diet. Mix it into pancake or muffin batter or other baked goods.

• Avoid red meat. It may increase your risk for colon and prostate cancer. Do not eat red

■ *Your Health* ■

meat more than three times a week—and choose lean cuts.

● **Drink fresh water.** You need adequate hydration. But forget about the eight-glasses-a-day rule.

Better: Drink enough so that your urine is clear to straw-colored, whether that's four or 12 glasses a day.

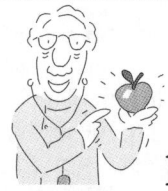

Simple Way to Boost Health

Consider taking 200 micrograms of selenium daily. The mineral enhances immunity... diminishes the adverse effects of drugs and alcohol in the body...and helps to protect against heart disease and some types of cancer, including colorectal, lung and prostate.

Julian Spallholz, PhD, professor of nutritional biochemistry, Texas Tech University, Lubbock.

How to Strengthen Your Immune System Easily

Jamison Starbuck, ND, naturopathic physician in family practice and lecturer at the University of Montana, both in Missoula. She is past president of the American Association of Naturopathic Physicians and a contributing editor to *The Alternative Advisor: The Complete Guide to Natural Therapies and Alternative Treatments* (Time Life).

Strengthening the immune system is a popular concept these days. But if you're like many of my patients, you don't even know what comprises the immune system—much less if yours needs help.

In conventional medical parlance, the "immune system" consists of white blood cells, the lymphatic system, adenoids, thymus, spleen, tonsils and parts of the mucous membranes of the gastrointestinal and respiratory tract. As your body's disease-fighting system, these organs and tissues are activated whenever you encounter microorganisms, foreign substances, such as soot, and/or allergens, such as pollen and animal dander. But your immune health is affected not only by blood cells and lymph tissue but also by emotional stress, physical activity, nutrition and liver function.

Symptoms of a flagging immune system can include chronic fatigue, frequent colds, flu or sinus infections. If you've had two or more of these symptoms for one week per month for three months or more, consider trying the following immune-boosting protocol. *Strategies...*

● **See your doctor to rule out disease.** Ask for a physical exam and lab tests, including a complete blood count...a blood chemistry panel, including cholesterol and glucose levels...a thyroid panel, which measures levels of thyroid-stimulating hormone (TSH) and the thyroid hormones T3 and T4...and an erythrocyte sedimentation rate (ESR) test—a marker of inflammation and illness.

● **Get enough vitamins.** The liver needs hefty supplies of vitamins A, C and E to give your immune system the energy it needs to keep you well. Dark-green veggies, such as spinach, kale and broccoli, as well as orange-colored fruit, such as mango, cantaloupe and apricots, are rich in vitamins A and C. Nuts and soy are high in vitamin E. Nourish your immune system by consuming four vegetables, three fruits, two whole-grain or legume servings and 64 ounces of water daily. Sugar is an immune system depressant, so avoid cola, sweetened cereal, juice and desserts. Eat no more than one serving of sweetened food per day.

● **Choose gentle exercise.** If your immune system is fatigued, shun strenuous exercise, such as jogging, tennis and cycling. These activities stress the muscles and bones, which can just increase inflammation. Instead, walk or swim and/or perform yoga or tai chi.

● **Keep your mood balanced and upbeat.** Avoid disturbing situations whenever possible. Decline social invitations that are not enjoyable. Choose to watch comedies or romances instead of violent films. Solve disputes or misunderstandings right away rather than letting them stew.

● **Take medicinal mushroom extracts.** In Asia, mushrooms have long been used as an immune-enhancing medicine. Modern studies confirm this benefit. My favorite mushrooms include cordyceps, maitake, reishi and shiitake. They are available in powdered or liquid form. The mushroom extracts are safe to use for six months, but, if you suffer a chronic illness, check with your doctor first. For the appropriate dosage, follow the directions on the label.

How to Stay Healthy: Recommendations from Six Prominent Doctors

Robert Abel, Jr., MD, clinical professor of ophthalmology at Thomas Jefferson University Hospital, Philadelphia. He is author of *The Eye Care Revolution* (Kensington).

Samuel Meyers, MD, clinical professor of medicine at Mount Sinai School of Medicine, New York City.

Gail Saltz, MD, assistant professor of psychiatry at New York Presbyterian Hospital and a psychoanalyst in private practice, both in New York City.

Kenneth Offit, MD, MPH, chief of the clinical genetics service at Memorial Sloan-Kettering Cancer Center in New York City.

Sheldon G. Sheps, MD, emeritus professor of medicine at Mayo Medical School, Rochester, MN.

Lisa Meserole, ND, RD, adjunct faculty member of nutrition and botanical medicine and the former head of nutrition at Bastyr University, Seattle.

What's the best way to create a comprehensive strategy for staying healthy? *Leading specialists—experts in heart disease, cancer prevention, eye health and more —give their recommendations below...*

OPHTHALMOLOGIST
Robert Abel, Jr., MD

• **Wear sunglasses outdoors**—even in the winter. This is the best way to minimize eye damage from ultraviolet (UV) light. Consistently wearing sunglasses that block UV rays will halve your risk for cataracts and macular degeneration—the leading causes of vision loss in adults.

If you're taking diuretics or antibiotics: Sunglasses are especially important because these drugs increase photosensitivity, which makes the eye lens much more vulnerable to UV damage.

• **Drink more water.** The body's blood supply does not feed the lens of the eye, so drinking lots of water to flush toxins can reduce the risk for cataracts.

• **Eat cold-water fish three times weekly.** Salmon, tuna, mackerel and sardines are the best dietary sources of *docosahexaenoic acid* (DHA), a long-chain fatty acid that rebuilds damaged cell membranes in the retina and may improve night vision.

If you don't eat fish: Take a fish oil supplement containing 500 milligrams (mg) of supplemental DHA daily...or consume 500 mg of supplemental algae, which is also rich in DHA.

GASTROENTEROLOGIST
Samuel Meyers, MD

• **Eat 30 grams (g) of fiber daily, and limit your fat intake to 30% of total calories.** These two changes alone could substantially reduce your risk for colon cancer and precancerous colon polyps.

Helpful: Start the day with All-Bran, 100% Bran, Raisin Bran or some other whole-grain cereal. Each of these cereals contains at least 8 g of fiber per serving. Other high-fiber foods include strawberries (3 g per cup) and sweet potatoes (4 g per potato).

• **Cook meats and fish thoroughly.** More than 90% of supermarket chicken is contaminated with disease-causing bacteria. Safe food preparation will prevent most cases of infection caused by *Salmonella, Shigella* and *Campylobacter*—and eliminate millions of doctor visits annually. Use a food thermometer to ensure that meats are cooked to 160°F and poultry to 180°F. Never let raw meat juices drip on foods.

• **Get a colonoscopy.** After a baseline test at age 50, repeat the screening at least once every five years. About 150,000 new cases of colon cancer are diagnosed each year. Most could be prevented—or treated early—with proper screening.

If you have a family history of colon cancer: Get your first colonoscopy 10 years before the earliest age at which a family member got the disease. Repeat the test every one to three years, following your doctor's advice.

■ *Your Health* ■

PSYCHIATRIST
Gail Saltz, MD

•**Get help if you suffer from depression**—even if you've had it for only a few weeks. One in 10 Americans suffers from depression. However, most of those people never seek help because they're embarrassed…or they wait so long that the depression becomes resistant to treatment. If you feel symptoms, such as difficulty sleeping, loss of appetite, difficulty concentrating or hopelessness, for more than two weeks, see a mental-health professional. If you have thoughts of harming yourself, seek help immediately.

•**Look for negative patterns in your life.** Don't spend another year making the same bad decisions…sabotaging work success…or failing at relationships.

Break the cycle by reviewing all aspects of your life—family, friends, work, leisure, etc. If things are going poorly, ask yourself why. Look for behaviors that may be setting you back. It is the first step to finding healthier ways to live your life.

•**Acknowledge that you're not perfect.** We all experience anger, frustration and anxiety from time to time. You'll suffer more if you believe that these and other "negative" emotions are somehow abnormal.

When things don't go smoothly, regroup and move forward…and remember to appreciate the good things in your life, such as your health or loving relationships. It's impossible to be happy when your expectations are too high.

GENETIC ONCOLOGIST
Kenneth Offit, MD, MPH

•**Ask family members about their cancer histories.** Find out as much as you can about your relatives' medical histories. Family history is one of the most important risk factors for breast, colon, prostate and other common types of cancer.

Example: If you have a strong family history of breast cancer, your risk of getting it could be 20 times higher than that of someone without the family history.

Knowing that cancer runs in the family will alert you to take the necessary steps to protect yourself. This includes getting regular screening tests and eating a more healthful diet.

Important: Family history goes beyond your parents, siblings or other first-degree relatives. You also need to know the cancer histories of grandparents, aunts and uncles.

•**Do not give up on mammograms.** In reevaluating the previous studies, researchers recently questioned if women who received regular mammograms were less likely to die from breast cancer than women who did not get them. The preponderance of evidence, however, still supports the use of mammograms as a screening technique.

About 47 million American women ages 40 or older should be receiving mammograms. Deaths resulting from breast cancer could be reduced by up to 30% with regular screening. Get tested annually.

CARDIOLOGIST
Sheldon G. Sheps, MD

•**Eat to lower blood pressure.** The DASH (Dietary Approaches to Stop Hypertension) diet is now the gold standard for preventing or reducing high blood pressure. It includes seven to eight daily grain servings…four to five servings each of fruits and vegetables…two to three servings of low-fat dairy…two servings of meat, poultry or fish…and four to five weekly servings of legumes, nuts or seeds. People who follow the diet are less likely to suffer from heart disease, stroke, osteoporosis or kidney stones.

Important: The newly revised DASH diet limits sodium intake to 1,500 mg per day. In sodium-sensitive individuals, reducing sodium can prevent blood pressure in the high end of the prehypertension range (130–139/85–89) from progressing to true hypertension (140/90 or above)…and may reduce your need for medication if you already have hypertension.

•**Set modest weight-loss goals.** If you're overweight, losing as little as 10 pounds may be enough to lower blood pressure by five points. Losing up to 10% of your body weight is often enough to lower blood pressure to a healthful range.

Helpful: Physical activity promotes weight loss and lowers blood pressure—and you don't have to set aside "extra" time to do it.

Incorporate more activity into your daily life by walking the halls at work...parking farther away from the entrance...and taking stairs instead of elevators. You'll get substantial health benefits as long as all forms of physical activity add up to at least 30 minutes daily.

• **Practice slow, deep breathing** for 15 minutes most days. It has the same benefits as other meditative techniques—lowering blood pressure...slowing the heart rate...reducing stress hormones, etc.

• **Don't forget the dangers of secondhand smoke.** Everyone knows that smoking contributes to heart disease, cancer and other serious illnesses. Secondhand smoke will also increase the risk for these ailments, but few people take the necessary steps to avoid prolonged exposure.

NATUROPATHIC PHYSICIAN
Lisa Meserole, ND, RD

• **Eat organic,** locally produced foods. Even so-called "safe" levels of pesticides, herbicides, hormones and other chemicals in commercially grown produce and meats may increase the risk for cancer and other serious diseases.

In recent years, studies have shown a 50% drop in the sperm counts of American men...probably due to environmental toxins. Eating organic foods won't eliminate your exposure to toxins, but it will help minimize the amount you ingest.

• **Personalize your health decisions.** In addition to adopting new habits to improve your overall health, it's important to address specific medical conditions.

Suppose you get frequent sinus infections. Resolve to eat more vitamin C–rich foods to help the mucous membranes function effectively...keep the air moisturized with a humidifier...and exercise daily to improve immunity.

• **Balance work with play.** Don't try to do everything. Psychological stress is at epidemic levels in this country. Stress damages blood vessels, raises blood pressure and makes it hard to think clearly and make intelligent, life-affirming decisions. Relaxing isn't a luxury—you need it for your health. Make time each day for humor and love.

The Best in Natural Healing

Cranberries Protect Against Disease

Cranberries top the list of disease-fighting foods. Ounce for ounce, they contain more beneficial compounds than other nutritional powerhouses, like broccoli and blueberries. Fresh and dried cranberries provide the greatest antioxidant protection against heart disease and cancer, followed by cranberry sauce and cranberry juice.

Good idea: Eat one-half cup of fresh or dried cranberries daily.

Joe A. Vinson, PhD, professor of chemistry, University of Scranton.

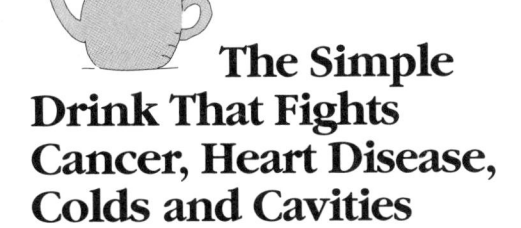

The Simple Drink That Fights Cancer, Heart Disease, Colds and Cavities

Lester A. Mitscher, PhD, distinguished professor of medicinal chemistry at University of Kansas, Lawrence. In 2000, Dr. Mitscher won the American Chemical Society's lifetime achievement award for his work with teas and antibiotic resistance. He is coauthor of *The Green Tea Book: China's Fountain of Youth* (Avery).

You know that green tea is good for you. But did you know that green *and* black teas help ward off many types of cancer, fight heart disease and colds, even prevent cavities?

A Chinese emperor first touted the health benefits of green tea more than 4,000 years ago. *Here's what the latest scientific research shows...*

WHY TEA HELPS

Green and black teas are made from the leaves of the *Camellia sinensis* plant. The leaves contain *catechins,* antioxidants that block the action of free radicals (harmful molecules).

The most powerful catechin is *epigallocatechin gallate* (EGCG). A study conducted at the University of Shizuoka in Japan showed that the antioxidant power of EGCG in green

■ *Your Health* ■

tea was 200 times stronger than that of vitamin E, another antioxidant.

Green tea is made from fresh, young leaves, which are steamed right away to preserve catechins and then dried. Black tea contains about half the catechins as green tea because it undergoes more processing before leaves are dried.

SPECIFIC BENEFITS

The health benefits of catechins found in tea include...

•**Reducing risk of certain types of cancer,** including cancers of the lung, breast and digestive tract. In a University of Minnesota study of more than 35,000 women over eight years, those who drank two or more cups of green or black tea daily had a 10% lower risk of developing any cancer than those who seldom drank tea.

•**Reducing heart disease** by blocking the formation of plaque in the coronary arteries. A four-year study conducted at Harvard Medical School indicated that participants who drank 14 cups or more of green or black tea weekly had a 44% lower death rate after a heart attack than people who didn't drink tea.

•**Fewer colds and other illnesses.** Tea prevents free radicals from undermining the immune system. In a 2002 report, researchers at Toyama Medical and Pharmaceutical University in Japan confirmed reports that catechins in green tea extract inhibit the growth of the influenza virus. Scientists at the Health Science Center of the State University of New York in Syracuse, reviewed this literature and concluded that green tea enhances immunity.

•**Building bone density.** One study of more than 1,000 participants indicated that drinking two or more cups of tea a day for at least six years strengthened bone density.

•**Preventing cavities** by blocking growth of *Streptococcus mutans,* bacterium associated with dental plaque.

•**Aiding digestion** by fostering the growth of beneficial bacteria in the intestines.

HOW MUCH TEA?

Aim for four cups of green tea or six cups of black tea daily. Expensive teas may taste better, but they don't necessarily provide more health benefits.

Brew tea for three minutes to ensure the release of antioxidants. Longer steeping only produces more tannins, which taste bitter.

Iced tea yields the same benefits, but antioxidants degrade with time, so drink the tea soon after brewing.

Tea contains less caffeine than coffee—up to 30 milligrams (mg) per cup of green tea...up to 90 mg for black, versus 160 mg for brewed coffee. People who are sensitive to caffeine may prefer decaffeinated tea. The process that removes caffeine from tea does not interfere with its health benefits.

Alternative: Try caffeine-free green tea capsules, available at health food stores. Look for a brand that is organic, free of preservatives and has an expiration date to ensure freshness. The usual dose is two 250-mg capsules daily.

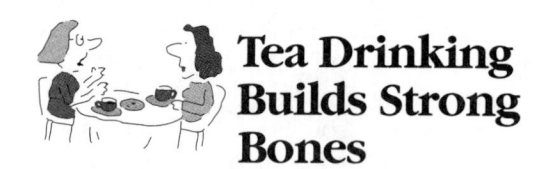

Tea Drinking Builds Strong Bones

In a recent finding, the lumbar spine and hipbones in people who averaged two cups of tea a day for six years were an average of 2% denser than those of people who did not drink tea. After 10 years, bone density among tea drinkers was 6% greater.

Theory: Fluoride and chemical compounds in tea called *flavonoids* enhance bone density. Black, green and oolong tea all offer the same benefit.

Chang Chin Jen, MD, director, diabetes and obesity research center, National Cheng Kung University Hospital, Taiwan.

Better Tea Drinking

Herbal tea has long been touted for helping to fight heart disease and cancer. But recent research now indicates that herbal teas made out of dried citrus fruit contain a high acid content that will dissolve tooth enamel.

If you drink citrus teas: Have no more than three cups per day, and drink it with meals. High salivary flow produced when eating helps neutralize acids. Rinse your mouth with water after each cup.

Paul Brunton, PhD, senior lecturer in integrative restorative care, University Dental Hospital of Manchester, England.

When Herbs Are Safer Than Drugs

Ethan Russo, MD, clinical assistant professor of medicine at the University of Washington School of Medicine in Seattle. Dr. Russo is an adjunct professor of pharmaceutical sciences at the University of Montana and a neurologist in private practice, both in Missoula. He is also author of the *Handbook of Psychotropic Herbs: A Scientific Analysis of Herbal Remedies for Psychiatric Conditions* (Haworth).

Each year, an estimated 100,000 Americans die from side effects caused by prescription medications. That's nearly 20 times the death rate caused by illegal drugs.

Why so many deaths? Ironically, one contributing factor is the US government's drug-approval process. To maximize the effectiveness of drugs, the Food and Drug Administration approves many medications based on studies performed at high dosages.

New study: Dosage and usage instructions for 20% of prescription medications are corrected *after* they become available to consumers. In most cases, that means lowering the recommended dosage or adding warnings for certain patients.

Even at low dosages, some drugs cause side effects and pose a risk for dangerous interactions when they are taken along with other medications.

Good news: In many cases, centuries-old herbal remedies can be just as effective, much safer and less expensive than prescription and over-the-counter (OTC) drugs.

Here are some herbal alternatives for five common conditions*...

ACUTE PAIN

Most people who suffer a sprain, muscle strain or some other acute injury take an OTC pain reliever, such as aspirin or *acetaminophen*. The prescription Cox-2 inhibitors *rofecoxib* (Vioxx) and *celecoxib* (Celebrex) are also popular options.

However, aspirin can cause gastrointestinal bleeding, while acetaminophen can damage the liver when taken with alcohol. And, the drugs rofecoxib and celecoxib have been linked to heart attack.

Alternative: *Bromelain* is an enzyme found in pineapple. Bromelain offers effective relief for various types of inflammation and pain, including arthritis.

Reliable brand: Now Foods' Bromelain. Take 2,000 gelatin dissolving units (GDU) as needed between meals.

Caution: Do not confuse this remedy with *bromaline*, a decongestant.

DEPRESSION

Fluoxetine (Prozac), *sertraline* (Zoloft) and other selective serotonin reuptake inhibitors (SSRIs) are among the most widely prescribed medications in America.

While these drugs generally produce fewer side effects than older antidepressants, they can cause drowsiness, constipation, insomnia, anxiety, tremor and reduced sex drive. On average, one in five people stop taking SSRIs because of side effects.

Alternative: *St. John's wort* fights mild to moderate depression. In Germany, doctors prescribe this well-known herb nearly eight times as often as prescription antidepressants.

So why is recent research questioning the effectiveness of St. John's wort? Ninety percent of the treatment failures with St. John's wort are attributable to inadequate dosing or inadequate preparations. Ideally, 300-milligram (mg) capsules should be taken three times daily.

Reliable brands: Kira and Movana.

*Check with your doctor before stopping a prescription drug or taking any of these products.

■ *Your Health* ■

INSOMNIA

Zolpidem (Ambien) is a popular and effective drug for insomnia. However, it can cause daytime drowsiness, constipation and dry mouth. Doctors also commonly prescribe *diazepam* (Valium) for insomnia, but it is highly addictive.

Alternative: *German chamomile* contains *apigenin,* an antianxiety agent that has a calming effect without causing drowsiness. It can be used during waking hours to curb anxiety or at night as a sleep aid.

Add one teaspoon of German chamomile powder to boiling water and drink as a tea 30 minutes before bedtime—or whenever you feel anxious. German chamomile is also available in capsules.

Reliable brand: Nature's Way Chamomile Extract. Take one to two 125-mg capsules as they are needed.

MIGRAINE

In rare cases, *sumatriptan* (Imitrex), the popular prescription drug used to treat migraines, has been associated with heart attacks and transient spikes in blood pressure.

Alternative: Studies show that *feverfew* helps prevent and treat migraine. The herb is believed to interrupt the inflammatory process that triggers headaches.

Reliable brand: MygraFew by Nature's Way. Take one 600-microgram tablet daily to prevent migraine.

MOTION SICKNESS

The popular OTC treatment *dimenhydrinate* (Dramamine) should be used carefully. It often causes drowsiness, which can be dangerous—especially if you're driving or operating machinery.

Alternative: *Ginger* is effective for motion sickness as well as nausea.

Reliable brand: Nature's Way capsules, containing powdered gingerroot. Take two to four 550-mg capsules as needed.

Bonus: When taken at the same dosage, ginger also helps relieve headaches.

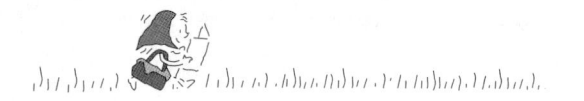

Oregano Oil May Replace Antibiotics

Oregano oil extract destroys the deadly *Staphylococcus* bacterium as effectively as the strongest antibiotic.

Bonus: The extract may provide an alternative treatment for antibiotic-resistant organisms. However, it has not yet been tested in humans.

Focus on Alternative and Complementary Therapies, Peninsula Medical School, Universities of Exeter and Plymouth, 25 Victoria Park Rd., Exeter EX2 4NT, UK.

Are You Aging Too Fast?

Roy Walford, MD, professor of pathology at the University of California at Los Angeles School of Medicine. Dr. Walford is recognized internationally as one of the top experts in the field of gerontology and is a pioneer of the life-extension movement. He has published more than 350 scientific articles and six books, including *Beyond the 120 Year Diet: How to Double Your Vital Years* (Four Walls Eight Windows).

Self-tests are an easy way to help determine your *functional* age—a measurement of how a person actually functions, rather than how many years he/she has been alive.

●**Elasticity test.** This measures the degree of deterioration of the connective tissue under the skin, a sign of aging.

Pinch the skin on the back of your hand between your thumb and forefinger for five seconds, then time how long it takes to flatten out completely.

Up to age 50, it will take about five seconds ...by age 60, the average time is 10 to 15 seconds...by age 70, the typical time will be 35 to 55 seconds.

●**Static balance test.** How long can you stand on one leg with your eyes closed before falling over?

Perform this test either barefoot or wearing low-heeled shoes. Stand on a hard surface (not a rug) with both feet together and close your eyes. Lift your foot six inches off the ground, bending your knee at about a 45-degree angle. (If you're right-handed, stand on your left leg. Left-handers should stand on the right leg.) Have a friend close by to catch you in case you fall. Do the test three times, and calculate the average.

On average, a 100% decline occurs from age 20 to age 80. Most young people are able to stand 30 seconds or more. Few older people will be able to hold the pose longer than a few seconds.

If your self-test results do not fall within the normal range for your age, consult your doctor for specific advice on how to minimize the effects of aging.

Think Positively and Live Longer

People who view aging as a positive experience live an average of seven-and-a-half years longer than those who look at it negatively, according to a recent study. In any given year, other studies indicate pessimists have a risk of death 19% greater than average. The power of optimism is even greater than that of lower blood pressure or reduced cholesterol—each of which lengthens a life by about four years, according to some studies.

Becca R. Levy, PhD, assistant professor of epidemiology, Yale School of Public Health, New Haven, CT, and leader of a study of 660 people over age 50, published in the *Journal of Personality and Social Psychology*.

The Wrinkle-Cure Diet— What to Eat to Look Much Younger

Nicholas Perricone, MD, dermatologist and adjunct professor of medicine at the College of Human Medicine, Michigan State University, East Lansing. He is best-selling author of *The Perricone Prescription* (HarperResource) and *The Wrinkle Cure* (Warner).

Most people think that wrinkles are an inevitable part of getting older. *This is not necessarily so.*

Wrinkles happen when low-grade cellular inflammation—caused by pollution, too much sun, poor nutrition and by-products of the body's metabolism—triggers the release of *activator protein 1* (AP-1) and other chemicals that destroy collagen, the connective tissue that makes skin supple and elastic.

Improving your diet can prevent wrinkles and minimize the ones you have already. The key is to avoid inflammatory foods and to eat foods that block the inflammatory process. Most of these good foods also boost general health and help prevent cancer, heart disease and other illnesses.

PROTEIN

Protein is an essential component for repairing cells, including the collagen cells. Without enough of it, people quickly lose skin tone. The optimal amount is 65 grams (g) each day for women and 80 g for men. I recommend that people have three meals and two snacks a day —each of which should include protein.

Examples: Just four ounces of roasted chicken breast delivers about 31 g of protein... one-half cup of navy beans has 7 g...four ounces of baked salmon has 22 g.

Animal protein—from chicken, eggs, pork, lean beef, fish, etc.—provides more amino acids, a component of protein essential for cell repair, and is more readily absorbed than plant protein. Vegetarians should supplement their diets with protein powders and soy foods, such as tempeh and tofu.

SALMON

In addition to high-quality protein that aids in skin repair, fish contains essential fatty acids (EFAs) that block inflammation. Fish is also the best dietary source of *dimethylaminoethanol* (DMAE), which prevents metabolic by-products (free radicals) from damaging skin cells.

Recommended: Eat fish at least three times a week.

Salmon—either canned or fresh—contains the most protective compounds. Eating salmon twice a day can make skin look more radiant in just three days.

If you don't like fish: You can take capsules of fish oil or flaxseed oil two or three times a day. Or you can have four teaspoons of

■ *Your Health* ■

flaxseed oil daily. You also can grind up one tablespoon of flaxseed, and sprinkle it on food. After fish, it's the best dietary source of EFAs.

DARK GREEN VEGETABLES

The dark, leafy greens—such as arugula, romaine and spinach—and broccoli contain EFAs, carotenoids and other antioxidants that block inflammation.

Recommended: Eat green vegetables at least twice a day.

OLIVE OIL

Olive oil is rich in *polyphenols*, another type of antioxidant that blocks inflammation. It also contains a monounsaturated fat called *oleic acid*, which makes it easier for the EFAs in fish and other foods to penetrate cell membranes. You can cook with olive oil or use it to make salad dressings.

Recommended: Two tablespoons of olive oil daily. Extra virgin Spanish olive oil contains the largest amount of skin-protecting polyphenols. We don't know why Spanish oil is the most protective—it might be the soil or the particular type of tree.

LOW-GLYCEMIC FOODS

An important consideration in a skin-healthy diet is a food's glycemic index. The index rates foods on a scale of 1 to 100, depending on their effects on blood-sugar (glucose) levels. Blood-sugar control is important because sudden surges trigger an inflammatory response in the skin.

White bread, for example, has a very high glycemic index of 95, which means that it is quickly absorbed and floods the bloodstream with glucose, the form of sugar used by cells to produce energy.

Other high-glycemic foods: White rice, pasta, pretzels, candy, cake and other low-fiber starches.

Low-glycemic choices: Lentils, oatmeal (instant or regular), peanuts, nuts and most fruits and vegetables.

BERRIES

Fresh or frozen strawberries, raspberries, blueberries and blackberries are among the best sources of *anthocyanins*, compounds that block enzymes that degrade collagen as well as other connective tissue.

Recommended: One-quarter cup of berries every day.

ANTIOXIDANT SUPPLEMENTS

I advise most people to supplement their diets with 1,000 milligrams of vitamin C in divided doses and 400 international units of vitamin E daily.

Vitamin C capsules and powders are absorbed more readily than hard tablets. For vitamin E, take a capsule combination supplement that includes *tocotrienols* and *tocopherols*. Take vitamin E with meals for better absorption.

LOTS OF WATER

Water plumps up skin cells...reduces the concentration of inflammatory chemicals...and improves the body's absorption of vitamins and minerals.

I avoid tap water, which is usually chlorinated and may contain unhealthy compounds like heavy metals. Treat yourself to spring water.

Recommended: At least eight glasses of water a day.

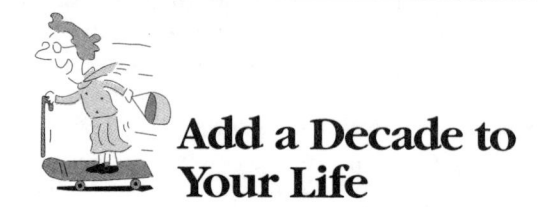

Add a Decade to Your Life

Healthful living can add an extra *decade* to your life. In what's believed to be the first study to quantify the life-extending benefits of a healthful lifestyle, researchers found that people who ate a vegetarian diet, exercised vigorously for at least 15 minutes three or more times every week, maintained an appropriate weight, never smoked and ate moderate amounts of nuts five times a week lived 10 years longer than people who didn't.

Gary Fraser, MD, PhD, professor of epidemiology and medicine, Loma Linda University, Loma Linda, CA.

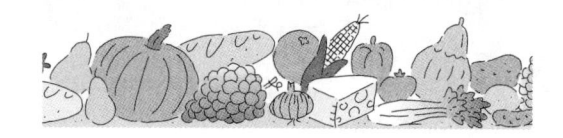

The Best in Natural Healing

Natural Treatment For Alzheimer's

Aromatherapy may decrease agitation from Alzheimer's. In a recent study, applying lemon balm to the face and arms helped ease agitation in up to 60% of patients treated, compared with only 14% who received the placebo cream. The lemon balm group was also more sociable with others and better able to perform constructive activities.

Elaine K. Perry, PhD, senior scientist at Newcastle General Hospital, Newcastle upon Tyne, England. Her study was published in *The Journal of Clinical Psychiatry*.

Olive Oil Helps Prevent Cognitive Decline

Eat to fight cognitive decline by including monounsaturated fats, such as olive oil, in your diet—instead of saturated fats, such as butter and other animal fats.

Recent study: Elderly Southern Italians consuming a typical Mediterranean diet were less likely to develop age-related cognitive problems if they consumed large amounts of olive oil—the oil with the most monounsaturated fat per ounce.

Also: Unsaturated fats work to lower LDL (bad) cholesterol levels while helping to raise HDL (good) cholesterol.

Vincenzo Solfrizzi, MD, PhD, specialist in geriatric medicine, department of geriatrics, Center for Aging Brain, University of Bari-Policlinico, Bari, Italy.

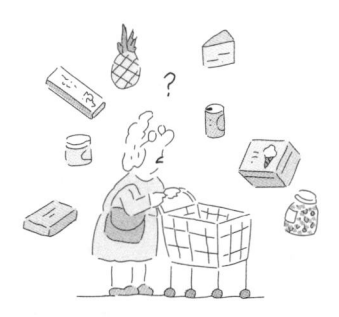

Tired? Forgetful? You May Need More B Vitamins

Michael Hirt, MD, assistant clinical professor of medicine at the University of California, Los Angeles School of Medicine, and medical director of the Center for Integrative Medicine at Encino-Tarzana Regional Medical Center in Encino, CA.

By now, everyone should recognize that folate (folic acid) prevents birth defects when taken by pregnant women.

But now there's strong evidence that folate and other B vitamins provide many additional benefits. In fact, B vitamins do a better job of protecting an adult's *overall* health than any other vitamin.

A new study of more than 9,000 Americans shows that people with the highest dietary intake of folate—400 micrograms (mcg) a day—have an 86% lower risk for heart attack and a 79% lower risk for stroke than those with the lowest intake (100 mcg).

Evidence also suggests that a high intake of folate may decrease the risk of developing colon and breast cancers. In addition, B vitamins may help prevent Alzheimer's disease as well as other memory problems older adults experience.

How can one nutrient provide so many health benefits? *Michael Hirt, MD, one of only a handful of US physicians board certified in nutrition, answers this question and more...*

•**What is the function of B vitamins?** There are seven different B vitamins. In addition to folate, there are B-1 (thiamine), B-2 (riboflavin), B-3 (niacin), B-5 (pantothenic acid), B-6 (pyridoxine) and B-12 (cobalamin).

Each of these vitamins is critical for optimum health. Collectively, they play an important role in how our bodies metabolize sugar, fat and protein and in the production of energy.

B vitamins also aid the functioning of the nerves and brain chemistry and boost immunity.

•**Why is folate so important in protecting the heart?** Folate helps lower blood levels of the amino acid homocysteine. A high level of homocysteine (above 10) is a risk factor for heart disease and stroke.

Low-fat diets, regular exercise and other heart-healthy actions don't affect the body's homocysteine levels. Getting enough folate is the only way to lower homocysteine.

•**Is that why flour-containing foods are fortified with folate?** No. This practice was mandated in 1998 to prevent birth defects. Along with vitamin B-12, folate is essential for synthesis of DNA—the genetic molecule that "instructs" cells how to form and act.

If a pregnant woman doesn't get enough folate, fetal DNA can't multiply properly. That can result in spina bifida, a neural tube defect in which the spinal bones and spinal cord don't fuse correctly as the body forms.

Fortifying flour with folate helps to ensure that all women receive enough folate in their diets to prevent spina bifida. Every woman of childbearing age should consume 400 mcg to 800 mcg of folate daily.

•**What about the other B vitamins?** Vitamin B-12 is probably second to folate in therapeutic power. In large doses prescribed by a physician, vitamin B-12 can help to ease symptoms of low-grade depression, chronic fatigue, chronic pain, dust, pollen and other allergies and the mood swings of premenstrual syndrome (PMS). Vitamin B-12 can also help control the side effects of psychoactive medications, such as those used to treat Parkinson's disease and schizophrenia.

•**Which foods contain high levels of B vitamins?** Some of the best sources of B vitamins are whole grains, beans, peas and vegetables. Since most Americans don't eat a lot of these foods, they usually consume less than the government's recommended dietary intake of B vitamins.

Helpful: Everyone should be sure to get a blood test every two years to check for any B vitamin deficiencies.

•**Is low dietary intake the sole cause of a deficiency?** No. Stress depletes the body of B vitamins, so a hectic lifestyle can cause a deficiency.

Also, cooking vegetables—one of the best sources of these nutrients—reduces B vitamin content. To avoid this problem, you can steam your vegetables—which destroys fewer vitamins—or even better, eat them raw.

Older adults—particularly those over age 65—are at risk for a deficiency of vitamin B-12 no matter how much they get in their diets.

As the stomach lining ages, its ability to absorb B-12 decreases. This condition causes a deficiency that can usually be corrected with a B-12 injection or a tablet that dissolves under the tongue.

•**Should all adults take a B vitamin supplement?** Yes. Because these vitamins help lower levels of homocysteine in the blood, we would see a dramatic decrease in the incidence of heart disease in this country.

Each year, more than 500,000 Americans die from heart disease—many of those lives would be saved if everyone included a B vitamin in their supplement regimen.

•**What do you look for in a B vitamin supplement?** I recommend a B-complex supplement that contains 100% of the recommended daily intake, or daily value (DV), of each of the seven B vitamins. Be sure to check the label.

Important: Under certain conditions, you should take more than the DV of vitamin B-12. For example, I recommend supplementing your B-complex intake for a total of 100 mcg to 200 mcg of vitamin B-12 if blood tests determine that you have difficulty absorbing the nutrient…if you're over age 65…or if you have frequent indigestion, which can indicate an inflammation of the stomach that decreases absorption of B-12.

•**Is it possible to consume too much in B vitamins?** Yes. More than 200 milligrams (mg) daily of vitamin B-3 (niacin), which may be prescribed to lower cholesterol levels, can cause skin flushing and dangerously high levels of liver enzymes.

With vitamin B-6, which can be taken to alleviate PMS symptoms, you should never take more than 25 mg a day without a doctor's supervision. Taken on a daily basis, high levels of vitamin B-6 can cause permanent nerve damage.

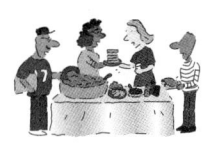

Smart Food Choices Boost Brainpower

Arthur Winter, MD, neurosurgeon and director of the New Jersey Neurological Institute in Livingston. He is coauthor, with his wife, science writer Ruth Winter, of *Smart Food: Diet and Nutrition for Maximum Brain Power* (Griffin Trade).

Everyone knows that diet has a profound effect on weight, as well as risk for heart disease, cancer and many other serious illnesses. But very few people recognize the impact that food has on brain function.

Brain chemicals known as neurotransmitters carry messages that alter both mood and the ability to think. One such neurotransmitter, *serotonin,* is the body's natural antidepressant. Another, *cholecystokinin,* aids memory.

Research now shows that you can influence neurotransmitter activity through food choices. By eating the right foods, you can improve memory, maintain alertness throughout the day and soothe anxiety.

Situation: Mental fatigue causes you to lose your focus during an intensely competitive round of bridge.

What to eat: There's nothing like caffeine to reverse a sinking mental performance or snap you out of fatigue. But you must consume a considerable amount for the best effect—150 milligrams (mg) to 600 mg for a 150-pound person. Six ounces of coffee contains about 100 mg of caffeine.

Natural forms of sugar also act as mental boosters because they increase blood sugar levels. Glucose, found in grapes, oranges and corn, is a fast-acting form of natural sugar. It takes only two minutes to raise blood sugar.

Fructose, found in many fruits and vegetables, is slow acting—it takes about 25 minutes to increase blood sugar—but its energy effect is longer lasting. Munch on fresh fruits and crudités throughout your game to stave off mental fatigue.

Situation: You face a day-long seminar. You need both mental alertness and endurance.

What to eat: Protein is key. It provides the building blocks for *norepinephrine* and *dopamine*—neurotransmitters that help you maintain your mental edge.

Eating any type of breakfast helps increase concentration and performance. A protein-rich breakfast enhances those benefits.

Best protein sources: Eggs, fish, meat, yogurt, cheese and milk.

Everyone experiences a decline in alertness about two hours after lunch. The bigger the lunch, the bigger the drop-off. If you must stay in high gear, consider skipping lunch.

If midday fasting doesn't work for you, opt for easy-to-digest protein choices, such as tuna or egg salad.

Carbohydrates elevate levels of the amino acid *tryptophan,* which helps to produce the calming neurotransmitter serotonin. Loading up on protein and limiting carbohydrates, such as pasta and french fries, will help to minimize post-lunch drowsiness.

Situation: You are giving a presentation at work. You need quick recall.

What to eat: Cholecystokinin is a neurotransmitter that improves memory by releasing tryptophan and another amino acid called *phenylalanine.* However, timing is everything if you want to achieve cholecystokinin's optimal effect.

Review your presentation *before* you eat. Immediately after you finish memorizing the material, have a snack or meal that contains cholecystokinin-releasing foods to help you memorize what you have just learned.

Foods that release cholecystokinin include milk, nuts and rice.

Situation: You feel cranky and out of sorts.

What to eat: Foods rich in the omega-3 fatty acids—salmon, trout, herring, walnuts, canola oil, soybeans and flaxseed oil—help to curb depression.

Chocolate, which boosts levels of serotonin, also eases a depressed mood.

For a calming effect, it's best to choose foods that contain tryptophan. It's found in turkey, bananas and peanuts.

■ *Your Health* ■

Little-Known Benefit of Watermelon

Watermelon is a good source of the cancer-fighting antioxidant *lycopene*. They have 60% more lycopene than raw tomatoes. The body needs a little fat to absorb lycopene, so consider having watermelon for dessert after a meal that includes some fat.

Penelope Perkins-Veazie, PhD, plant physiologist, US Department of Agriculture, Agricultural Research Service, Lane, OK.

Cancer-Fighting Condiment

Turmeric contains curcumin, a compound that has been found in lab tests to slow progression of some forms of cancer—particularly of the colon, esophagus, mouth and skin. Turmeric is often used in Indian dishes, like rice and curries, and is also used in pickles.

Bandaru S. Reddy, PhD, chief, division of nutritional carcinogenesis, Institute for Cancer Prevention, 1 Dana Rd., Valhalla, NY 10595.

New Benefits of Broccoli

Broccoli fights ulcers and may even prevent stomach cancer. *Sulforaphane,* in broccoli and broccoli sprouts, often kills *Helicobacter pylori,* which causes stomach ulcers and sometimes stomach cancer. Research has been done on mice and human cells in the laboratory, not on people, so scientists do not know how much broccoli is needed for a protective effect. Further research is in the planning stages.

Jed Fahey, faculty research associate, Johns Hopkins University School of Medicine, Baltimore, and leader of the sulforaphane study, reported in *Proceedings of the National Academy of Sciences.*

Another Natural Cancer Fighter

Preliminary evidence suggests that *mistletoe extract* (Iscar) helps to fight all types of cancer—most effectively as a complement to conventional treatment, including chemotherapy and radiation. In several studies, cancer patients who took mistletoe extract to augment their regular treatment survived an average of 40% longer than people who relied on conventional therapies alone.

Mistletoe extract is now the most widely used adjunct cancer treatment in Germany.

Self-defense: Ask your doctor about taking mistletoe extract as part of your cancer treatment program.

Ronald Grossarth-Maticek, MD, PhD, head, Institute for Preventive Medicine, University for Peace of the United Nations, Heidelberg, Germany.

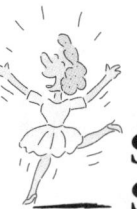

Stop Pain Fast with Self-Hypnosis

Bruce N. Eimer, PhD, clinical psychologist and hypnotherapist in private practice in Philadelphia. He is author of *Hypnotize Yourself Out of Pain Now! A Powerful, User-Friendly Program for Anyone Searching for Immediate Pain Relief* (New Harbinger).

As a clinical psychologist, I have specialized for 18 years in treating people with chronic pain.

However, only after a car accident left me in severe, unrelenting pain did I come to fully appreciate the power of hypnosis to pick up where drugs, physical therapy and surgery leave off.

WHY HYPNOSIS?

Hypnosis is an altered state of consciousness. It magnifies your ability to focus and temporarily sharpens your concentration.

All hypnosis is *self*-hypnosis. Even if the state is achieved with the help of an expert, you can become hypnotized only if *you* allow yourself to be.*

The nature of hypnosis makes it helpful for chronic pain. It is a state of concentrated attention, which in itself can reduce pain and emotional anguish associated with physical suffering. It also eases tension and curbs insomnia.

ENTERING THE HYPNOTIC STATE

The first step in hypnosis is called *induction*. In this process, you employ techniques that focus your attention (on the ticking of a metronome or the sound of a voice, for example) and provide suggestions to deepen your relaxation.

Try this two-minute induction method, which many people find effective...

Raise one hand. Concentrate on a single finger, with your eyes open (staring at the finger) or closed (imagining it). Then, let the other fingers fade away from your awareness.

As you continue to concentrate, feel your hand and arm start to grow heavier. Lower your arm slowly, and allow yourself to enter into a comfortable state of relaxation.

By the time your hand comes all the way down and is resting in your lap or on the armrest of your chair, your eyes should be closed and you should feel relaxed. Focus on your breathing. Feel your belly expand with each inhalation and contract as you exhale.

To relax more deeply, close your eyes and imagine you are walking down a set of 20 stairs. Feel the thick, plush carpeting beneath your feet as well as the smooth, polished wood of the handrail.

With each step, you fall into a deeper state of relaxation. At the bottom of the stairs, you find a door. Open it, and "enter" the place where you feel the most happy, content and pleased (a balmy beach, a peaceful mountain meadow or a sidewalk café in Paris). Imagine this "favorite place" in rich detail, and stay there as long as you want.

To emerge from the hypnotic state, walk back up the stairs, feeling more awake with each step. When you reach the top, you'll feel alert and refreshed.

*To locate a qualified clinical hypnosis practitioner in your area, contact the American Society of Clinical Hypnosis (630-980-4740 or *www.asch.net*).

The more often you repeat the induction, the better you will get at it. Practice at least twice a day, for 10 minutes each time.

USING THE HYPNOTIC STATE

After you have practiced induction daily for three weeks, you should be able to elicit deep relaxation at will and go to your "favorite place" whenever you need a stress break or a respite from pain.

Once you have mastered the induction process, the following techniques can be added. Practice the technique of your choice for 10 minutes daily.

•**Distraction.** Most people naturally cope with pain by focusing their attention elsewhere. For a simple distraction technique, rub the fingers of one hand together. Concentrate on the sensations in your fingers, the texture of the skin and the temperature.

Do this *before* inducing the hypnotic state. This will give your subconscious the suggestion that you can distract yourself the same way whenever you feel discomfort. After the first month, you'll find that even when you are in your normal waking state, you'll be able to divert your attention away from pain more effectively.

•**Dissociation.** This is perhaps the most powerful way to cope with severe pain. Your pain is not gone, but your subconscious mind takes over the task of feeling the pain while your conscious mind is relaxed.

Practice this technique by visualizing your shadow. It moves with you and is attached to your body, but it is not inside your body. While in a hypnotic state, imagine your shadow... then visualize yourself merging with it.

Put the pain in your shadow. Then imagine yourself floating away from the shadow and the pain. The pain is in your shadow, but not in your body.

•**Self-suggestion.** This technique helps to develop attitudes and beliefs that strengthen your ability to cope with pain.

Choose messages that have particular meaning for you, and write them in a journal or on index cards. Repeat one to yourself three times before inducing the hypnotic state.

■ Your Health ■

Some helpful self-suggestions...

- *I am in charge.*
- *I can manage the pain. I can stand this.*
- *Whenever I feel stressed, I accept the feelings and stay calm.*
- *I take satisfaction every day in handling my problems better and better.*

Lower Your Cholesterol Without Drugs

Robert E. Kowalski, medical journalist and author of The New 8-Week Cholesterol Cure: The Ultimate Program for Preventing Heart Disease *(Quill). He is editor of* Diet-Heart Newsletter, *Box 2039, Venice, CA 90294, www.thehealthyheart.net.*

It is possible to lower your cholesterol without medication. *Below, Robert E. Kowalski, author of* The New 8-Week Cholesterol Cure, *discusses his recommendations for reducing cholesterol naturally...*

•**How is your cholesterol level these days?** I'm a shining example of how successful "secondary prevention" can be. When I left the hospital after my first bypass operation in 1978, the doctors basically told me, "We've fixed the problem—now go out and enjoy your life."

Six years later, I was back in the hospital for another bypass. That's when I started to research cholesterol and came up with the idea of controlling my cholesterol through a diet low in fat and high in oat bran—plus daily doses of the vitamin niacin.

My total cholesterol dropped from 269 to 184 in only *eight weeks*. And, angiograms show that my coronary vessels are clear.

•**What is your current advice for people who are at risk for heart disease?** Start by taking a daily multivitamin supplement, along with an additional 1,000 micrograms (mcg) of folic acid...6 milligrams (mg) of vitamin B-6* and 500 mcg of vitamin B-12.

These B-vitamins "normalize" blood levels of *homocysteine*—an amino acid that is as much a predictor of heart attack risk as is high cholesterol.

Ask your doctor to check your cholesterol levels—including total cholesterol, LDL (bad) cholesterol and HDL (good) cholesterol. Make sure he/she checks your triglyceride levels also.

These numbers indicate your risk for coronary artery disease. Regardless of your age, try to get your total cholesterol below 200—ideally 160 to 180—with an LDL level that's no higher than 100.

•**What if a person's total cholesterol exceeds 200?** You can lower your cholesterol level by about 10% simply by eating oat bran. When you eat one cup of oat bran (the equivalent of three bran muffins) or one and a half cups of oatmeal each day, the bran binds with bile in your digestive tract. The bile is then excreted in bowel movements.

Since bile contains cholesterol, more blood cholesterol must then be used up to make additional bile. Other foods high in soluble fiber, such as dried beans, raisins, prunes and figs, also help eliminate bile.

•**What other dietary approaches do you suggest?** You can reduce your blood cholesterol by another 10% by taking a cholesterol-blocking substance called *phytosterol*. When you take phytosterol before eating a meal containing animal products, phytosterol molecules occupy the cholesterol receptors in your intestines. This prevents cholesterol from passing into your bloodstream.

A company called Endurance Products sells a 400-mg phytosterol pill.

Cost: $55* for 400 tablets. (To order, call 800-483-2532 or visit *www.endur.com*.)

I recommend taking one or two tablets, 30 minutes prior to each meal. If you're eating eggs, take one tablet per egg yolk.

•**What about soy foods?** Eating soy can yield another 10% drop in cholesterol, but you have got to consume a fair amount—25 grams of soy protein a day. That's the equivalent of three eight-ounce glasses of soy milk, plus soy nut snacks.

If you adopt all these approaches, you'll make a real dent in your cholesterol level. The other step is to cut back on dietary fat.

*This is a very small amount, so look for B-6 in a vitamin mixture.

*Price subject to change.

• **Does this mean cutting out *all* fat?** No. You can eat all the fish you want, especially fatty fish, since it contains the heart-protective omega-3 fatty acids. Also, use as much olive oil and canola oil as you want.

Just be sure to cut back on trans fat (referred to on food labels as "hydrogenated" or "partially hydrogenated" fat or vegetable oil). Saturated fat, too, should be limited.

Trans fat not only raises levels of total and LDL cholesterol, but also lowers levels of protective HDL cholesterol.

Another huge source of trans fat is fast-food restaurants, which fry their products in hydrogenated fat. Have fast food no more than once a week. Never is best.

To reduce your intake of saturated fat, substitute avocados, nuts or peanut butter for meat whenever possible. Consume skim milk instead of low-fat milk products. Remove skin from chicken. And eat only lean cuts of meat.

If you plan on eating hamburgers or meat loaf, pick out a piece of lean London broil or top round at your supermarket and ask the butcher to trim the fat before grinding it. You'll have ground beef that's only 5% fat—the same fat content as skinless chicken breast. Regular ground beef is 15% to 30% fat.

• **Where does niacin come into the picture?** If your cholesterol is in the mid-200s or higher, bite the bullet and talk to your doctor about taking cholesterol-lowering medication.

I'm no doctor, but I prefer niacin, a vitamin of the B-complex group, to statin drugs—for several reasons. First, statins are expensive, and not everyone has insurance that covers the cost. Second, we know next to nothing about the long-term side effects of statins. Finally, while statins lower LDL and total cholesterol, they don't affect HDLs, triglycerides or other cholesterol "subfractions."

Niacin lowers total and LDL cholesterol *and* triglycerides. It also raises HDL and lowers levels of two other dangerous particles—lipoprotein subfraction alpha, or lp(a) cholesterol, and small, dense LDL cholesterol, both of which are especially prone to lodging in artery walls.

Niacin does have a downside. You have to take it three times a day (typically one 500-mg tablet with each meal) and have your liver enzymes checked *every six months,* since the high dosage required for cholesterol reduction can cause liver disturbances.

Niacin can also cause flushing, but a new form called Enduracin (also from Endurance Products) virtually eliminates that problem.

A new therapy that combines statins and niacin is also showing promise in clinical trials. In one recent study of heart patients at the University of Washington, the results of this approach virtually halted the progression of heart disease. Statin drugs alone did not.

Drinking Water Protects the Heart

In a recent finding, men who drank at least five glasses of water a day had a 54% lower chance of dying from a heart attack than men who drank only two glasses a day. Women drinking five glasses of water per day had a 41% lower risk. Other liquids—such as tea, juice, coffee and milk—did not have the same protective effect.

Jacqueline Chan, DrPH, researcher, Adventist Health Studies, School of Public Health, Loma Linda University, Loma Linda, CA.

Eggs Can Be Part of a Heart-Healthy Diet

One large egg contains approximately three-quarters of the 300-milligram (mg) daily cholesterol limit set by the American Heart Association. You can safely eat one egg a day as long as you limit your consumption of other cholesterol-containing foods.

Helpful: Choose nonfat or 1% dairy products...eat at least one vegetarian meal a day...choose fish and lean meat, such as chicken without the skin or very lean ground beef...choose medium eggs, which contain about 25

■ *Your Health* ■

mg less cholesterol than large ones...or use egg whites or egg substitutes, both of which have no cholesterol.

Alice H. Lichtenstein, DSc, vice-chair, nutrition committee, American Heart Association, Dallas.

Chocolate Is Good For the Heart

A bit of chocolate may be good for the heart. Chocolate contains flavonoids—antioxidant compounds also found in fruits and vegetables that protect against heart disease. Dark chocolate contains more flavonoids than milk chocolate.

Francene Steinberg, PhD, RD, assistant professor of nutrition, University of California, Davis.

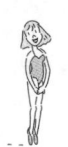

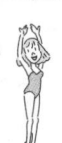

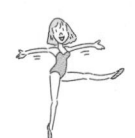

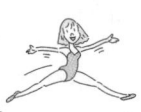

Exercise Lowers Cholesterol

Exercise lowers cholesterol danger even when it doesn't improve the balance of cholesterol in the blood. It takes vigorous exercise to increase the good (HDL) cholesterol...and exercise alone can't lower bad (LDL) cholesterol. But even a little exercise can change the number and size of particles that carry cholesterol throughout the bloodstream. Cholesterol is more likely to clog arteries when carried by small, dense protein particles. Exercise increases the number of larger, fluffy, cholesterol-carrying particles—which are less likely to block arteries.

William E. Kraus, MD, associate professor of medicine and cell biology, Duke University Medical Center, Durham, NC, and leader of a study of 111 sedentary and overweight men and women, published in The New England Journal of Medicine.

Honey May Protect Against Heart Disease

Honey contains the same levels of antioxidants as many fruits and vegetables. It inhibits the oxidation of cholesterol in the blood, a process that can lead to heart attack and stroke. In a recent study, participants who drank four tablespoons of honey in 16 ounces of water showed a significant improvement in the antioxidant levels in their blood.

Helpful: Use honey in tea, coffee or in any beverage that you would normally sweeten with sugar.

Nicki J. Engeseth, PhD, assistant professor of food science and human nutrition at University of Illinois, Urbana-Champaign.

Vitamins After Heart Surgery

Vitamins help keep arteries open after coronary angioplasty. After angioplasty, many patients experience *restenosis,* in which the surgically opened vessels narrow again and require more surgery within six months. But recent research found that taking a high-dose combination of folic acid and the vitamins B-12 and B-6 daily for six months reduced incidence of restenosis by 48%.

Caution: High doses of vitamins should only be taken under a doctor's supervision.

Guido Schnyder, MD, assistant professor, cardiology division, University of California San Diego Medical Center, and leader of two restenosis studies of more than 500 patients ages 29 to 84, reported in The Journal of the American Medical Association.

Cut Stroke Risk Easily

Cut stroke risk by 15% by taking daily vitamin supplements. Multivitamin users who also took additional supplements of the antioxidant vitamins A, C or E were less likely to suffer a stroke than those who took only a multivitamin or no vitamins at all. Researchers have yet to identify the reason for this effect.

Margaret L. Watkins, MPH, epidemiologist, National Center on Birth Defects and Developmental Disabilities, Centers for Disease Control and Prevention, Atlanta.

Folate Lowers Risk of Stroke

People who consume at least 300 micrograms (mcg) of folate a day have a 20% lower risk of stroke and 13% lower risk of cardiovascular disease than people who take less than 136 mcg a day. Current guidelines call for consuming 400 mcg a day. Folate is found in citrus fruits...leafy, green vegetables...beans and grain products... and nutritional supplements.

Jiang He, MD, PhD, associate professor of epidemiology, Tulane School of Public Health and Tropical Medicine in New Orleans, and coauthor of a study of 9,764 adults, ages 25 to 74, reported in *Stroke*.

Use Ginger to Ease Arthritic Knee Pain

Among arthritis patients taking 225 milligrams of a ginger extract twice a day, 63% reported less pain while standing and after walking 50 feet.

Theory: Ginger contains *salicylates,* the same anti-inflammatory compounds that are found in aspirin.

When taken in high doses, aspirin, unlike ginger, can cause stomach irritation. Ginger extract is available in most drugstores and health food stores.

Roy D. Altman, MD, professor of medicine and chief, division of rheumatology and immunology, University of Miami School of Medicine.

The Best in Natural Healing

Secrets of Avoiding Digestive Problems

Raphael Kellman, MD, Kellman Center for Progressive Medicine, New York City. He is author of *Gut Reactions* (Broadway).

Ulcers...heartburn...gastric reflux...bowel disease. More than half of all American adults have been diagnosed with these or other problems of the digestive tract.

Gastrointestinal (GI) problems prompt more doctors' visits than any other medical condition except the common cold. But few sufferers are getting effective treatment.

Now there's evidence that GI problems contribute to heart disease, arthritis and some neurological problems, such as dementia.

Sound hard to believe? Researchers have determined that the gut (30 feet of tube that runs from your mouth to your anus) contains two-thirds of your body's disease-fighting immune cells. It acts as the "gatekeeper" to your overall health.

In one study recently published in the British medical journal *Lancet,* patients with congestive heart failure were found to have high blood levels of *endotoxins,* proteins derived from bacteria that are normally confined to the gut. Irritation or inflammation of the intestinal wall causes bacteria and their toxins to pass into the bloodstream and spread throughout the body. This triggers inflammatory reactions that can lead to heart disease, arthritis and autoimmune disease.

ARE YOU HURTING YOUR GUT?

Digestive problems often result from some of the very treatments and dietary practices that people follow to help ensure their gastrointestinal and overall health.

Example: Americans spend more than $1 billion a year on over-the-counter (OTC) antacids in an attempt to curb heartburn and stomach upset.

Problem: Prolonged use of antacids reduces stomach acid levels, causing an imbalance in the microbes in the digestive tract. This not only allows stomach viruses and infections to

■ *Your Health* ■

flourish, but also blocks the absorption of calcium, zinc and magnesium.

Better than OTC antacids: Deglycyrrhizinated licorice (DGL) root. Licorice root makes the intestinal lining more resistant to food-borne illnesses and inhibits growth of the *Helicobacter pylori* (H. pylori) bacterium, a leading cause of ulcer formation. Ask your physician about taking one 500-milligram (mg) tablet of DGL root 30 minutes before each meal.

NATURAL HEALING

Herbal and dietary regimens can prevent and heal most common gastrointestinal disorders. Unlike most prescription and OTC drugs, the natural approach treats the cause of the problem rather than the symptoms. Natural treatments are also usually safer than medication.*

•**Gastroesophageal reflux disease or GERD.** This happens whenever stomach acid backs up into the esophagus, causing a burning sensation in the chest.

What to do: Take just one 1,000-microgram (mcg) tablet of vitamin B-12 and one 800-mcg tablet of folic acid daily. Avoid pasta and bread, as well as chocolate and coffee.

•**Ulcers.** Lesions in the stomach's mucous membrane bring on gnawing, cramping and severe pain.

What to do: Take 800 mcg of folic acid twice daily and 500 mg of DGL root 30 minutes before each meal. Take 2 grams (g) of the herb goldenseal twice daily for 14 days.

Helpful: Cabbage juice promotes healing of ulcers by building the stomach's mucosal lining. Drink two glasses daily.

To mix up your own: In a juice machine, blend two cups of chopped cabbage with four celery sticks and two carrots.

•**Heartburn and indigestion.** This causes gas, bloating, belching and stomach malaise.

What to do: Take 4 g of the amino acid *L-glutamine* three times a day and 500 mg of DGL root 30 minutes before each meal. Take 1,000 mg of mastic (an oil derived from tree sap) twice daily. Drink ginger tea after meals. Avoid the OTC nonsteroidal anti-inflammatory drugs (NSAIDs), which can worsen symptoms.

Note: My clinical experience shows that patients who suffer from GERD, ulcers and/or heartburn often benefit from short-term use of high-dose vitamin A. Consult your doctor for advice on dosage. Too much vitamin A can cause liver toxicity and birth defects.

•**Irritable bowel syndrome.** This causes diarrhea and/or constipation, excessive gas and GI pain.

What to do: Drink peppermint, lemon balm or ginger tea to reduce gas. Avoid wheat products. Instead, gradually increase your consumption of oat and rice products. Apples, legumes, raisins and grapes can exacerbate gas problems.

•**Crohn's disease.** This causes severe abdominal pain, bloody bowel movements, fever and rectal bleeding.

What to do: Take one 800-mcg tablet of folic acid a day, along with a dietary fiber supplement. Take a 500-mg tablet of DGL root 30 minutes before each meal. Take 2 g of fish oil or flaxseed oil three times daily and 2 g of the bioflavonoid *quercetin* and 4 g of L-glutamine twice daily with meals. In addition, take 2 g of goldenseal twice daily with meals for 14 days. Avoid any foods containing hydrogenated fat, such as margarine, cookies, cakes and most processed snack products.

EXERCISING YOUR GUT

Just as aerobic exercise strengthens your heart, your gut also needs a daily workout to ensure proper functioning. This is true even if you do not have gastrointestinal problems.

Proper physical activity stimulates blood flow and keeps the neurotransmitters lining the intestinal wall healthy and active.

I also recommend practicing deep breathing or yoga or doing sit-ups or stomach crunches for about 10 minutes a day.

Helpful: While lying on your back, massage your stomach area twice a day for approximately 10 minutes.

---

*Caution: Do not stop taking your current medication or begin the regimens described above without your doctor's approval. Also, some herbs and high doses of vitamins can be dangerous for pregnant women.

Kidney Stones and Soy Foods Don't Mix

Kidney stone sufferers should avoid soy foods, including soy milk and soy nuts. Such foods contain *oxalate,* an acid found in plant foods, at levels up to 40 times higher than what's considered safe for stone sufferers. Oxalate binds to calcium, producing the sharp crystals that comprise kidney stones. Other stone-promoting foods include spinach and rhubarb, which have high oxalate levels.

Linda K. Massey, PhD, RD, professor of human nutrition, Washington State University, Spokane. Her study was published in the *Journal of Agriculture and Food Chemistry.*

If You Have a Food Allergy...

Food-allergy sufferers can lower their risk for a serious attack by 30% by avoiding aspirin, alcohol and ACE inhibitors. In a recent study, patients who had suffered anaphylactic shock—a severe allergic reaction—were more likely to have consumed one of these three agents immediately prior to the attack.

Theory: These substances make the intestine more permeable, increasing the food allergen's access to the blood.

Denise-Anne Moneret-Vautrin, MD, head, department of internal medicine, clinical immunology and allergology, University Hospital, Nancy, France.

Traffic Trap

Attacks of hay fever and asthma are often triggered by clouds of pollen and mold stirred up by passing cars and trucks.

Recent finding: Twelve percent of airborne allergens near roads come from dust kicked up by traffic. And up to 70% of those dust particles are small enough to be inhaled and trigger a subsequent hay fever or asthma attack.

Ann G. Miguel, PhD, research scientist, California Institute of Technology, Pasadena. Her two-year study was published in *Environmental Science and Technology.*

Moderate Wine Drinking May Prevent the Common Cold

In a recent study, people who drank eight to 14 glasses of wine per week were half as likely to come down with a cold as the nondrinkers. Red wine was more protective than white. Beer and hard liquor had no effect.

Caution: More than one alcoholic beverage daily increases breast cancer risk.

Miguel A. Hernan, MD, DrPH, instructor in epidemiology, Harvard School of Public Health, Boston. His one-year study of 4,287 men and women was published in the *American Journal of Epidemiology.*

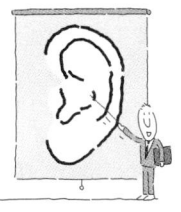

How to Reverse Hearing Loss

Partial hearing loss can often be reversed by eliminating dairy products from your diet. Anecdotal evidence shows that some patients who stop eating dairy products and foods that are rich in whey, such as many breads and pastries, may experience significant improvements in hearing.

Theory: Age-related hearing loss may be caused by an allergic response to a protein in dairy and whey products.

If you suffer from age-related hearing loss: See an ear and hearing specialist (otologist). As a three-week trial, you might also want to eliminate from your diet all dairy products as

■ Your Health ■

well as manufactured foods containing whey or milk protein.

Robert A. Anderson, MD, president and acting executive director, American Board of Holistic Medicine, East Wenatchee, WA.

Canned or Fresh Produce?

Canned or frozen produce can be more nutritious than fresh. Nutrients in fresh fruits and vegetables often are depleted during shipping and storage. New technology allows canned and frozen produce to retain their nutrients for at least several months and keeps many fruits and vegetables fresh tasting. Buy fresh produce if you will be eating it within two or three days. Otherwise, choose frozen or canned.

Melanie Polk, RD, director of nutrition education, American Institute for Cancer Research, Washington, DC.

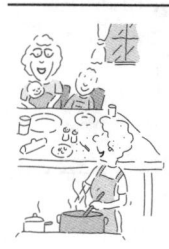

Cook Tomatoes For More Lycopene

Tomatoes cooked for two, 15 and 30 minutes contained 54%, 171% and 164% more of the antioxidant lycopene than did uncooked tomatoes. However, vitamin C levels fell 10%, 15% and 29%, respectively. But that's not as important, because, unlike lycopene, you can get vitamin C from many sources other than tomatoes.

Rui Hai Liu, MD, PhD, assistant professor and food scientist, Cornell University, Ithaca, NY.

Potassium Warning

Unless you exercise enough to have heavy loss of fluids and minerals from sweating, potassium supplements, in the form of sports drinks, pills or powder, are unnecessary and can cause harm.

Potassium can irritate the esophagus, stomach lining and small intestine, and it may cause an irregular heart rate. You can get all the potassium you need—and you can't possibly get too much—from foods.

Some good sources: Fruits, particularly figs, oranges, bananas and cantaloupe...vegetables, including potatoes, beets and radishes...any meat or seafood.

Michael Mogadam, MD, clinical associate professor of medicine, George Washington University, Washington, DC, and in private practice, Alexandria, VA.

Get More Vitamin C from Orange Juice

Ready-to-drink orange juice loses half of its vitamin C one week after opening. In fact, vitamin C levels begin to drop immediately after opening—regardless of the expiration date.

Reason: Once open, the juice is exposed to oxygen, which destroys vitamin C. Oxygen can also pass through wax and plastic containers.

Better: Drink orange juice that's made from canned concentrate. Because juice from concentrate contains higher vitamin C levels, it can be used for up to 14 days after preparation.

Carol S. Johnston, PhD, RD, professor of nutrition, Arizona State University East, Tempe.

Sweet Sleep Aid

Eat a handful of cherries one hour before bedtime. They contain lots of *melatonin,* the naturally occurring sleep agent.

Better: Juice made from cherry concentrate contains 10 times more melatonin than the whole fruit.

University of Texas Health Science Center located in San Antonio.

Your Health

6
Strictly Personal

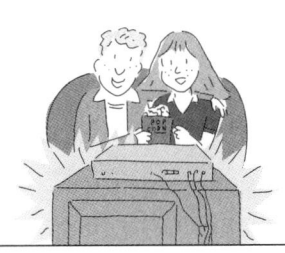

Best Ways to Boost Your Sexual Fitness

Don't allow advancing age to interfere with your sex life. Many sexual problems can be eliminated with a program that emphasizes diet and physical fitness.

Everyone knows that some medical conditions, including diabetes and hormone deficiency, can cause sexual difficulties ranging from impotence to lack of desire. It is also well known that many drugs, including antidepressants and blood pressure drugs, often produce unwanted sexual side effects.

If you experience sexual difficulties, see your doctor for a thorough evaluation to rule out a treatable medical condition. But you should also be aware that a significant number of sexual difficulties are *not* linked to a medical condition or medication. *For these cases, keeping your body fit—with proper diet, exercise and rest—is the best solution...*

EAT SMART

Excessive dietary fat and cholesterol produce artery-clogging plaque that not only increases your risk for heart attack and stroke but also restricts blood flow to the genitalia. This can hinder a man's ability to achieve or maintain an erection and may also reduce vaginal and clitoral sensitivity in women.

Self-defense: Consume no more than 30% of your daily calories as fat. Avoid saturated fat and trans-fats (abundant in fried foods and commercially baked goods). Choose unsaturated fats, found in olive and flaxseed oils, nuts and fish.

Avoid sugary snacks and high-fat fast food. Opt instead for whole-grain breads and pastas, fresh vegetables and fruits and proteins,

---

Robert N. Butler, MD, professor of geriatrics and adult development at Mount Sinai Medical Center and president and CEO of the International Longevity Center-USA, *www.ilcusa.org,* a nonprofit research and education organization focused on longevity, both in New York City. Dr. Butler was founding director of the National Institute on Aging. He is coauthor of *The New Love and Sex After 60* (Ballantine).

including beans, lean beef, fish, skim milk and low-fat cheese.

A multivitamin can help to offset nutritional deficiencies. Most older adults should choose one without iron, since a reasonably balanced diet provides adequate amounts of iron. Excess iron levels have been shown to contribute to heart disease.

Important: Overindulging in alcohol can dampen sexual appetite and diminish sexual performance. Although alcohol lowers inhibitions, it's known to depress physical arousal.

Eating until you're uncomfortably full can leave you feeling too bloated and sluggish for sex. To avoid unnecessarily straining the heart, it's advisable to postpone sex for a few hours following a heavy meal.

A heart attack during sex is extremely uncommon. According to a study conducted at Harvard University, the risk for heart attack during sex among people who have coronary disease is 20 in one million.

A Japanese study found that when heart attacks do occur, the victims are usually men engaged in illicit sex following an eating or drinking binge.

GET MORE EXERCISE

For the stamina and flexibility required to enjoy sex, you need to exercise. Brisk walking usually provides the best overall workout for people age 60 or older. Aim for 10,000 steps each day, five to six days every week (2,000 steps equals roughly one mile).

If that sounds daunting, consider that even relatively inactive adults average 3,500 steps a day. Simple changes—taking the stairs instead of the elevator or walking rather than driving to a store, for example—can add to that number substantially. That means a two- or three-mile walk may be all that's required to reach your overall goal.

To stay motivated: Recruit a walking partner or join a walking club...and keep track of your miles with an electronic pedometer.

Supplement daily walks with strengthening and stretching exercises. If back pain prevents you from enjoying sex, toning the back and stomach muscles can help. Try crunches to strengthen the upper abdominal muscles...leg lifts to work the lower abs...and swimming to strengthen the back and shoulders.

SLEEP MORE

At least half of all adults over age 50 suffer from sleep disturbances. Insomnia, illness, pain or frequent nighttime trips to the bathroom can interfere with sleep cycles, depriving you of sufficient rapid eye movement (REM) sleep—the kind associated with dreaming. Chronic sleep deprivation can leave you too exhausted for sex and may also lead to a deficiency of important hormones, including human growth hormone, which helps keep your body lean, fit and energized.

Self-defense: Limit or eliminate naps and caffeine, particularly after the late afternoon. Exercise at least two hours before bedtime. Retire to a dark, quiet room at the same time each evening.

Ease yourself into slumber with a proven relaxation technique, such as deep breathing, meditation or a massage from your partner. If arthritis or muscle pain keeps you awake, ask your doctor about taking *acetaminophen* or aspirin before bed.

Caution: Overuse of acetaminophen may cause liver damage. Aspirin can cause stomach irritation. To minimize these risks, always take these drugs with a full glass of water.

Avoid sedative-hypnotics, such as *zolpidem* (Ambien) and *zaleplon* (Sonata), except to treat short-term sleeplessness caused by jet lag, for example, or grief over the passing of a loved one. If used for more than four consecutive nights, these sleep aids can trigger "rebound insomnia." Rather than inducing sleep, they heighten restlessness, leaving you more awake than ever.

Important: After age 60, it's common to experience a sleep pattern that occurs when you fall asleep at dusk and awaken before dawn. This can disrupt your sex life, particularly if your partner maintains a traditional sleep schedule.

Fortunately, this problem can usually be reversed with regular exposure to the late-afternoon sun. Aim to get about 30 minutes of sun *without sunscreen* between 4 pm and 6 pm. This will not only correct sleep patterns, but also help prevent osteoporosis by triggering production of vitamin D in your skin.

Warning: Avoid unprotected sun exposure between 10 am and 2 pm, when harmful ultraviolet rays are most intense.

ADDITIONAL STRATEGIES

Improved nutrition, exercise and rest typically lead to more satisfying sex within a matter of weeks. *For more immediate results...*

- **Use visual, tactile stimulation.** Men, especially, are aroused by sexual images and touch. Dim the lights and watch a steamy movie. Women may want to put on sexy lingerie. Share a gentle massage or engage in mutual stimulation.

- **Fantasize.** Imagining sexy scenarios can heighten arousal for both partners. Interestingly, however, one study showed that men's ability to fantasize may diminish with age. This may explain why men tend to rely on sexy pictures, videos and other visual aids.

- **Use lubricants.** Postmenopausal women, especially, may find their enjoyment of sex hampered by vaginal dryness. Water-based lubricants, such as Astroglide, can help. Oil-based lubricants may lead to vaginal infections.

- **Plan around arthritis pain.** Taking a hot shower before sex can help reduce joint pain and stiffness. So can taking your pain medication 30 minutes before sex. If you suffer from osteoarthritis, try to have sex in the morning, before joints have a chance to stiffen or become inflamed. If you have rheumatoid arthritis, sex in the late afternoon or evening may be preferable, since symptoms often subside with physical activity.

- **Vary times and positions.** Don't get stuck in the rut of always having sex at night, in the missionary position. If you or your partner are too tired for sex at night, plan a morning or afternoon sex date. If one of you has a heart condition, hip or back pain, let that person take the bottom position, which requires less vigorous movement.

- **Practice seduction.** Good sex starts in the brain, which means it should begin hours before you actually arrive in the bedroom. Throughout the day, shower your partner with caresses, kisses and other outward signs of affection. Genuine intimacy is really the most effective aphrodisiac.

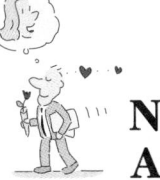

Natural Aphrodisiacs

Chris D. Meletis, ND, dean of naturopathic medicine and chief medical officer at the National College of Naturopathic Medicine in Portland, OR. He is author of seven books, including *Better Sex Naturally* (HarperResource), *Complete Guide to Safe Herbs* (DK Publishing) and *Instant Guide to Drug–Herb Interactions* (DK Publishing).

Men troubled by an erectile dysfunction (impotence) often assume that *sildenafil* (Viagra) is the answer. A woman who suffers from low libido may think that testosterone cream is the most effective way to boost her flagging desire.

While both of these approaches may offer a temporary solution, they will not remedy the underlying causes of these problems. Discovering and curing the cause of a sexual problem can be the key to long-term enjoyment of sex.

To identify the cause, I perform a detailed medical history and then order diagnostic tests, including a prostate-specific antigen (PSA) test for men and a Pap test for women.

In addition to low levels of testosterone, a hormone that fuels sex drive in both men *and* women, there are a number of possible scenarios. These include circulation problems that inhibit blood flow to the genitals...psychological stress, which diminishes interest in sex ...and insomnia, which steals the vitality necessary to pursue sexual activity.

After unraveling the clues, I rely on safe, natural medications, such as herbs* to trigger the healing process.

ERECTILE DYSFUNCTION

More than half of men over age 40 have some degree of erectile failure, according to one recent study. The condition can be caused by a variety of health problems, such as poor

---

*The Food and Drug Administration does not regulate herbal supplements. Check with your physician before taking any of these products. They can interact with prescription medications.

■ *Your Health* ■

circulation or nerve damage. For this reason, it's important to see your primary-care physician for a diagnosis. *The most effective herbal treatment for optimal erectile function…*

●**Ginkgo biloba.** An erection depends on healthy blood flow to the penis. Clogged arteries reduce circulation, which compromises a man's ability to achieve an erection. The herb *ginkgo biloba* dilates blood vessels, improving circulation and helping restore erections.

In a recent study, 78% of men with erectile dysfunction who took the herb regained their ability to have erections.

Good news for women: Women who use ginkgo biloba may experience longer, more intense orgasms.

People most likely to benefit from ginkgo biloba have circulatory symptoms, such as dizziness, varicose veins, cold hands or feet and/or high blood pressure.

Typical use: 40 milligrams (mg), three times daily. Look for a formula containing 24% *flavonglycosides,* the active ingredient.

Ginkgo should not be taken by anyone who uses blood-thinning medication, such as aspirin, antidepressants known as MAO inhibitors or anyone who has had a stroke or has a tendency to bleed or bruise easily.

INHIBITED SEXUAL DESIRE

A flagging libido can plague both men and women. *Fortunately, both sexes can benefit from the following…*

●**Ginseng.** This herb energizes the body, helping it respond better to almost any health problem. It also boosts the production of sex hormones, such as testosterone in men and women, to enhance sexual response.

People likely to get the most benefit from ginseng have anxiety, blood sugar problems, fatigue, high levels of stress, menopausal symptoms or frequent infections like colds.

Typical use: Look for a product that contains *ginsenoside Rg1,* the active ingredient. Take 10 mg, twice daily.

Ginseng is a stimulant, and it is not recommended for people with high blood pressure or anyone taking medication for diabetes, bipolar disorder or heart disease.

FOR WOMEN ONLY

Hormone levels play an important role in a woman's sexual health and emotional involvement during sex. Too little estrogen can thin the vaginal walls, causing painful intercourse. Too little testosterone reduces sex drive. Too little progesterone or too much prolactin can lead to anxiety and depression.

The following herbs* can help to regulate female hormones…

●**Black cohosh.** This herb helps regulate hormones by controlling the secretions of the pituitary gland, which help balance estrogen and progesterone production. This can enhance a woman's interest in sex and help with vaginal lubrication.

Typical use: 500 mg, twice daily. Or, if you use a standardized tablet, take 2 mg of *27-deoxyacteine,* the active ingredient.

●**Dong quai.** The herb *angelica sinensis* is most commonly known by its Chinese name, dong quai. It balances estrogen levels and can enhance sexual pleasure.

Typical use: 500 mg, twice daily.

Helpful: Consider taking a formula that combines black cohosh and dong quai—particularly if you have PMS or are menopausal. Dong quai can increase energy and improve mood, while black cohosh helps reduce PMS symptoms, such as bloating, and menopausal problems, such as hot flashes.

DANGEROUS NATURAL REMEDIES

Stay away from…

●**Damiana.** Derived from the leaves of a shrub found in the Southwest US and Mexico, this herb has many possible side effects, including diarrhea, vomiting, heart palpitations and anxiety. Use it *only* under the supervision of a doctor or naturopathic physician.**

●**Spanish Fly.** This beetle is pulverized and eaten. It contains the chemical *cantharidin,* which can damage your heart, kidneys, stomach and intestines—or even kill you.

*Pregnant or lactating women should *not* use these.

**To locate a naturopathic physician in your area, contact the American Association of Naturopathic Physicians (866-538-2267 or *www.naturopathic.org*).

Sex Makes You Look Younger

People who have loving sex at least three times per week look more than 10 years younger than the average adult.

Possible reasons: Sex is pleasurable and produces feel-good chemicals...and loving couples like to look their best for each other.

David J. Weeks, PhD, clinical neuropsychologist at Royal Edinburgh Hospital, Scotland, and leader of a 10-year study of 3,500 people ages 18 to 102, published in *Sexual and Relationship Therapy*.

Working Out Can Improve Your Sex Life

In a recent study, men who rode a stationary bicycle for one hour, three times a week for eight weeks reported better erections and more satisfying sex than sedentary men. Exercise improves the ability of blood vessels to dilate, which allows greater blood flow to the penis.

Helpful: Men who are not able to take *sildenafil* (Viagra) may benefit from this type of exercise regimen. Check with your doctor.

Romualdo Belardinelli, MD, director, cardiac rehabilitation program, Lancisi Heart Institute, Ancona, Italy.

Biking Can Cause Sexual Dysfunction in Women

The front part of the bicycle seat, called the nose, can press against the perineum—which contains nerves and arteries leading to the genitals. Over time, this can cause numbness and sexual dysfunction in women as well as impotence in men.

Self-defense: Limit cycling to three hours a week. And, sit upright while biking to relieve pressure on the perineum. Finally, stand up frequently when you are riding.

Also: Consider a seat without a protruding nose. Split-seat, or "noseless," bike saddles are designed to ease pressure on the perineum.

Cost: About $70, at most bike shops.

Irwin Goldstein, MD, director, Institute for Sexual Medicine, Boston University School of Medicine.

More from Irwin Goldstein...

Daily Exercise Protects Against Impotency

Men who burned 200 calories every day through physical activity—the equivalent of a brisk two-mile walk—were less likely than sedentary men to become impotent, a new study has found. Moderate daily exercise delays the normal, age-related slowdown in the production of testosterone, which is necessary for erections.

Good daily exercise: Walking, jogging or swimming.

Caution: Men who bicycle for more than three hours per week have a higher risk for erectile dysfunction.

Also from Irwin Goldstein...

Better Than Viagra

A new competitor to Viagra is even more effective. *Vardenafil* (Levitra) works by blocking the same enzyme (PDE-5) as Viagra—but Levitra works faster and stays in the system longer.

Result: Lower doses to achieve the same effect—five, 10 or 20 milligrams (mg) of Levitra, versus 25, 50 or 100 mg of Viagra.

Levitra had excellent safety and efficacy in premarket tests. It was recently approved by the FDA.

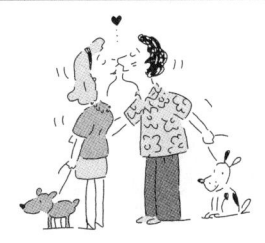

■ *Your Health* ■

Impotence/Cardiovascular Disease Link

Impotence is often an early sign of cardiovascular disease. In a recent study, 30% of men with erectile dysfunction were at high risk for heart attack, 37% had high cholesterol, 24% were diabetic and 17% had high blood pressure.

Theory: The same fatty buildup in the arteries (atherosclerosis) that reduces blood flow to the penis, resulting in an inability to achieve erection, is also responsible for the narrowing of coronary arteries that feed the heart.

If you are impotent: Ask your doctor to also test you for cardiovascular disease.

Hemant Solomon, MD, cardiology research fellow, Stanford University Medical Center, Palo Alto, CA.

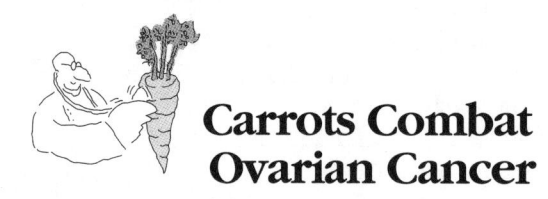

Carrots Combat Ovarian Cancer

In a new finding, women who ate just four carrot sticks at least five times a week halved their risk for ovarian cancer.

Theory: Beta carotene, the nutrient found in carrots that gives them their orange color, helps prevent cancer with its potent antioxidant properties.

Good news: Other orange-colored foods, including apricots, sweet potatoes, cantaloupe, butternut squash and pumpkin, are also high in beta carotene.

Daniel W. Cramer, MD, professor of obstetrics and gynecology, Harvard Medical School and Brigham and Women's Hospital, both in Boston. His study was published in the International Journal of Cancer.

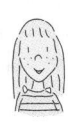

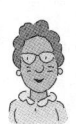

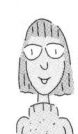

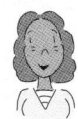

Grape Juice as a Breast Cancer Preventive

Purple grape juice may help prevent breast cancer. In addition to improving heart health, *polyphenols,* antioxidant plant compounds found in fruits and vegetables (and their juices), may also inhibit the growth of breast cancer cells. Further studies are needed to confirm the beneficial effects of grape juice and to determine if it can help prevent other cancers. In the meantime, researchers say this finding confirms that plant foods, including fruits and vegetables (and their juices), are an important component of a healthful diet.

Keith W. Singletary, PhD, professor of nutrition, University of Illinois at Urbana-Champaign.

Better Breast Cancer Detection

Mammography plus ultrasound helps detect small cancers in dense breast tissue, which occurs in almost half of women. In the densest breast tissue, mammograms alone detect less than half of all invasive tumors. Adding ultrasound raises the detection rate to 97%.

Thomas M. Kolb, MD, radiologist in private practice, New York City, and leader of a study of breast cancer detection in 11,220 women, published in Radiology.

More Accurate Mammograms

The accuracy of mammograms is affected by breast positioning during the procedure. The ability of the mammogram to find cancer when it is present can range from 84% to 66%, depending on how the breasts are positioned. Breasts are improperly positioned in about one-third of all screenings.

Self-defense: Help the technician to get an accurate picture by leaning forward and allowing the entire breast to be compressed.

Stephen H. Taplin, MD, MPH, associate director of preventive-care research and senior investigator, Center for Health Studies, Group Health Cooperative, Seattle.

Mammograms Can Help Predict Stroke Risk

Women whose mammograms indicated calcification of the blood vessels of the breast had a 40% higher chance for ischemic stroke than women with normal vessels.

Theory: Calcium buildup may indicate a generalized hardening of the arteries.

Self-defense: If calcifications are visible, ask your doctor to assess your risk for cardiovascular disease.

Carlos Iribarren, MD, PhD, research scientist, division of research, Kaiser Permanente, Oakland, CA.

HRT and Breast Cancer Risk

John R. Lee, MD, Sebastopol, CA–based family practitioner who pioneered the study and use of natural progesterone. Recently retired, Dr. Lee is coauthor of *What Your Doctor May Not Tell You About Breast Cancer: How Hormone Balance Can Help Save Your Life* (Warner).

Medical experts have recently done an about-face on the supposed health advantages of hormone-replacement therapy (HRT). This shift in thinking is long overdue. For more than 20 years, I have been warning women about the potential dangers of hormones. Now there's mounting evidence that even the standard HRT regimen can cause breast cancer.

THE ESTROGEN FACTOR

The problem is, doctors are prescribing the wrong hormone. Conventional wisdom has held that menopause is caused by estrogen deficiency. This belief was supported by the fact that supplemental estrogen alleviated hot flashes in menopausal women. However, the majority of women going through menopause are deficient in progesterone—*not* estrogen.

Why is progesterone so important? To begin with, it is just as critical as estrogen in preventing osteoporosis. Estrogen slows down bone loss, but progesterone is responsible for the formation of new bone tissue. In addition, progesterone works to counteract the breast cancer–promoting effect of estrogen.

That's why maintaining a proper balance of these two hormones is so important. Ideally, a woman's ratio of progesterone to estrogen should be between 200:1 and 300:1. If this ratio drops below 200:1—meaning there's too little progesterone—*estrogen dominance* results. Symptoms of this dangerous condition include difficulty sleeping, anxiety, headaches, increased body fat, swollen or tender breasts, bloating, fatigue, irritability and diminished sex drive.

Even more ominous, estrogen dominance activates the normally dormant cancer-causing gene Bcl-2.

A statistical link between estrogen dominance and breast cancer is now beginning to emerge. In one recent study of 3,000 breast cancer patients, more than 99% had estrogen dominance. Among healthy women, the majority did *not* have estrogen dominance.

DANGERS OF HRT

Many women on HRT have a progesterone/estrogen ratio far lower than it should be. *This occurs for two reasons...*

•**HRT increases estrogen levels**—often unnecessarily. As a recent *Lancet* article pointed out, even in the minority of instances where women *do* require estrogen supplements, the necessary dose is usually just 0.25 milligram (mg)—four to eight times less than the 1 mg to 2 mg that is typically prescribed.

•**HRT supplements contain no natural progesterone.** Instead, they use a synthetic progesterone, called progestin. Progestin does not provide as much protection against uterine cancer as does natural progesterone. What is

■ *Your Health* ■

more, progestin does *not* have progesterone's protective effect against breast cancer.

While progesterone benefits a woman's body by building up bone, contributing to the normal function of blood clotting and blood sugar levels, progestin has a long list of toxic side effects, including increased risk for stroke, fluid retention, epilepsy and asthma.

Many women *not* on HRT may also be at increased risk for breast cancer due to estrogen dominance caused by...

• Birth control pills, which can block the body's production of progesterone.

• Working a night shift under artificial light and sleeping during the day. Doing so inhibits progesterone production.

• A diet high in sugar and starches or low in green, leafy vegetables.

• Prolonged stress, which increases the sensitivity of the body's estrogen receptors.

• Eating meat from cattle that have been given estrogen supplements to boost their weight.

STABILIZING HORMONE LEVELS

Every woman should get her estrogen and progesterone levels tested—and discuss the results with her doctor.

Blood tests do *not* accurately reflect the level of active hormones. A saliva test,* which measures the amount of "free," or biologically active, hormones in the body, is essential for an accurate reading.

If testing reveals a progesterone/estrogen ratio below 200:1, I recommend using a topical progesterone cream, which enters the bloodstream more efficiently than pills.

The cream, which can be applied to your palms, chest and neck, is sold over the counter. It costs about $12 to $30. Look for the key words like "progesterone" or "natural progesterone." The cream is sold under many brand names, including Awakening Woman, FemGest, Natra Gest and Renewed Balance.

Most postmenopausal women must use 15 mg to 20 mg of cream every day (which is equivalent to about one-quarter teaspoon) for several months before regaining their progesterone/estrogen balance.

After three months, have your progesterone and estrogen levels tested again to make sure you're taking an adequate dose.

If saliva tests reveal low levels of progesterone *and* estrogen, ask your doctor about supplementing the progesterone cream with oral estrogen. Start with a dose of 0.25 mg daily (half a 0.5 mg estrogen pill, currently the lowest dose you can get). Have another saliva test done after three months to recheck your hormone levels.

Alternatives to Hormone Replacement

Menopausal women concerned about hormone replacement therapy should consider these alternatives...

• **Traditional remedies** for hot flashes and night sweats, such as black cohosh, licorice, red clover and chasteberry.

• **Estradiol and progesterone** (best administered in a cream base)—prescription medicines identical to the hormones produced in the body.

• **Soy-rich foods or ground flaxseed**—sprinkle over cereal, mix in a smoothie, etc.

Also helpful: Avoid alcohol and spicy foods, which can trigger hot flashes...dress in layers that you can take off during a hot flash.

Andrew L. Rubman, ND, associate professor of clinical medicine, College of Naturopathic Medicine, University of Bridgeport, CT. He is consultant to the North American Menopause Society in Cleveland.

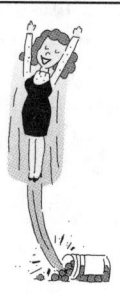

---

*To obtain a mail-order saliva test, contact Aeron Life Cycles Lab (800-631-7900 or *www.aeron.com*)...Great Smokies Diagnostic Lab (800-522-4762 or *www.gsdl.com*)...or ZRT Lab (503-466-2445 or *www.salivatest.com*). *Typical cost:* $50 and up.

Postmenopausal Breathing Remedy

Postmenopausal women often have breathing difficulties, such as partial respiratory obstruction, during sleep. This has been linked to the sharp decline of female hormone levels, particularly *progesterone,* after menopause. The synthetic hormone *medroxyprogesterone* eases the problem by stimulating breathing, improving oxygen saturation and lowering high levels of carbon monoxide in the lungs. The benefits continue for up to three weeks after treatment. Postmenopausal women who suffer from nighttime breathing difficulties should check with their physicians to see if they are candidates for short-term treatment with this hormone.

Tarja Saaresranta, MD, PhD, pulmonologist, sleep research unit, University of Turku, Finland.

Menstrual Cycle Red Flag

Lighter-than-usual menstruation for more than two cycles could indicate an overactive thyroid. See your doctor for a blood test if your period suddenly becomes lighter and you experience weight loss, trembling or palpitations. Left untreated, hyperthyroidism can lead to osteoporosis and heart disease.

Paul W. Ladenson, MD, director, division of endocrinology and metabolism, Johns Hopkins University, Baltimore.

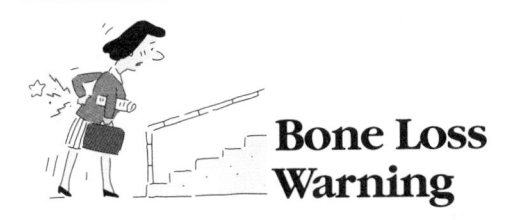

Bone Loss Warning

Irregular menstrual cycles may signal a hormonal shortage that could lead to osteoporosis. *Amenorrhea*—the absence of a menstrual period for three months or more—may mean a deficiency of estrogen and other reproductive hormones. These hormones help maintain bone density. Most women don't consider the condition serious enough to warrant medical attention, leading to a delay in treatment that can result in further bone loss.

Lawrence M. Nelson, MD, reproductive endocrinologist, National Institutes of Health, Bethesda, MD, and investigator of a study of 48 women published in *Obstetrics & Gynecology.*

Beware of Diagnosing Your Own Yeast Infections

In a recent finding, only about half the women treating themselves with over-the-counter remedies actually had vaginal yeast infections. The rest of the women had either another type of infection or no infection at all.

Problem: If left untreated, certain types of vaginal infections, such as trichomonas and bacterial vaginosis, can lead to infertility and make women more susceptible to AIDS.

Women experiencing vaginal itching, burning or irritation should consult their physicians.

Daron Ferris, MD, professor of obstetrics/gynecology and family medicine, Medical College of Georgia in Augusta. His study of 95 women was published in *Obstetrics & Gynecology.*

Best Therapies for Prostate Cancer

Robert G. Uzzo, MD, urological oncologist, Fox Chase Cancer Center and assistant professor of medicine, Temple University School of Medicine, both in Philadelphia.

Prostate cancer is the second most common cancer in men (after skin cancer). Even so, there's still controversy over how aggressively to treat a prostate malignancy—or even *whether* to treat it.

Unlike most cancers, prostate cancer tends to grow gradually, often over decades. Older men with prostate cancer that's confined to the gland are statistically more likely to die from other causes than from the cancer itself.

■ *Your Health* ■

Yet some prostate cancers do grow quickly. Even cancers that are initially slow growing can progress and become fatal. In fact, prostate cancer is the second leading cause of cancer death in men. The challenge is knowing when treatment is necessary—and choosing a treatment that is most likely to be effective.

KEY DIAGNOSTIC TESTS

Once a biopsy of the prostate is performed and cancer cells are discovered, the appropriate treatment depends on how aggressive the cells are likely to act. *Three main factors to consider prior to treatment...*

•**Prostate-specific antigen (PSA).** It's a protein produced by the prostate gland and detected in the blood. Elevated levels suggest that cancer cells are present. A normal PSA is below 4 nanograms per milliliter (ng/ml) of blood. A level between 5 and 10 suggests that prostate cancer cells *may* be present...a level above 10 is a strong warning sign. The higher the PSA, the higher the probability that cancer cells have spread outside of the gland.

Important: An elevated PSA reading can also be caused by an enlarged or infected prostate. In addition, there is evidence to suggest that a recent ejaculation may temporarily elevate a PSA reading. Also, a small percentage of men with a normal PSA will still have cancer. Therefore, all men should have a digital rectal exam in addition to a PSA test to detect the presence of prostate cancer.

•**Gleason score.** If your PSA is abnormal (typically above 4 ng/ml), your doctor should perform a needle biopsy of the prostate to look for cancer. Multiple biopsies (typically six to 12) are taken from the prostate. Cancer cells are graded based on a system called the Gleason score, which ranges from 2 (least aggressive) to 10 (most aggressive).

Gleason scores ranging from 2 to 4 typically indicate the cancer is growing slowly and may not need immediate treatment. Scores from 8 to 10 indicate a fast-growing tumor that requires immediate attention. Scores in the middle range can indicate either slow- or fast-growing tumors.

•**Staging.** Prostate cancer is staged by digital rectal exam as well as a CT scan and/or a bone scan when appropriate. This determines where the cancer is located—and whether it has spread beyond the prostate gland.

A prostate malignancy is assigned one of four stages, with stage 1 being a very early cancer and stage 4 being the most advanced.

TREATMENT OPTIONS

Controversy exists regarding the best treatment for localized prostate cancer. There have been no head-to-head, randomized trials comparing the two main treatment options—surgery or radiation—for prostate cancer. The treatments appear to have roughly equal survival rates for early-stage cancers over the short term, but no long-term data comparing the two are available.

"Watchful waiting" is also a reasonable strategy for older men with cancers that are unlikely to grow or spread quickly.

•**Surgery.** Surgically removing the prostate gland—a procedure called *radical prostatectomy*—is often recommended for men with localized prostate cancer. Many physicians, including myself, feel it's the best choice overall.

During this procedure, the surgeon makes a small incision below the navel. The entire gland and some of the tissue surrounding it are removed. Nearby lymph nodes will also be removed and checked for cancer.

"Nerve-sparing" radical prostatectomy is recommended for most patients. If the bundles of nerves on either side of the prostate gland are cancer free, the surgeon will attempt to leave them intact while removing the gland. This decreases a man's chances of suffering from impotence after surgery.

Some men who have surgery, even if it is nerve-sparing, become impotent. The drug *sildenafil* (Viagra) helps in some cases, but not all. The surgery may also cause urinary dribbling for several weeks following surgery. While most men don't have a long-term problem, 5% to 10% of men may never regain total urinary control.

Important: Choose a surgeon who performs at least 50 nerve-sparing surgeries a year.

•**Radiation therapy.** Men who are too frail to have surgery for prostate cancer—or who do not want to undergo the discomfort and lengthy recovery time—may be candidates for radiation treatments. *Two radiation options...*

- External beam radiation is delivered from outside the body and targeted at the prostate. This treatment is generally well-tolerated. However, like surgery, it can cause complications, including impotence and diarrhea, which typically clear up in the long term.

Outpatient treatments are usually given five days a week for five to seven weeks.

It is important to look for a hospital that offers the intensity-modulated radiation therapy (IMRT), which gives higher doses of radiation to the prostate gland while minimizing the amount given to nearby healthy tissues.

- Radioactive seeds are inserted into the prostate gland with fine needles. The rice-sized seeds, made with iodine-125 or palladium-103, are directly implanted into the prostate gland to deliver high doses of radiation to the prostate. What's the advantage of using seeds rather than external radiation? Patients only have to come to the hospital once, when the seeds are inserted.

Current data suggest that the seeds tend to work only when there's a relatively low volume of cancer cells and the PSA and Gleason scores are in the low to moderate ranges. If these numbers are high, external beam radiation may be a better choice. The long-term risk for impotence is about the same as with surgery.

- **Hormone therapy.** Hormone treatment includes oral or injected medications or surgical removal of the testicles (orchiectomy). These therapies lower the production of testosterone and/or block the effects of testosterone and other male hormones (androgens). Lowering androgen levels can slow the growth of cancer —but it isn't a cure.

Hormone therapy is mainly used when the cancer has spread beyond the prostate gland. It may also be used in combination with radiation in men who have aggressive tumors with a high Gleason score. The hormone treatments can frequently cause cancers to go into remission for several years.

- **Watchful waiting.** Most prostate cancers progress over years, not months. Men in their 70s and older whose life expectancy is less than 10 years because of other medical conditions may be advised by their physicians to defer medical treatment if the cancer is expected to grow slowly and isn't causing symptoms.

A man will typically be advised to have PSA tests twice annually to determine if the volume of cancer cells is increasing. He should also have regular physical exams.

Prostate Cancer Fighter

Compounds in soy called *isoflavones* inhibit the growth and spread of prostate tumors.

Helpful: Prostate cancer patients should consume 150 milligrams (mg) to 200 mg of isoflavones daily. One cup of soy milk contains 20 mg to 40 mg isoflavones...one-half cup of tofu contains 35 mg to 40 mg...and one-half cup of soy nuts contains about 170 mg.

Important: Check with your doctor before making any changes to your diet.

Jin-Rong Zhou, PhD, assistant professor of surgery at Harvard Medical School, Boston.

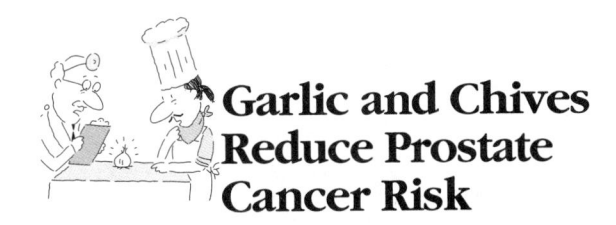

Garlic and Chives Reduce Prostate Cancer Risk

Members of the *allium* family, garlic and chives, are rich in *flavonols,* plant substances known to have antitumor effects. They have previously been shown to help prevent cancer of the stomach, colon and esophagus.

Recent finding: Men who ate 10 grams (g) of these herbs (approximately three cloves of garlic) a day had half the rate of prostate cancer as did men who ate only 2.2 g per day. Onions, leeks and shallots are also beneficial.

Ann W. Hsing, PhD, investigator, division of cancer epidemiology and genetics, National Cancer Institute in Rockville, MD. Her study was published in the *Journal of the National Cancer Institute.*

■ *Your Health* ■

Reverse Prostate Cancer

A low-fat diet may reverse prostate cancer. Eating a 10%-fat vegan diet, in combination with moderate exercise, meditation and yoga, reduces levels of prostate-specific antigen (PSA) in men with early-stage nonaggressive prostate cancer. Be sure to consult your doctor before making changes to your diet.

Dean Ornish, MD, clinical professor of medicine, University of California, San Francisco, and leader of a study of 84 men with prostate cancer, reported at the International Scientific Conference on Complementary, Alternative and Integrative Medicine Research.

Better Prostate Cancer Detection

During the typical prostate biopsy, six samples of suspicious cells are taken. However, this technique misses up to one in seven prostate malignancies. New research suggests that taking 10 to 12 cell samples uncovers 14% more cancers. Additional samples mean higher lab fees, but the new technique could save money and worry by eliminating the need for follow-up biopsies.

If scheduled for a prostate biopsy: Ask your doctor about testing more samples.

Robert Bahnson, MD, professor and director, division of urology, Ohio State University Medical Center, Columbus.

The Best Prostate Cancer Surgery

The best surgery for prostate cancer can cure without devastating side effects. Unlike traditional surgery, *nerve-sparing*—or anatomic—radical prostatectomy preserves continence and potency in up to 90% of men with localized cancer. Not all insurance pays for this surgery. Some patients pay $20,000 and up for it. Ask about a surgeon's track record regarding cancer control, incontinence and impotence.

Patrick Walsh, MD, professor of urology and director of the Brady Urological Institute, Johns Hopkins Medical Institutions, Baltimore. He is author of *Dr. Patrick Walsh's Guide to Surviving Prostate Cancer* (Warner).

Getting Help for Drug Or Alcohol Addiction

Penelope Ziegler, MD, medical director, William J. Farley Center, 5477 Mooretown Rd., Williamsburg, VA 23188, and head of the treatment section, American Academy of Addiction Psychiatry.

Find help for drug or alcohol addiction as close to home as possible. Recovery affects the whole family, and effective programs include family participation. Check with your insurance provider first. Most plans have approved programs that they will cover, at least in part. Some may give you a choice...others have exclusive agreements with a single center. Most insurers require you to try outpatient programs first—allowing residential treatment only if the outpatient approach fails.

Among the top treatment centers for adults addicted to alcohol or drugs are the Betty Ford Center in Rancho Mirage, CA, and Father Martin's Ashley in Havre de Grace, MD. For adolescents, the Caron Foundation in Wernersville, PA, has an outstanding program. Among the top centers for treating addiction with accompanying psychiatric problems are the William J. Farley Center in Williamsburg, VA, and Silver Hill Hospital in New Canaan, CT.

To find a facility: Go to the Substance Abuse & Mental Health Services Administration Web site at *www.findtreatment.samhsa.gov/facilitylocatordoc.htm.*

Your Money

7

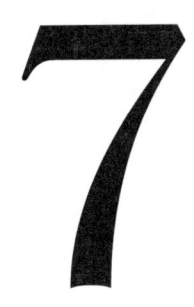

Money Matters

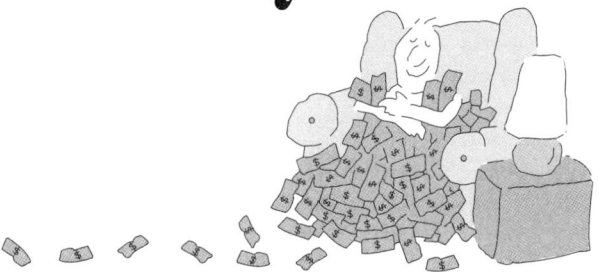

Secrets of Shrewd Money Management in a Volatile Economy

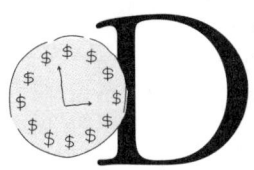

Despite the repeated blows that many stock market investors have endured, it's important to avoid the temptation to get out of stocks completely. All long-term investors need the growth potential of common stocks to preserve their purchasing power against inflation.

True, retirees do need to focus on income, selecting more dividend-paying stocks and mutual funds that invest in them. But it's a mistake to go too heavily into fixed-income investments. Today you would need a king's ransom in capital to provide a living income just from bond yield.

MONEY-MANAGEMENT KEYS

•**Maintain adequate diversification.** The important lesson to be learned from the past few years is the need to diversify. Those who were invested in 60% stocks and 40% bonds lost only 10% between January 2000 and the end of August 2002. *How they were invested...*

Stocks: 15% large-cap growth, 15% large-cap value, 15% small- and medium-cap growth and value and 15% international.

Bonds: 15% municipals, 10% US Treasury and 15% corporate.

•**Get out of debt—and stay out.** If you have credit card bills, develop a program to pay down that debt as soon as possible.

Unfortunately, many older people who were making progress paying down their mortgages have been tempted to give it all up and take out large home-equity loans at today's low rates. Do not be tempted. Never take out a home-equity loan simply to buy things like stocks (which

---

Jonathan D. Pond, CPA, president, Financial Planning Information, Inc. at 9 Galen St., Watertown, MA 02472, www.jonathanpond.com. He is author of many books on personal finance, most recently Your Money Matters: 21 Tips for Achieving Financial Security in the 21st Century *(Perigee). He also is host of www.yourfinancialroadmap.com, an investment and financial planning Web site.*

97

Your Money

can lose value) or a new car (which rapidly depreciates).

• **Beware of real estate.** Many people have been pulling money out of stocks and putting it into real estate, buying a larger house or a second home.

Caution: The real estate market may slow down in some areas as long-term interest rates rise. And values have already been driven up in the most desirable vacation and retirement areas. You can't "buy low" in today's market—and if real estate prices plummet, you won't be able to "sell high" either.

Smarter strategy now: Trade down. Take a fat profit on your big house and move to something smaller with lower property taxes and reduced maintenance costs. Take advantage of the $250,000 (for singles) or $500,000 (for couples) exemption from capital gains taxes on your profit, and use those funds to boost your retirement savings to make up for stock market losses.

• **Keep a cash cushion.** Everyone needs a cash reserve in case of unanticipated expenditures that can wreak havoc with your retirement budget. People underestimate emergency outlays—a new roof, car repairs, a big rise in property taxes, a child in financial trouble, etc.—by as much as $10,000 to $15,000 a year.

Solution: Keep money that is likely to be needed in the next few years in safe short-term investments, such as money market funds, Treasury bills and CDs. Each year, set aside funds for taxes and the other known future liabilities, such as the need for a new car.

• **Don't be afraid to dip into principal.** That's why you have stocks to provide growth.

Example: In the 28% tax bracket, to get $1,000 cash to spend, you would have to earn $1,390 in other income, such as interest. It would cost you only $1,181 after taxes to take that amount from gains on a stock. And now, dividends on stock provide greater after-tax income than other types of ordinary income.

• **Don't overinsure.** Those age 65 or older should buy Medigap insurance to pick up where Medicare leaves off if they opt for traditional Medicare coverage. But don't buy a policy with features you don't need and won't use, and don't buy Medigap if you're in a Medicare HMO.

Long-term-care insurance: The need for this type of insurance is a function of your age, wealth and family situation.

If you have less than $500,000 in assets, you can't afford it. If you have assets of more than $1 million (single) or $1.5 million (married), you can afford to pay for any care you might need. If you decide you need long-term-care insurance, comparison shop. Policies are cheaper and more readily available the younger you are.

Optimum age to purchase: In your 50s. As you get older, you may develop health problems that make you ineligible for coverage.

• **Pay more attention to taxes.** Under current law, bond yields and stock dividends are more heavily taxed than capital gains. So, as you near retirement, it makes more sense, tax-wise, to keep growth stocks and mutual funds *outside of* traditional retirement accounts from which distributions will be taxed as ordinary income.

Consider converting traditional IRAs to Roth IRAs. Money you put into a Roth is not tax deductible. But money you take out of a Roth is tax free when certain conditions are met.

Converting to a Roth IRA makes sense even in your 50s, 60s or 70s, provided you have outside funds to pay the taxes that become due immediately upon conversion *and* that you plan to hold the Roth IRA for at least 10 years to make up for the initial tax bite.

• **Aim to earn a little**—not necessarily a lot—more and spend a little less. Be conscious of small expenses or savings that can add up over the years. For example, putting taxable bonds in your tax-deferred accounts and stocks in a taxable account could add 1% to 3% to your after-tax return each year. In this market, that can make a big difference.

Don't pay higher-than-necessary fees for professional fund management.

Best: Buy only no-load funds that have low expense ratios.

To do a bit better: Corporate bonds look attractive. As the economy improves, consider putting 5% to 10% of your bond portfolio into high-yield corporate bond funds.

Also look at short (two to three years) and ultra-short (one year or less) bond funds.

I also like Treasury Inflation Protected Securities (TIPS), which adjust returns upward with inflation. You must pay taxes on the interest each year even though you don't collect it until maturity, but that is a small price to pay for inflation protection.

Ginnie Mae funds also have been paying higher yields.

As a result of today's modest investment returns, it's important to revisit the question of how much you can safely withdraw each year from your retirement funds. During the boom years of the late 1990s, we used to say 5% to 6% was OK. In today's investment climate, it's prudent to restrict withdrawals to 4% a year.

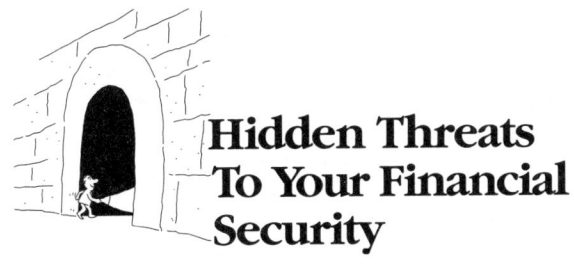

Hidden Threats To Your Financial Security

Ric Edelman, CFS, chairman of the financial planning firm Edelman Financial Services, 12450 Fair Lakes Circle, Fairfax, VA 22033. He is author of several books, including *Ordinary People, Extraordinary Wealth* and *Financial Security in Troubled Times* (both from Harper).

There are always threats to financial well-being—job loss, a serious accident, disability, etc.

Here are the most common gaps in household safety nets—and how to close them…

TOO LITTLE CASH

The first rule of financial planning is to build a "rainy day" fund to tide you over in the event of job loss or anything else that stops the checks from coming in. Many people forgot this rule in the 1990s, when money in the bank earned 2% while tech stocks seemed to double overnight.

Strategy: Keep a cash reserve at your bank or credit union, in a money market mutual fund or even in US Treasury bills. The reserve should be big enough to cover three months' take-home pay—six months' is preferable. For extra safety, keep cash or traveler's checks on hand to cover two weeks of expenses.

TOO SMALL A MORTGAGE

Conventional wisdom says to pay off your mortgage quickly so your home isn't at risk if you lose your job.

In reality, if you *were* to lose your job, you would be in a better position to hold on to your home if you owed a large sum than if you had paid off the mortgage.

If you lose your job *after* paying off your mortgage and then try to borrow against the equity in your home, the lender can turn you down. Home-equity loans are based on income, not the value of your home.

Strategy: Obtain a home-equity loan or refinance to a larger mortgage while you are still working. The less equity you have tied up in your house and the more you have to invest in things other than real estate, the more of each monthly payment goes toward interest, not principal. And mortgage interest payments are tax deductible.

Opt for a 30-year term with monthly payments, rather than a shorter term with biweekly payments. This will keep costs down while allowing you to have a bigger mortgage.

INADEQUATE LIFE INSURANCE

Most Americans are woefully underinsured. According to the American Council of Life Insurers, the average American household has just $196,200 in life insurance.

Test the adequacy of your existing protection with my "cut-in-half-and-drop-a-zero" formula.

Example: If family wage earners have a total of $300,000 in life insurance, first divide that number by two, to $150,000. Then drop a zero, to $15,000. Your $300,000 policy will generate about $15,000 a year in income for your family. If you were to die, could your family get by on $15,000 a year?

Strategy: Figure out how much in support your family would really require if you died. Assuming that your spouse continues working, all that should be necessary is enough income to get your children through their high school and college years.

Which type is the best? Term insurance is cheaper, but it has no cash value. Permanent

Your Money

cash-value insurance provides coverage that will never go away.

If you only want to provide for your kids until they finish college, term is usually best. If you want to make sure that your spouse will be protected for life, consider cash-value insurance. Deciding between term and cash-value insurance is complex. Consult a professional financial planner.

Warning: Since September 11, some agents have been pushing "double-indemnity" riders. These riders double your coverage if you die in an accident—but they also boost your costs significantly.

Better: Your family's needs are the same, no matter how you die. Buy as much coverage as you can afford. Avoid double-indemnity riders.

Editor's note: To compare term life insurance costs, visit *www.reliaquote.com.* For both life and disability insurance quotes, check out *www.insure.com.*

NO DISABILITY COVERAGE

Every homeowner's policy includes fire coverage, yet there is only one chance in 1,200 that your home will burn down. Only 15% of all American workers have disability-income protection—even though there is one chance in eight that you will suffer a long-term disability (one that lasts more than 90 days) before age 65. Since 1960, frequency of death from serious illness has decreased by 32%—but frequency of disability has increased by 55%.

Thanks to air bags, you are less likely to be killed in an auto accident—but more likely to be injured severely enough that you will need to spend an extended time away from work.

Few people have disability insurance outside of employer-sponsored plans. The typical employer disability policy provides only two-thirds of the coverage you need.

Annual premiums for disability insurance bought in the private market can run 1% to 3% of your annual salary. My clients complain that's too much. I say, "If you can't afford the premium, how will you afford the loss of income if you're disabled?"

Good news: If you buy your own policy, benefit payments are not taxable, as they are under an employer-sponsored policy.

VULNERABILITY TO LAWSUITS

You don't have to work in a high-risk profession, such as medicine, to be sued. Your dog could bite the postman. A neighbor could fall on your front steps.

Liability coverage on auto or homeowner's policies rarely exceeds $500,000. An umbrella policy linked to your home and/or auto policy protects you from nearly any kind of liability and even pays your legal expenses.

Cost: Usually less than $250 per year for $1 million in coverage. Add more until coverage roughly equals your net worth.

NOT HAVING A WILL

Only 41% of adult Americans have a will. Among Americans with children, just 34% have a will. Yet you need a will to ensure that your property will be distributed as you wish.

People think that creating a will is complicated, but your lawyer will take care of the legalese for you.

Where to Get Money for An Emergency

William J. Cafero, certified investment management analyst and senior personal financial consultant at Ernst & Young in New York City, *www.ey.com.*

Need to raise some cash for an impending layoff, medical procedure or another unforeseen emergency? *Here are nine ways, starting with the most desirable...*

PERSONAL GIFTS

Anyone can give you a tax-free gift of up to $11,000. Friends and relatives can multiply that amount by giving you and your spouse separate gifts.

PERSONAL LOANS

Loans from friends and family members are the most cost-effective way to borrow. The loan can be for any amount, and the lender does not have to charge interest. However, he/she probably should, since he will be taxed *as if* he received the applicable federal rate, regardless of whether or not you paid interest.

For more information, search under "Applicable Federal Rate" at *www.irs.gov*. Use an attorney, and put the loan agreement in writing.

HOME EQUITY

●**Refinancing allows you to tap your home's equity.** Today's low rates may allow you to increase the size of your mortgage without increasing monthly payments. You might, for example, be able to borrow as much as $130,000 against your home even though you only need $100,000 for your mortgage.

Caution: A bank is unlikely to let you refinance if you have lost your job. Even if you do get a loan while unemployed, it may be at a higher interest rate.

●**Home-equity loans can be taken in addition to your primary mortgage,** typically at a fixed level above the prime interest rate, with a term of five to 20 years.

Bonus: Generally, there are no closing costs …interest is tax deductible on loans of up to $100,000…and it takes only a week to set up.

Caution: Carrying a larger debt increases your risk of default, which increases your risk of foreclosure.

●**Home-equity lines of credit also use your residence as collateral.** The interest on up to $100,000 is tax deductible. You don't pay interest until you use the credit line and then only on the money you tap. You also can borrow again if you repay the loan before the line expires.

Caution: Lines of credit and certain home-equity loans have variable interest rates. If the prime rate rises, so will your rate.

INVESTMENT LOANS

●**Margin loans** allow you to borrow up to 50% of the value of your securities portfolio from your brokerage firm (up to 90% on US government securities). There is no check of credit, so you can get the money in about a day. You can even add the interest payments to the loan balance instead of paying each month.

Caution: If your portfolio declines in value, reducing your collateral, you will face a margin call. You will have to put up cash or sell securities to cover the account.

Best: Borrow only 30%. Leave yourself a cushion of about 20%.

●**Sell long-term investments,** especially underperforming stocks or real estate.

Caution: Selling property takes time. Commissions, closing costs and taxes will reduce the proceeds.

●**Borrow against whole and universal life insurance policies.** The money is tax free, and you never have to pay it back. You will be charged interest on the loan. And, if you don't repay, the amount owed will be deducted from the death benefit.

●**Borrow from retirement accounts,** including 401(k)s. Generally, the loan must be repaid in equal monthly payments plus interest over a period of up to five years. If you can repay the loan quickly, a 401(k) loan is a cheap, easy way to get cash.

But remember—money borrowed for any length of time retards asset growth.

If you change jobs, the entire loan becomes due within 90 days, depending on the plan sponsor. If you can't repay it, the loan will be considered a taxable distribution, which is subject to a 10% penalty if you are younger than age 59½.

To Avoid Big Money Mistakes…Ignore Your Intuition

Morton Davis, PhD, professor emeritus of mathematics, City College of New York in New York City. He is author of *The Math of Money: Making Mathematical Sense of Your Personal Finances* (Copernicus).

From paying off the mortgage to buying stock—most people make the big money decisions based on intuition. Yet they seldom look at the numbers. To demonstrate how intuition can lead *anyone* astray, I have applied principles of mathematics to four situations.

AT THE APPLIANCE STORE

You buy a dishwasher for $600 and agree to pay 13 consecutive monthly payments of $50—

Your Money

$650 in all. You figure that if you're paying $50 in interest for a one-year loan, your interest rate is going to be 8.33% ($50 ÷ $600 = 8.33%).

Reality: If the loan really were for one year at that interest rate, you would be able to keep the money for a full year before repaying any part of it.

Instead, your first payment, including interest and principal, is due immediately, and you must make additional payments each month until the loan is paid off. Worse still, you owe interest for the full year on the original $600 you borrowed—even though the amount you owe diminishes each month. Even in your final payment, which reduces the unpaid balance of the loan to zero, you are paying interest on the full $600. The effective interest rate goes up each month as the unpaid balance declines.

My calculations show the real annual rate of interest on that loan—repaid month-by-month—is 17.36%.

With each payment, you borrowed money for an average of six months. Yet you paid for a one-year loan—about double the nominal interest rate of 8.33%. Using a credit card that had a rate of 17% or less would have been a better strategy.

ON YOUR MORTGAGE

You decide to shop around for a 30-year mortgage. With a fixed-rate, 8% mortgage for $100,000, your monthly payment would be $714. For most people, paying as much in the early years as in the later years is difficult because they have less earning power when they are starting out.

Strategy: Shop around for an "escalator" mortgage, which evens out the burden of payments for most people. With a 30-year $100,000 escalator mortgage, your first year's payments would be $571 a month. Payments would climb by 2% each year over the life of the loan. The weighted average interest rate would be 8%.

Intuition says this is a bad deal because your payments will keep getting larger, eventually climbing above the $714 a month you would have paid.

Reality: When adjusted for inflation, payments that are made in later years, though larger, are worth much less in today's dollars than payments that are made today.

Note: If you easily can afford your payments now and expect to have less income in the later years, you might do better with a standard mortgage.

IN THE STOCK MARKET

Investment experts talk about "undervalued" stocks. The idea is that these stocks can be bought at bargain prices now—and sold at a profit when they return to their "proper" prices.

Reality: The only "proper" price for a stock is what an investor will pay for it. Growth and value managers expend great effort calculating what a stock *might* sell for next month or next year, yet active investment managers seldom beat the market.

Strategy: Put the majority of your investments in a low-cost, broad-market index fund. You won't have to worry that a given stock is overvalued, undervalued or fairly valued.

AT THE CASINO

People naturally are averse to risk. They want the odds on their side when they bet on anything. Yet they can bet against the odds and still win.

In a casino, the house always has an edge. The mathematical "Law of Large Numbers" says that when the odds are against you, the longer you bet, the more certain you are to lose. This is why casinos limit the size of bets. A casino is more apt to make money if a patron makes many small bets than if he/she makes one large one.

Strategy: Put the Law of Large Numbers on your side by limiting the number of bets. If you bet $500 in one shot instead of small increments, the odds are virtually even that you will double your money. Win or lose, walk out of the casino.

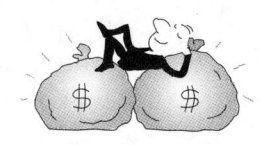

Money Matters

How to Choose an Internet Bank

Check out an Internet bank carefully before using it. Look at the *About Us* section on the bank's site for its history, physical location and phone numbers. If you are considering opening an account, confirm that the institution is insured by the Federal Deposit Insurance Corporation (877-275-3342 or *www.fdic.gov*). Beware of Web sites whose offers are significantly better than those of other banks... and those using a name or Internet address similar to that of a well-known financial institution. These could be signs of a fraudulent site.

Jay Rosenstein, editor, *FDIC Consumer News*, 801 17 St. NW, Washington, DC 20434.

Check-Writing Alert

Some of the checks you write are clearing faster than ever before. It used to take up to two weeks before funds actually were debited—but major companies, such as American Express and Wal-Mart, have started converting checks into electronic fund transfers. Using the account and bank information on your check, the money is then moved from your checking account to the company's account within 24 hours of receiving the check. If the funds are not available, you can be charged for overdrawing. Be sure to check your billing statement for notices of this new policy.

Hal Morris, veteran Las Vegas–based consumer affairs journalist who writes widely about scams, schemes and rip-offs. He is also a former bank director.

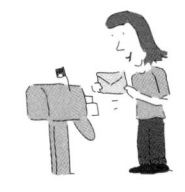

On-Line Banking Dangers

Edward Mrkvicka, Jr., president, Reliance Enterprises, Inc., national financial consulting firm, 22115 O'Connell Rd., Marengo, IL 60152, and author of *Your Bank Is Ripping You Off* (St. Martin's).

If you bank on-line or are looking for an on-line bank, don't get caught up in these sneaky traps...

•**Some banks may offer no-fee checking to attract customers,** then start charging fees within a year.

•**On-line banking may not be secure**—if you don't have a firewall on your PC, a hacker could obtain your account information.

•**When on-line banks merge,** depositors may lose access to funds for a week or more.

•**Some on-line banks charge odd fees.**

Example: A fee if you sign up for on-line bill payment but don't use it.

•**Scammers create Web sites with Web addresses similar to those of some legitimate banks,** then collect personal data, such as account and Social Security numbers, from customers who make errors when typing the bank's Web address.

When You Prefer To Be Billed By Mail...

To cut their costs, more companies are offering on-line billing. A notice is put in billing statements months in advance. Bills are sent via E-mail or posted on secure Web sites. These firms, which include insurers and telecommunications companies, may charge their customers between $12 and $48 a year to mail bills.

If you prefer to be billed by mail: Negotiate with the company's customer service department. Say that you're being penalized for not having a computer or Internet access at home. If negotiations fail, switch companies.

Elizabeth Robertson, senior analyst with TowerGroup, 63 Kendrick St., Needham, MA 02494, a research and advisory firm that specializes in assessing the impact of technology on financial services.

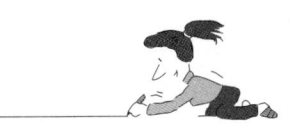

■ *Your Money* ■ ■

Before You Cosign…

Cosigning a loan makes you personally liable for the full amount of the loan. A lender can—and will—come after you if the person for whom you cosign misses a payment. Your credit rating can be damaged by his/her late payments.

Self-defense: Carefully review the risks document that lenders are required to give everyone who cosigns. Agree with the cosigner that he will give you early notice of any late payments or other troubles, so you can work directly with the lender to set up a payment plan if necessary.

Steve Rhode, president and cofounder of Myvesta.org, a financial management organization in Rockville, MD.

More from Steve Rhode…

Credit Card Alert

Watch out—credit card companies can and do change payment dates. Check your credit card statements carefully to avoid penalties.

Trap: Some issuers are now specifying an exact time when payment is due in addition to a date. Your payment must be received by a specific hour or you are charged a late fee.

Caution: If you're using an automatic bill-paying service, be sure to revise the due dates when they change.

Easy Way to Get a Better Credit Card Deal

Get a better credit card deal simply by asking for it. Most companies will lower interest rates or reduce annual fees for customers who maintain good credit records. When you call your card issuer, be specific about what you want—a lower interest rate, lower annual fee, more frequent-flier miles, etc.

Greg McBride, CFA, senior financial analyst, Bankrate.com, 11811 US Hwy. One, North Palm Beach, FL 33408.

Improve Your Credit Report

Lenders examining your credit report are most concerned if any credit card account or personal line of credit (excluding a home-equity loan) exceeds 50% of its limit. If consolidating has pushed you past the 50% mark, ask the card issuer to increase your credit line to bring it back under 50%. Otherwise, consider splitting the debt among two or more cards. Lenders also hold it against you if you have opened several credit accounts within the past 12 months. If your credit is good, dormant accounts on your report can actually help you get future loans. These records help lenders see how you used credit in the past.

Gerri Detweiler, president of Ultimate Credit Solutions Inc., a consumer credit assistance organization, Sarasota, FL, *www.ultimatecredit.com*. She is author of *The Ultimate Credit Handbook* (Plume).

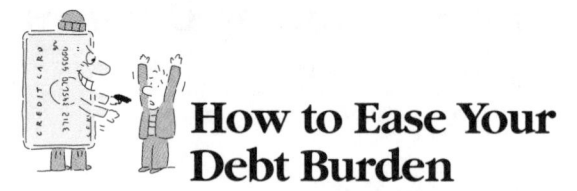

How to Ease Your Debt Burden

Scott Kays, CFP, principal at Kays Financial Advisory Corp., Atlanta, *www.scottkays.com*, and author of *Achieving Your Financial Potential* (Doubleday).

Financial services companies are making big money in their campaign to "help" us manage our debt. *Here are the moves that make sense for you and the ones that don't…*

BEST MOVES

•**Negotiate with your credit card companies.** You may be able to lower interest rates and stretch out repayment schedules. Pay off high-interest debt first.

•**Take out a home-equity loan** if your need is short-term and you don't want to refinance your mortgage. Rates average 5.25%, but you can do better if your credit is good. Interest may be tax deductible, and there may be no closing costs.

Risk: As with a mortgage, if you fail to make the payments, the lender can foreclose.

Money Matters

•**Refinance your mortgage.** If your home's value has risen, you can cash out some of the equity to pay off short-term debt.

Example: You purchased your home for $100,000 and borrowed 80% of the value, or $80,000. When you refinance, your home is appraised at $130,000 and you've paid off $3,000 of the mortgage. You may now borrow $104,000—80% of the *higher* value. If you use $77,000 to pay off the old mortgage, you can cash out $27,000. Your monthly payment may even be lower, depending on the new mortgage rate.

•**Refinance your car loan.** Use your car's value as collateral for a personal loan from a bank or credit union. The rate will be 7% to 8%, versus 14% for a personal unsecured loan.

Caution: You might have trouble buying a new car if you owe more on the old one than it is worth.

WORST MOVES

•**Taking a debt-consolidation loan.** If you need one because your credit history is poor, be wary of offers advertised on the Internet or through direct mail. The interest rate will probably be higher than those on your credit cards—possibly as high as 22%.

Even when your monthly payment is lower, you will end up paying more because of the longer term of the loan.

Debt consolidators who promise to "take care of everything" typically attach a service fee to your monthly payments—about 10% of the amount paid.

Better: If you are a credit card "junkie," get help from a nonprofit community organization that provides free debt consolidation and management advice.

Good resource: Consumer Credit Counseling Service (888-577-2227 or *www.cccs.org*).

•**Making frequent balance transfers** from high-interest credit cards to cards with low initial teaser rates. At some point, credit card issuers will no longer let you transfer balances.

Result: You will look like a bad credit risk and may be stuck with high-interest cards in the future.

If you choose to transfer a balance: Ask the old credit card company to note that the account has been "closed at customer's request" so that it doesn't look as if the creditor closed it.

When Choosing a Debt Consolidator...

Before using a debt consolidator see if any complaints have been filed against it with the Better Business Bureau and/or your state's attorney general.

Red flags: Make sure the firm isn't making unrealistic claims, such as that it will settle debts for less than 30 cents on the dollar...or your credit record won't be hurt by using the service.

Also: The firm should not guarantee to eliminate all of your debts. There is no way that such a promise can be made before working with you.

Caution: A firm that wants complete payment up front is not necessarily a scam. But be careful.

Mory Brenner, Esq., national debt consultant, Pittsfield, MA, *www.debtworkout.com*.

It Pays to Use a Mortgage Broker

Keith Gumbinger, vice president of HSH Associates, financial publishers of mortgage information, Butler, NJ.

Approximately two out of every three home loans are arranged by a mortgage broker.

Mortgage brokers typically work with dozens of financial institutions. They can offer a wider menu of options than individual lenders can, such as mortgage products that might not be available in your area or obscure types of loans that might prove advantageous to you.

Your Money

A borrower with poor credit who might never get a loan from a bank or savings and loan directly often can find one through a mortgage broker.

FINDING A MORTGAGE BROKER

Be careful when choosing a mortgage broker. This industry is poorly regulated. Brokers may offer come-on rates or provide inadequate documentation of loan terms. Some scam artists demand up-front fees, then walk away with your money.

•**Start with recommendations.** Ask for suggestions from friends and family. Also talk to bank lending officers and other lenders to find out what sort of mortgage is typical for someone in your situation.

Helpful: The National Association of Mortgage Brokers maintains a database of its members on its Web site, *www.namb.org.* Just type in your area or zip code to find a listing of local brokers.

•**Ask brokers for references.** Find out what kind of experiences other borrowers have had with the broker. How responsive was he/she? Were there any problems with the process or outcome?

•**Do a background check.** Contact your local Better Business Bureau and state mortgage broker association to find out if a broker has been the subject of any complaints. The National Association of Mortgage Brokers also lists state groups on its Web site.

Other good sources for general mortgage information: Fannie Mae, 800-732-6643 or *www.homepath.com...www.mortgagecalc.com...*or my company, HSH Associates, *www.hsh.com.*

SECURING THE LOAN

Don't expect a broker to give you more than one quote. While he may, his job is to find you the best rate for the kind of mortgage you want.

By law, a broker has to give you a written estimate of closing costs after you apply for a mortgage. Many also will give you an estimate beforehand if you ask.

Important: Don't forget to ask about the commission. Most mortgage brokers take less than 1% of the loan as a fee. But if you have bad credit or other circumstances that make getting a mortgage difficult, you will probably have to pay more.

PROTECTING YOUR RIGHTS

•**Ask a lawyer to look over any contracts** before you sign them.

•**Know who is processing the loan** and how to contact that person. Don't depend on the broker to see that the loan is processed in a timely fashion.

Double-Check Your Mortgage Escrow Account

Escrow is used to pay insurance and property taxes through your mortgage payment.

Trap I: Some banks hold more funds than called for—authorities recently required one bank to pay refunds to 40,000 home owners.

Trap II: Some banks hold too little, leaving home owners facing a big surprise tax or insurance payments.

Self-defense: Add up your annual property tax and insurance bills and then divide by 12 to see what your monthly escrow payment should be. Next, read your loan agreement to find the details of how escrow is handled. Check your monthly payment to be sure it matches what your calculations indicate.

This Old House, 1185 Avenue of the Americas, 27th Flr., New York City 10036.

How to Handle a Mortgage Buyout

If your mortgage is bought out by another lender, make these smart moves...

•**Pay with paper checks until the transfer is complete**—electronic payments could go astray when the first lender cashes out.

Money Matters

• **If you accidentally send a payment to your old mortgage holder,** you have 60 days from the transferral to redirect your payment. You can't be charged a late fee during that time.

• **After the transferral,** if the new servicer makes a mistake and sends a statement for too much money, pay the larger amount and sort out the problem later—if you pay less, the new servicer may charge you late fees or even start foreclosure.

• **Label any complaint** *Qualified written request under Section 6 of the Real Estate Settlement Procedures Act.* This gives the servicer 60 business days to fix the problem.

Terrell Kelley, residential mortgage specialist, Mortgage Monitor Financial Services at 1372 Summer St., Stamford, CT 06905.

Save 50% When Refinancing

Home owners typically are charged for a new title search and title-insurance policy when they refinance. Reissue-rate or other discount title insurance can save you as much as 50% when refinancing.

However, title insurers don't advertise these reduced-rate policies—you have to ask. And, they are not available in every state or for every transaction.

James R. Maher, executive vice president of American Land Title Association, Washington, DC.

Extra Deduction For Refinancing

Low interest rates are motivating many home owners to refinance their mortgages. A tax deduction for "points," or loan fees, can make a refinancing even more attractive.

Normally points incurred on a refinancing must be deducted over the life of the loan. *But there are two exceptions...*

• **If the new home loan is used in part to finance improvements to the home,** an allocable portion of the points is deductible.

• **When a home is refinanced for a second time,** any remaining undeducted points from the prior refinancing may become fully deductible.

Details: IRS Publication 936, *Home Mortgage Interest Deduction.*

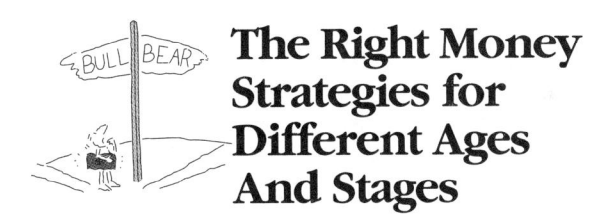

The Right Money Strategies for Different Ages And Stages

Gary Schatsky, JD, president of The Objective Advice Group in New York City, *www.objectiveadvice.com,* and chairman emeritus of the National Association of Personal Financial Advisors. *Worth* has named him one of the country's best financial planners every year since 1997.

The stock market is still uncertain...tax laws have changed dramatically...and the economy is on its way to recovery. Now is the time to evaluate and strengthen your financial position.

Here are the strategies I'm suggesting to my clients at various life stages...

IN YOUR 30s AND 40s

• **Start a 529 plan.** These state-sponsored investment vehicles, exempt from federal tax on gains, are my favorite way to save for a child's education.

Benefits: No limit on annual contributions... high maximum lifetime contribution—$250,000 in some states...you retain control of the money even after the child turns 18.

New York has the best plan in the country. I recommend it even to nonresidents for its great management (TIAA-CREF, 800-842-2252) and low expenses. Fidelity (800-343-3548) and Vanguard (800-523-7731) also offer good plans in several states.

Your Money

Questions to ask about 529s...

• How flexible is the plan? The plan should allow the money to be used at any accredited college in any state...and allow for transfers to a sibling or relative if the child decides not to go to college. If you don't use 529 money for qualified educational purposes, you'll have to pay taxes on withdrawals, plus a 10% penalty.

• Does the plan offer a break on state income taxes for residents? Investing in your own state's plan may entitle you to significant benefits.

• Who manages the plan? Most states use one investment management company, which offers aggressive, moderate and conservative portfolio allocations based on a child's age.

For comparisons of state plans: Go to www.savingforcollege.com...or www.morningstar.com/centers/529.html.

Caution: Having a 529 plan could limit your child's eligibility for financial aid.

• **Put conservative investments in retirement accounts.** Conventional wisdom says retirement accounts should be filled with stocks because they have the best long-term returns. That is tax-inefficient.

In the past several years, if your tech stocks got clobbered and you lost a large part of your IRA, you had no ability to reduce your taxes by writing off the loss.

Outside of your tax shelter, use the Tax Code to enhance your rate of return.

Example: A 40-year-old client who has a $2 million portfolio—with $1 million in taxable accounts and $1 million in retirement accounts—was comfortable with an allocation of 75% equities and 25% bonds. Most of the stock was in the retirement-account allocation.

Strategy: We shifted half of his retirement-account money into bonds and increased the equity positions in his regular accounts, leaving him the identical stock/bond ratio. Since 2001, the equities in his portfolio decreased 10%, a loss of $50,000. But he was able to write off most of that against capital gains and wound up saving $10,000 in taxes.

For a client wanting more income, I might have also put in the retirement portfolio other tax-inefficient, but low-risk, investments, such as high-dividend stocks or real estate investment trusts.

IN YOUR 50s

• **Limit ownership of your company's stock to 20% of your portfolio.** You already have a substantial investment in your company by way of your paycheck. *To determine if you own too much company stock...*

• Study your company's financial statements, annual reports and quarterly SEC filings. Before you invest, assess the company's prospects for profit and growth as you would for any stock.

• Check with your 401(k) administrator to learn the rules governing your company stock. Are there circumstances in which you would be unable to sell?

• Check if any mutual funds you own invest heavily in your company. Top holdings are listed in the prospectus and quarterly reports. Buy additional shares of the stock if it is attractive...you don't own too much of it...and the stock is offered at a discount, such as through stock-option plans.

If you leave a job: Roll your 401(k) into an IRA to give yourself more control over retirement assets—even if the holdings are 100% in company stock.

Example: Ex-Enron employees who left their stock in the company's plan were temporarily banned from selling. They watched helplessly as the value of their holdings took a big plunge. With a rollover IRA, they could have sold shares immediately.

• **Take advantage of new "catch-up" provisions for retirement savings.** Annual contributions to most tax-advantaged accounts are increased through 2006. *After that, increases will be indexed for inflation...*

• IRAs. Those age 50 or over can contribute $3,500...$4,500 in 2005...$5,000 in 2006...and $6,000 in 2008. For others, contributions are limited to $3,000...$4,000 starting in 2005...$5,000 starting in 2008.

• 401(k)s and 403(b)s. The maximum contribution for one person is $12,000 in 2003 and $13,000 in 2004. It will increase by $1,000 a year before reaching a maximum of $15,000 in 2006. Those age 50 or older can contribute the normal amount *plus* an additional $2,000 in 2003...$3,000 in 2004...$4,000 in 2005...$5,000 in 2006.

Money Matters

IN YOUR 60s

•**Decide whether to pay off your mortgage.** Simply determine whether the after-tax cost of your mortgage is more than the interest rate you could earn on a top-quality, low- to moderate-risk investment. If it is, consider prepaying your mortgage.

Examples: One client in the 30% tax bracket, including state and local taxes, had an 8% mortgage. His after-tax rate was 5.6%.* He had a large sum of money that he intended to invest in bonds. I told him to pay down his mortgage instead, because the conservative, fixed-income instruments that he had in mind could not pay 5.6% on an after-tax basis.

Another client in the 40% tax bracket, including state and local taxes, had a 6.5% mortgage. His after-tax rate was 3.9%. He had a small amount of money in bonds, and he thought he might need this within the next few years. I suggested he keep making his monthly mortgage payments and leave the money in the bond fund. It would give him liquidity while letting him earn roughly the same after-tax rate he paid on his mortgage.

•**"Test-drive" retirement.** Many people assume that once they retire, they can live comfortably on 70% of their current income. Try it for a year. If you find you don't mind living on less, you might be able to retire sooner than you planned. However, many new retirees find their expenses spike for two or three years because they are traveling more and buying big-ticket items.

Also, rent a home for several months in the retirement location to which you would like to move. Do you enjoy the amenities in the new location? Do you miss family and friends more than you thought you would?

IN RETIREMENT

Many strategies from other life stages apply here as well—keeping the more conservative investments in your tax-sheltered accounts... limiting your holdings of company stock...even strategies for investing in 529 plans—in this case, on behalf of your grandchildren.

One additional strategy: Gradually reduce equity exposure. Shift into bonds or short-term investments. While life expectancies are rising, your investment time horizon is still shorter than when you were working. And with less income to replenish your assets, your risk tolerance should be lower.

*After-tax rate = mortgage rate x (1 - tax rate).

More from Gary Schatsky...

How Safe Is Your Money?

With some banks and brokerages suffering large losses, regulatory scrutiny and criminal investigations, many investors worry about what would happen if their financial institutions failed.

While there is no protection against market losses, most financial institutions are covered by insurance...

•**Banks.** Most people realize that the Federal Deposit Insurance Corporation (FDIC) will insure up to $100,000 per traditional account. Investments in stocks, bonds, mutual funds and annuities that are sold by banks or affiliated broker-dealers are *not* FDIC insured.

Regarding traditional bank accounts, make sure your bank, credit union or savings and loan carries FDIC protection. If you want to keep more than $100,000 at one bank, divide the money among several accounts under different titles (individual, joint, trust or IRA). Go to *www.fdic.gov/index.html* for details.

•**Brokerages.** Accounts are insured by the Securities Investor Protection Corporation (SIPC). If your brokerage fails, each account is protected for up to $500,000 in securities and $100,000 in cash. Mutual funds held by your brokerage are covered by the brokerage's insurance.

Many large brokerages will supplement SIPC with private insurance. Some, such as Merrill Lynch & Co. and Smith Barney Citigroup, have bank charters, so they provide their customers with FDIC insurance for uninvested cash in customer accounts.

•**Mutual funds.** In the unlikely event that there is an outright theft by the management company, investors will not be compensated, but they can sue. If a fund company fails, the assets it manages would likely be transferred to a third party to administer. To be safe, diversify among several fund families.

■ *Your Money* ■ ■

For a Simpler Divorce...

Collaborative law for divorce is a simpler, much less expensive and less emotionally charged way of ending a marriage. The husband and wife each have a lawyer. The couple and their lawyers sign an agreement to dissolve the marriage without litigation. If they fail to do so, the contract provides that the lawyers must withdraw from the case before it goes to court. This provides a big incentive to settle, since the couple would have to start all over again with new attorneys. Collaborative law will cost about $1,000 to $4,000 per spouse, depending on the complexity of the case. Nearly 3,000 lawyers in 25 states now offer it.

More information: International Academy of Collaborative Professionals' Web site, *www.collabgroup.com*.

Jennifer Jackson, JD, board member, Web master and editor, *Collaborative Review*, and chair, International Academy of Collaborative Professionals, San Francisco.

Postnuptial Agreement Basics

Arlene G. Dubin, Esq., partner, Sonnenschein Nath & Rosenthal, 30 Rockefeller Plaza, New York City 10112, and author of *Prenups for Lovers: A Romantic Guide to Prenuptial Agreements* (Villard).

A postnuptial agreement determines how assets would be divided upon death or divorce. It is similar to a prenuptial agreement but is drawn up *during* a marriage. You may need a postnuptial agreement to protect against your spouse's creditors...provide for children from a previous marriage...amend a prenuptial agreement...or address a change in circumstances (e.g., you sell your business or leave your job). Be straightforward about your concerns, and solicit your spouse's input. In addition, remain open-minded and ready to compromise.

Helpful: Each spouse should have a lawyer, and the agreement should be arranged for both spouses' best interests—and their children's best interests.

Caution: A postnuptial agreement should specify which state controls it—marriage contracts are governed by state law.

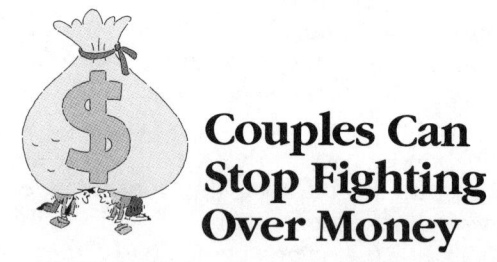

Couples Can Stop Fighting Over Money

David Bach, founder and CEO, Finish Rich, Inc., financial education company, 424 W. Broadway, New York City 10012, *www.finishrich.com*. He is author of *Smart Couples Finish Rich: 9 Steps to Creating a Rich Future for You and Your Partner* (Broadway).

When my wife and I got married five years ago, I was annoyed that she would spend part of every paycheck on new shoes.

Instead of getting into a shouting match, however, I questioned my own need to dictate what she spent. Was it so that I would feel more powerful in the relationship?

Eventually, I realized that I didn't care *what* she was buying. I was just concerned that we would not have enough money to protect ourselves. That realization allowed me to open a dialogue about our real money goals.

I have clients who have been married for 25 years who talk about money only during a credit squeeze. I urge them to discuss their financial situation. Secrets about debt and credit problems inevitably come out. Getting turned down for a mortgage because of a spouse's deception creates mistrust.

GET TO KNOW EACH OTHER ON A FINANCIAL LEVEL

•**Ask your partner about his/her money habits,** including spending patterns, use of financial advisers, credit history, insurance and investment philosophies. Find out how much your partner knows—or doesn't know—about money. If neither of you knows enough, enroll in a class at a local college.

Helpful: Get your credit report from Fair, Issac and Co., a leading credit-record scoring company, *www.myfico.com.*

Cost: $12.95.*

• **Talk about how your parents managed money.** Chances are, you each inherited attitudes about spending and saving.

Example: Your spouse may be very frugal because when he was a child, his father worked only sporadically, so his family struggled to make ends meet. You, on the other hand, may spend money freely because you grew up in a wealthy home.

• **Examine your values and goals.** When you think about your life and things that matter, what's most important to both of you?

Examples of values: Creativity...family ...freedom...friendship...security.

Examples of goals: To be debt-free... get a new car...give more to charity.

Make sure your goals are based on your values. Retiring with $1 million is a goal. The underlying value is security.

Helpful: My Web site, *www.finishrich.com/ resource/financialhealth.html,* has a questionnaire and checklists to help set goals and values.

• **Decide if your attitude toward money fits your situation as a couple.** *Discuss...*

• Retirement. How do we want to safeguard our future? Are we contributing the maximum to 401(k) plans and IRAs? Where can we cut back spending so we can save even more?

Aim to put aside 10% to 15% of each of your incomes or, in the case of 401(k)s, enough to get your employers' matching contributions. Invest for growth and income, especially if you are below age 50. Invest no more than 20% in your employers' stock, taking into account any shares held in your 401(k) plan.

Each spouse should have his/her own nest egg. Besides its psychological importance, this gives a couple two sources from which to borrow in the event of an emergency. If one spouse doesn't work, contribute the maximum ($3,000 in 2003 and 2004 or $3,500 if you are age 50 or older by year-end) to a traditional or Roth IRA in his name.

*Price subject to change.

• Security. How do we protect ourselves and our family? Do we have adequate and fairly priced life insurance? Enough money to cover medical emergencies, the death of a loved one or the loss of a job?

Determine how much of a cash cushion will make you comfortable—but always keep enough to cover at least three months of living expenses.

Decide what should be done if you become ill or incapacitated. Do you have disability insurance? Have you each drafted health care proxies?

• Dreams. How do we fulfill specific, deeply held desires that spring from our values and goals —such as taking a trip to Italy or buying a boat or collectibles? Devise a budget together to make your dreams come true.

DIVIDE FINANCIAL RESPONSIBILITIES

It is usually a bad idea to let one spouse take charge of all the finances. If he becomes incapacitated or dies, the other spouse may be lost. One newly widowed client paid her household bills throughout her entire marriage, but she had no idea about investments, which her husband handled.

No matter how you divide the responsibility, schedule a monthly "money date," so you are both aware of financial issues.

• **Establish a primary joint checking account to pay most of your bills.** Decide how much each spouse will contribute to pay monthly expenses.

• **Establish separate checking accounts.** Each spouse can use the money in his account for anything he wants. This averts many arguments and preserves financial privacy.

• **Maintain a joint investing account for common savings goals,** such as a house or vacation. You need not contribute the same amount, especially if one spouse earns more than the other. You may decide to contribute an equal percentage of your incomes.

REVISIT YOUR PRIORITIES

Examine your division of financial chores and money strategies every few years. Review the goals that money enables you to attain as a couple.

Bring in a third party—an accountant or a financial adviser—if you have trouble reaching a compromise.

Your Money

Teaching Grandkids About Money

Grandparents have more time than parents to be financial mentors—and more experience, too. *Here is how to make the most of those advantages...*

• **Have grandkids check the various toy store ads to compare prices** before you take them shopping.

• **Have them form financial goals**—such as getting an expensive toy—and show them how to save a percentage of their allowances each week until they have enough.

• **Go into business with grandchildren.**

Example: One grandmother and grandchild found stuffed toys and other collectibles in thrift shops, cleaned them and resold them at a profit.

Peggy Houser, certified financial planner, and Hassell Bradley Wright, freelance writer, both in Denver. They are coauthors of *How to Teach Children About Money* (Western Freelance Writing Services, Ltd.).

What Not to Say to Children About Money

When talking about money-related topics with your kids, it's best to avoid these common statements...

• **We can't afford it.** This is rarely true—if you do not want to buy a child something, say so and explain why.

• **Money is the root of all evil.** The Bible actually says that *love* of money—greed—is the root of all evil.

• **Time is money.** Time is simply time. If you constantly tell children not to waste even a single minute, you are then teaching them to value everything based on money.

• **Those people are disgustingly rich.** This makes wealth seem negative instead of showing that there can be good or bad ways of being affluent.

Eileen Gallo, PhD, psychotherapist specializing in money and family issues, Los Angeles, and coauthor of *Silver Spoon Kids: How Successful Parents Raise Responsible Children* (McGraw-Hill/Contemporary).

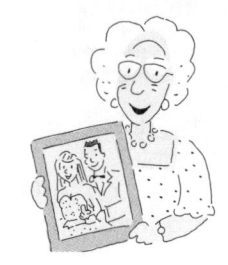

Protect Elderly Relatives from Financial Abuse

Paid caregiving by relatives can lead to financial abuse of the elderly. Some relatives will take money but do not provide proper care.

Self-defense: Discuss with your family what needs to be done and by whom. Write up an agreement that includes reasonable pay, weekly time off and regular vacation time for the caregiver. Include contingency plans in case care requirements change. Give power of attorney to someone other than the caregiver.

Denise Brown, publisher, *Caregiving,* Box 224, Park Ridge, IL 60068, *www.caregiving.com.*

■■ Your Money ■

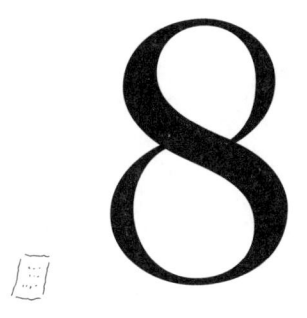

8

Insurance Savvy

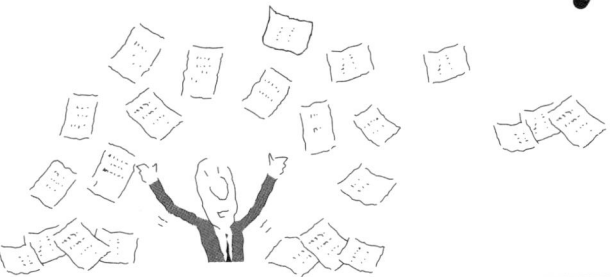

Life Insurance Checkup: Save Big Money Now

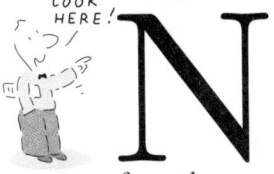

Now is the time to save big money by reviewing your life insurance policies that have been battered by the market. Intensified competition from the recession and longer life spans have brought down premiums.

TERM LIFE

•**Term life insurance** is for a specific period. The older you are when you initiate a policy, the higher the premium. But premiums may stay fixed for the term of a policy—from five up to 30 years. There is no savings (cash-value) component, and the death benefit is free from income tax.

Most people can save 20% or more on a 10-year level-premium policy if they shop around. That means big savings, since they will enjoy lower premiums for at least 10 years. There is no penalty to end a term policy—you just stop paying the premium. Rates may still decline. Comparison shop every two years.

CASH-VALUE

Checkups on whole, universal and variable life insurance begin with evaluating the cash value of your policy. The stock market decline might have left you with less cash value to borrow against in retirement. You may need to increase your premiums to get back on track. Talk to your insurance agent.

•**Whole life insurance** builds cash value and provides a death benefit. The policy stays in force for the client's lifetime, as long as the premiums—which are invested by the insurance company—are paid.

If you are shopping for insurance that builds cash value, put whole life at the top of your list. The 5% annual return most companies now pay beats returns on many investments.

Richard Newman, CPA, partner, Newman & Cohen, financial management and investment advisory firm, 2500 N. Military Trail, Boca Raton, FL 33431. He also has designed insurance products and lectured on insurance.

113

■ *Your Money* ■ ■

That return will increase as the dividends underlying your policy go up.

As with all cash-value life insurance plans, your investment grows tax free and the death benefit is exempt from income tax.

Because you can also borrow against its value, the policy provides a savings cushion in rocky times. Once you buy whole life, you are protected without ever having to renew the policy or take another physical exam as you age.

I recommend whole life to clients ages 25 to 40—those who have a need for life insurance and have plenty of time to build up significant cash value. For people who are just starting coverage and have less time to build up cash value, term insurance is often a better idea.

The insurance you should choose depends on your individual circumstances, goals and length of time to invest.

•**Universal life insurance** combines low-cost term insurance and a savings, or cash-value, component. The policyholder will earn tax-deferred money market rates on the cash value. This insurance also allows the insured to increase or decrease his/her coverage and premium levels.

Make sure that your policy has a guaranteed death benefit, or current market returns may leave you without one.

This type of whole life insurance puts your premiums in short-term investments. Returns partly or fully pay future policy premiums. But today's low interest rates have prevented some policies from earning enough to automatically pay those premiums. In fact, many policies with guaranteed minimum returns are near that level now.

If rates fall, there won't be enough income to pay the cost of the death benefit, so the premium might have to be increased. Talk to your agent.

Important: Too frequently, insurers notify customers after much of their cash value has been drawn down to pay premiums for the death benefit. By that time, clients may be in their 70s or 80s and don't have the years or the income to rebuild their cash value. Sometimes, they even lose their death benefits.

•**Variable universal life insurance** lets clients invest the policy's cash value in market portfolios that are selected by the owner from choices provided by the insurer. Cash values and death benefits rise and fall with investment performance.

In the 1990s, many insurance agents advised clients to put their premiums into a single variable life insurance policy stock fund. Many of those funds have been hit hard by the bear market, leaving policyholders with far less insurance protection because the cash value of the account has diminished.

If the investments made with your premiums have been decimated, don't automatically abandon the policy. You will lose the commission you paid to buy it. A commission is generally 90% to 95% of the first year's premium.

Better: Reconsider the allocation of your policy subaccounts. No matter how long your time horizon, you need bonds and cash as well as stocks. Carefully discuss the allocation with your agent or financial adviser.

If market losses have slashed the amount of life insurance you have and you need more, cover the gap with a low-cost term policy.

FINDING HELP

Go to an independent insurance agent to find out about policies from a wide range of companies. *Or contact these organizations for information...*

•**AccuTerm**—call 800-752-2999 or visit *www.accuterm.com*.

•**Insure.com**—call 800-556-9393 or visit *www.insure.com*.

If your agent never alerted you to problems in your insurance plan, find someone better. Talk to other insurance agents, financial planners and insurance consultants.

Be aware that while there are no tax penalties when switching policies, there might be penalties for surrendering your policy.

Ask insurance professionals these important questions...

•How much life insurance should I buy—and why?

•What type of policy do you recommend—and why? See how he/she addresses your risk tolerance and growth goals with affordable policy alternatives.

• What qualifications do you have for advising me on how to allocate my cash among sub-accounts within a variable life insurance policy? Check referrals. Ask attorneys, accountants and other insurance representatives if the agent delivers a valuable service.

Ideally, you want someone who is a Chartered Life Underwriter (CLU) or Certified Financial Planner (CFP).

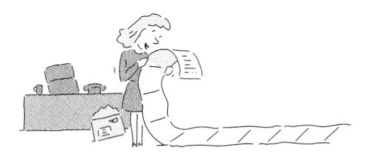

New Sales Gimmick for Whole Life Insurance

To lure customers away from low-cost term life insurance, insurers are selling whole life policies with *secondary guarantees*. These provide you with slow cash-value buildup and guarantee coverage for life, as long as you pay the premium.

Traps: They have little cash value in the early years, and they may not be attractive if interest rates rise.

Glenn Daily, fee-only insurance consultant, New York City, *www.glenndaily.com*.

Are You Missing a Life Insurance Policy?

Amy Danise, former editor and vice president, content development, Insure.com, insurance information and comparison Web site, East Hartford, CT.

An insurance company can't know that a policyholder has died if no one puts in a claim and the policy lapses. The insurer also is not legally obligated to find a beneficiary even if it knows that the insured has died.

To find a deceased's life insurance policy, look for...

• **Canceled checks.** See if any were written to pay premiums. If you can't find checks, ask the insured's bank for copies.

• **Credit card statements.** Check if insurance premiums were charged.

• **Probate court records.** A policy could show up as an asset of the estate.

Contact the policyholder's insurance agent, accountant, lawyer and any relatives familiar with his/her finances. Ask the insured's employer and any professional or trade associations to which the insured belonged if insurance was purchased.

If you locate the policy and premiums were paid up: The insurer will pay the beneficiary the death benefit once you prove the insured's death.

For unclaimed policies: Contact your state comptroller's department to claim the benefit.

More from Amy Danise...

Umbrella Policies Protect Against Lawsuits

Standard home and auto insurance policies won't protect you in the event of a major lawsuit. Still, 25% of all households with incomes above $100,000 don't have *umbrella policies*, which will cover personal injuries and property damage caused by you or a family member in excess of your standard coverage as well as the cost of legal defense.* Homeowner's and auto policies provide $100,000 to $300,000 in liability coverage. Umbrella coverage generally starts at $1 million, but lesser amounts may be available.

Cost per year: About $150 to $300 for the first million...$75 for the next million...$50 for each million thereafter. The higher your net worth, the more protection you need.

Example: If your assets are worth $1.3 million and the liability limit on your homeowner's policy is $300,000, the remaining $1 million should be covered under an umbrella policy. You must purchase homeowner's and auto insurance from the same firm to get an umbrella policy.

*Survey by the Chubb Group of Insurance Companies.

■ *Your Money* ■ ■

Better Home Insurance

Consider *guaranteed* replacement coverage—it can be the key to rebuilding your home if it is destroyed by a disaster.

An insurance firm requires your house to be insured for an amount based upon what it calculates to be replacement cost in the event of a total loss. If the claim and actual rebuilding cost are more than the amount of insurance, a guaranteed policy goes beyond a standard replacement policy to come up with the extra money.

Caution: There are some insurers that cap what they will pay even under guaranteed replacement coverage.

Robert Mackoul, president, Mackoul & Associates, insurance brokers, Long Beach, NY.

Insurance Trap If You Leave Home for More Than 30 Days

Many homeowner's insurance policies have an *abandonment* clause that excludes coverage if the owner leaves the premises unoccupied for 30 days or more. So if your home is robbed or damaged by a fire or flood on the 31st day you are away from it during a six-week vacation, you may have no insurance coverage at all.

Safety: Check your insurance policy's specific terms. If you will be away from home for an extended period, have someone spend a night in it once a week or so, or perform some other activity there sufficient to meet the policy's definition of occupancy. And keep proof of doing so.

Jens Jurgen, editor, TravelCompanions.com, Box 833, Amityville, NY 11701, www.travelcompanions.com.

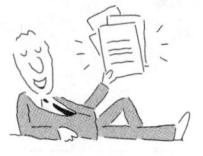

Lower Insurance Costs by Paying Bills on Time

The big auto and home insurers check credit ratings of new customers, and many check the credit ratings of existing customers. A good credit rating can mean lower insurance premiums. A poor credit history may result in much higher premiums—or in you being unable to obtain the insurance you want.

Jeanne Salvatore, vice president of consumer affairs, Insurance Information Institute, 110 William St., New York City 10038, www.iii.org.

Insurance Premiums Headed Up

Lee Rosenberg, CFP, founder and partner, ARS Financial Services, 500 N. Broadway, Jericho, NY 11753.

Squeezed by the terrorist attacks, a wave of natural disasters and losses on investments, insurers are boosting premiums. Renter's and homeowner's policy premiums are up by an average of 30% nationwide. Auto and casualty premiums have doubled.

To keep insurance costs down...

•**Shop around.** Ask friends and check out consumer guides, including *www.insurance.com* or 866-533-0227...*www.insure.com* or 800-556-9393.

•**Raise your deductible.** Going from $250 to $500 could save 12% a year.

•**Buy your home and auto policies from the same company** to cut premiums by 5% to 15%.

•**Enroll in a safe driving course** to save another 10%.

•**Beef up home security**—a smoke detector, burglar alarm and deadbolt locks can save you 5%, while a home sprinkler system can save 15% to 20%.

•**Get group coverage if possible.** Obtain member discounts through alumni and business associations.

Insurance Savvy

• **Stay loyal to your insurer.** Staying with the same insurer for three to five years may yield a 5% reduction…six years or more, 10%. This should happen automatically, but call the insurer to confirm.

• **Compare limits in your policy and the value of your possessions annually.** Eliminate unnecessary coverage.

Report All Car Accidents

Failing to report an accident to your insurer can sacrifice your auto coverage. If you have a minor accident, it might be tempting to settle the damages with cash and avoid making a claim, which could trigger a premium increase.

Problem: If the other driver or a passenger later files a medical or other claim, you might not be covered. Some auto insurers simply won't pay and will refuse to renew your policy if you fail to report an accident.

Safest: File an accident report with the police, and ask your insurance agent whether you should file a formal claim.

Eric Nicolaysen, insurance consultant with Nicolaysen Agency Inc., Chappaqua, NY.

Save 25% or More on Car Insurance

Robert Krughoff, president, Consumers' Checkbook, which publishes guides to consumer services, including insurance, in the Washington, DC, and San Francisco areas, *www.checkbook.org*.

Auto insurance rates are increasing as companies raise premiums to compensate for losses in their investment portfolios. Surprisingly, you often can save when the companies change their premium policies. Even if you secured a good rate in recent years, you might find a better one now.

SHOP AROUND

Shop for new quotes any time you buy a car, add a driver to your policy, change your commute or move to a new home.

• **Collect quotes for your specific circumstances** from at least three companies. *Have this information on hand when checking with insurers…*

• Copy of your current policy.

• Driving histories for each driver you insure.

• Your claims history.

• Vehicle identification number, make and model for each vehicle you insure.

• **Compare prices at…**

• *www.checkbook.org*

• *www.insurance.com*

• *www.insure.com*

• *www.insweb.com*

Compare the quotes you receive with the premium comparisons posted by many state departments of insurance. For links to their Web sites, go to the National Association of Insurance Commissioners Web site, *www.naic.org*.

You might save with insurers that sell directly to customers, such as Amica (800-242-6422 or *www.amica.com*)…or Geico (800-861-8380 or *www.geico.com*).

Caution: Price quotes typically are for married couples with clean driving records. Companies that offer the lowest rates for couples may have the highest rates for teenagers or people with blemished records.

Helpful: After gathering quotes, check the complaint histories of the companies you're considering. On their Web sites, many state departments of insurance rank the companies based on how many complaints consumers file against them. Also check out *www.insure.com*. Scroll down to "Insurance Company Guide," and insert "complaints" into the search box.

• **Ask your current agent if he/she can match your new quote.**

CUT COSTS

Once you decide on an insurer, you can further reduce your premium by…

• **Increasing deductibles.** If a $1,000 loss won't set you back too much, get a policy with a $1,000 deductible—or an even higher one if

■ *Your Money* ■ ■

you can afford it and your insurer allows it. Increasing a $100 deductible to $1,000 could reduce your total insurance premium by 25%.

•**Requesting specific discounts.** *They typically are available if you...*

•Have had a clean driving record for at least the past three years.

•Drive less than a certain number of miles per year. Companies use their own formulas, and mileage is just one variable.

•Insure more than one vehicle.

•Buy homeowner's and other insurance through the same company.

•Are a nonsmoker. Some insurance companies consider smoking an indicator of other risky behavior.

•Make your car harder to steal—by parking in a garage or adding antitheft devices.

•Have completed a defensive driving course.

•Earn good grades, if you are a student.

•**Keeping a clean credit record.** More companies are charging higher premiums for people with poor credit histories. Federal law generally allows this practice, but some states have placed limits on how insurance companies can use credit histories.

Helpful: If you are turned down for insurance or are told that your premiums are going up because of your credit report, you have the right to review the report. Report any mistakes to the insurance company and credit bureaus...and ask that corrections be made.

MORE WAYS TO REDUCE PREMIUMS

•**Drop collision coverage.** You may not need it if the annual cost is more than 6% of the car's value. Dropping collision can save you more than 25%.

•**Drop roadside assistance if you belong to an auto club,** such as AAA, or your car's manufacturer or lessor offers it. Eliminating it can save you more than $25 per year.

•**Drop rental reimbursement coverage.** You probably don't need it if you have a second car. This might save you $40 or more each year.

•**Check insurance rates before buying a new car.** Some cost less to insure than others. Premiums are higher for those that are stolen often, more costly to repair and/or easier to damage.

Example: The typical insurance bill for a Ford Explorer is likely to be 7% to 10% higher than that for a Ford Taurus.

•**File claims judiciously.** Before filing a claim, ask your agent how it will affect your premiums. Being involved in an accident, particularly one for which you may be responsible, may raise your rates by 20% or more.

LIABILITY COVERAGE

Buy an umbrella personal liability policy to protect your home, savings, other assets and future income in the event that claims against you exceed your auto liability limit. Premiums are usually $200 to $300 a year for $1 million in coverage for a family that has the legally required level of auto and homeowner's liability coverage.

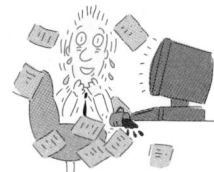

How to Get All the Medical Insurance You Are Due

Rhonda D. Orin, attorney, Anderson Kill & Olick, law firm specializing in representing policyholders against insurance companies, Washington, DC, and author of *Making Them Pay: How to Get the Most from Health Insurance and Managed Care* (Griffin).

To spot medical-claims errors and receive all the insurance payments to which you are entitled...

•**Get an itemized hospital bill,** and verify that you actually received all services listed.

•**If a claim is denied,** find out why—it may simply have been miscoded.

•**Ask for the surgeon's notes** on an operation if the insurer says charges are too high —they may show that your case was unusually complicated.

•**Get letters supporting your case** from all of your own doctors and from an outside physician verifying that the care you received was medically necessary.

When You Can't Resolve a Health Insurance Problem...

Vincent Riccardi, MD, president of American Medical Consumers, membership organization providing information, advice and advocacy, La Crescenta, CA, *www.medconsumer.com*.

If your insurer has refused to cover an expensive treatment for a disabling or life-threatening condition, consider bringing in an independent "patient advocate."

Advocates work with insurers, physicians and health facilities to help patients get what they need from the health care system. Because of their familiarity with medical and insurance procedures and their ability to prove the medical necessity of care, they often succeed where patients fail.

Initial consultations—during which the advocate reviews the case and may recommend certain steps to the patient—usually cost less than $100. If they are required to perform any additional work, patients pay an hourly fee or a percentage of the insurance reimbursement.

To find a patient advocate: Check with your employee benefits department—or search for "patient advocate" at *www.google.com* or another search engine. Advocates usually work by mail and phone.

Questions to ask before hiring an advocate...

•**How long have you or your company been in business?**

•**What similar cases have you handled**—and what were the outcomes?

•**Are you the person who would work on my case?** What are your credentials? (An MD or RN is best.)

Second Opinions and Your HMO

Get a second opinion if your health maintenance organization (HMO) denies medical benefits. Forty-two states and the District of Columbia have laws allowing HMO members to get second opinions from specialists unaffiliated with the HMO when care is denied. The HMO is required to pay for the second opinion. The US Supreme Court recently upheld the Illinois law, which is similar to those of most other states.

Charles Inlander, president, People's Medical Society, Box 868, Allentown, PA 18105, and author of *Take This Book to the Hospital with You* (St. Martin's).

More from Charles Inlander...

Higher Co-Pays at Certain Hospitals

Certain HMOs charge higher co-payments when patients go to more expensive hospitals. These "tiered" hospital plans have lists of favored hospitals, much as prescription-drug insurance plans list favored drugs and charge patients more if they use ones not on the list. Co-payments at preferred hospitals can be as high as $250 per day. Those at other hospitals are about $400 per day.

How to Minimize Health Insurance Costs

If you're looking to reduce health insurance costs, follow these practical tips...

•**Shop around for the best policy.** Benefits, premiums and restrictions vary widely.

•**Review policies annually** to be sure they still meet your needs.

•**Keep abreast of news affecting Medicare benefit changes and health care insurance**—new developments or legislation may change your needs.

Jeff Townsend, CRPC, RFP, CEA, financial planner specializing in retirement issues, Northglen, CO, and author of *The Master Plan: Retirement Strategies for the Best of Your Life* (Pendleton Clay).

■ *Your Money* ■ ■

Cheaper Long-Term-Care Insurance

Cut long-term-care insurance costs by buying only enough to cover what you cannot afford on your own. Your Social Security, pension and investment income may go a long way toward paying for nursing home care if you ever need it. Speak to an insurance broker experienced in long-term-care policies.

To keep costs low: Consider buying a policy that pays for only five years of nursing home care—the average stay is two-and-a-half years. Or buy a lifetime-benefit policy that does not start paying until one year after you meet eligibility requirements.

Lee Slavutin, MD, CPC, CLU, chairman, Stern Slavutin-2 Inc., life insurance and estate planning firm, 530 Fifth Ave., New York City 10036.

Check Your Long-Term-Care Coverage

In a recent national survey of people age 45 and older…

• **30% said that they had long-term-care health insurance,** even though the actual percentage is only 6%.

• **55% said Medicare pays for long stays in nursing homes,** when it doesn't.

• **75% either wrongly believed that Medicare pays for assisted living** or admitted they didn't know if it did.

• **Only 15% knew that a stay in a nursing home** costs an average of $4,600 per month.

Important: Review your options for long-term-care coverage—through an employer policy, AARP or private coverage. Smart planning can save your family tremendous costs in the long run.

Elinor Ginzler, manager, Independent Living/Long-Term Care/End-of-Life, AARP, Washington, DC.

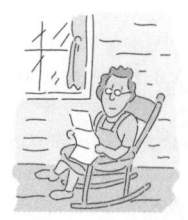

Nursing Home And Home-Health-Care Cost Danger

Robert M. Freedman, Esq., partner, Freedman and Fish, elder law attorneys, 521 Fifth Ave., New York City 10175.

Almost 70% of people who incur nursing home and home-health-care costs today have to pay them out-of-pocket or resort to Medicaid—which can cost them their homes or other valuable assets. Only 10% have their costs covered by insurance.

PAYMENT SOURCES

Medicaid	43.8%
Out-of-pocket	24.6%
Medicare	13.7%
Private insurance	10.3%
Other private sources	4.6%
Other public sources	2.9%

Important: Explore long-term-care insurance options while your health is still good and you are insurable.

If you have waited until it is too late to get insurance, be sure to consult with an elder law attorney about Medicaid.

▪▪ Your Money ▪

9

Tax Guide

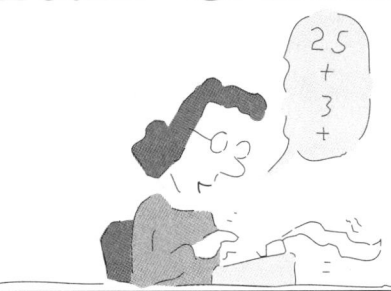

How to Profit from the New Tax Law

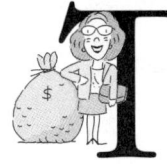

The new tax act,* which was signed into law by the president on May 28, 2003, is the third-biggest tax cut in our country's history. This tax benefits most people who pay taxes—rates are greatly reduced...tax brackets are shifted...and credits and deductions are increased.

Most of the changes were retroactive to January 1, 2003 and will last for years to come. There are hidden benefits in the new law, too. To get your fair share of the bounty—and more —you need to know where to look and what steps to take now. *Opportunities for profit...*

•**Review your withholding allowances.** While no action on your part was required to benefit from the new withholding tables, you may want to make adjustments to your withholding allowances in 2004 (file a new IRS

*The Jobs and Growth Tax Relief Reconciliation Act of 2003 (JGTRRA).

Form W-4) to take advantage of some of the new law's changes.

Impact: Even less tax will be withheld from your paycheck. *Scenarios under which you may want to make a change in your withholding include...*

•You had or will have a baby or adopt a child. In the summer of 2003, the government sent most families checks in the amount of $400/year per child. These checks reflected the increase in the child tax credit to $1,000 from $600. But checks only went to taxpayers who claimed the credit in 2002.

If your family expanded in 2003, you are entitled to the $400 added credit. You can create your own advance payment by reducing your withholding taxes accordingly.

•You use withholding to cover taxes on investments. If you intend wage withholding to

---

Barbara Weltman, attorney in Millwood, NY. She is editor and publisher of the on-line newsletter *Barbara Weltman's Big Ideas for Small Business, www.bwideas. com.* Ms. Weltman is author of numerous books, including *J.K. Lasser's Small Business Taxes* (Wiley) and *Bottom Line's Very Shrewd Money Book* (Bottom Line Books).

■ *Your Money* ■ ■

cover the taxes you'll owe on your capital gains and dividend income, you may want to reduce withholding. (See the following information on estimated taxes.)

REVIEW ESTIMATED TAXES

Many taxpayers pay income taxes through quarterly estimated tax payments. *You can reduce these payments in certain situations such as the following...*

•**You are an investor.** The new law drops the top tax rate on long-term capital gains to 15% from 20%. The tax rate on dividends has been cut to 15%. Formerly, dividend income was taxed at rates as high as 38.6%.

The new rates apply to sales or exchanges after May 5, 2003. In 2008, taxpayers in the lowest two tax brackets (10% and 15%) will pay no tax on long-term capital gains. Until then, their capital gains rates fall to 5% (from 10% or 8%).

The same rates apply to "qualified dividends," which are ordinary dividends paid by corporations after December 31, 2002, from earnings and profits.

Note: The dividends from real estate investment trusts and certain other dividends don't qualify for special tax rates.

•**You are self-employed or owner of a pass-through entity.** In these cases, business income is taxed on your own return at individual income tax rates. Since these rates have been cut, the tax on business profits is reduced accordingly. As a result of this, estimated taxes to cover liability for business profits can also be reduced.

In addition, if your business takes advantage of new increased first-year expensing ($100,000, up from $25,000) as well as bonus depreciation (50%), you will now be able to write off more of the expense of equipment purchases, further reducing your tax liability and the need for estimated tax payments.

Note: To avoid estimated tax penalties, keep estimated tax payments within a "safe harbor." You must pay at least 90% of your current tax liability or 100% of your prior-year liability (110% if your adjusted gross income in the prior year was $150,000 or more) to avoid penalty. But even if you fall short of the safe harbor, the cost is minimal—the current interest rate on underpayment of estimated tax is only 5%.

RETIREMENT PLAN SAVINGS

Many taxpayers find themselves short of the cash needed to fund an IRA or contribute to a 401(k) plan. The new law enables such taxpayers to put their tax cut to good use, creating added tax benefits.

Example: Say that because of the decline in tax rates and the increase in the child tax credit, you save $1,000 in taxes. If you contribute this money to a deductible IRA and you are in the 25% tax bracket, you save an additional $250.

Bonus: You may also be eligible for a tax credit for your contributions. The amount of the credit depends on your adjusted gross income. It is either 10%, 20% or 50% of up to $2,000 in contributions to an IRA or 401(k) or similar plan. This *retirement savings contributions credit* is in addition to any deduction or income deferral for making your IRA/401(k) contribution.

Strategy: If you participate in a 401(k) or similar plan, check with your plan administrator to see if you will be permitted to increase your 401(k) or other salary reduction contributions at midyear.

SEE A FINANCIAL PLANNER

In light of the changes affecting capital gains and dividends, it is vital to review your holdings both within IRAs and 401(k) accounts as well as in your personal portfolio. *Here are some guidelines...*

•**Municipal bonds.** Because the interest on municipal bonds is tax free, they may no longer be suitable investments now that your tax rate has dropped.

Your cutoff point: When the after-tax rate on taxable bonds is effectively paying you more than the tax-free interest on municipal bonds.

•**Dividend-paying stocks as well as stock mutual funds.** These generally should not be held within tax-deferred retirement accounts because you lose the benefit of the tax break on dividends. All the income distributed from these accounts is taxed as ordinary income, regardless of the source of that income.

•**Selling securities outside of retirement plans.** Where possible, make sure to hold on to securities for more than one year to qualify for favorable capital gains rates.

Strategy: Before rushing to make any new changes, discuss your holdings with a financial adviser. He/she will help you assess the impact of the new law on your existing investments and suggest alternatives to maximize the beneficial changes now in effect.

PROFITING EVEN MORE

Give appreciated property to children older than age 13 and to other relatives in the two lowest tax brackets.

Reason: They will now pay just 5% in tax when they sell the property (assuming it has been held for more than a year).

Other uses for tax savings: If you don't use tax savings to add to your retirement plans as discussed earlier, there are other ways to maximize the tax savings' effectiveness. *Here are two options to consider...*

•Contribute your savings to a 529 tuition savings plan or a Coverdell education savings account for a child or grandchild.

•Pay off consumer debt. You want to get rid of this debt because the interest you pay on it is not tax deductible.

More from Barbara Weltman...

Tax-Friendly States

The most tax-friendly states are South Dakota and Tennessee. They have the lowest overall tax burden...followed closely by Florida and Texas. Seven states have no personal income tax—Alaska, Florida, Nevada, South Dakota, Texas, Washington and Wyoming. Five have no sales tax—Alaska, Delaware, Montana, New Hampshire and Oregon. And 35 states (plus the District of Columbia) don't tax Social Security benefits.

More information: *www.taxsites.com.*

Learn About Taxes Before You Move

To learn a state's tax burden before moving there, log onto the US Census Web site at *www.census.gov.* In the alphabetical directory, click on "T" for taxes, and then on "State Government Tax Collections Data." You'll be presented with detailed information about the amount of taxes collected by each state (such as "taxes per capita") and a comparison to all other states. You'll also find links to other sources of state tax information, such as state tax rates by income level.

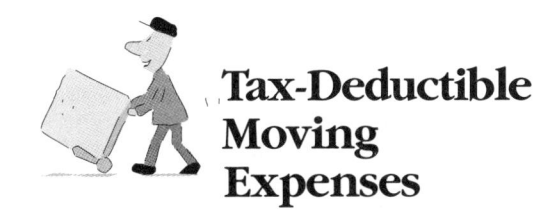

Tax-Deductible Moving Expenses

Tax treatment of moving expenses depends on how your company normally pays your expenses. A lump-sum payment will show up as part of your wages and salary on your W-2 form, and you will need receipts to back up your moving cost deductions. If your company reimburses you, the money will show up in box 12 of your W-2 form—separate from wages and salary—and won't be taxed.

Caution: Find out which moving expenses are deductible.

Examples: Costs of a moving van, gas and hotel stays are deductible—but meals and temporary rental housing are not.

David S. Rhine, CPA, regional director, family wealth planning, Sagemark Consulting, a division of Lincoln Financial Advisors Corp., a registered investment adviser in Rochelle Park, NJ.

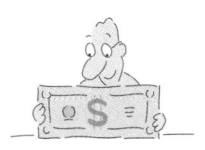

■ *Your Money* ■ ■

24 Sources of Tax-Free Income

Janice M. Johnson, JD, CPA, financial consultant, 301 E. 52 St., New York City 10022. She was previously with American Express.

You don't need fancy investment strategies or risky tax shelters to get tax-free income. *Here are two dozen straightforward ways...*

1. Home rentals of up to 14 days are tax free. If you rent out your home or second home for no more than 14 days, you don't have to report to the IRS the rent you receive.

Tactic: If a popular tournament, game or other attraction is scheduled near you, consider renting your home to an attendee and using the money you receive *tax free* to pay for your own vacation.

2. Roth IRAs allow withdrawals after age 59½ that are totally tax and penalty free. A Roth IRA that's set up early in life will earn compound investment returns for decades and will ultimately provide a tremendous tax-free payoff.

3. Gifts of all kinds are income tax free to the recipient. They can decrease or eliminate income taxes that a family is currently paying, as well, when income-producing property is given by a high-tax-bracket taxpayer to family members in low tax brackets, such as children over age 13.

Caution: Investment income above $1,500 of children under age 14 is taxed at their parent's top rate.

Gifts of up to $11,000 each can be made to as many recipients as you wish in 2003 and 2004 using the annual gift tax exclusion. The limitation is $22,000 for gifts made with a spouse.

4. Expense reimbursements from an employer are tax free. Negotiate for reimbursement from your employer if you currently incur out-of-pocket business costs—for items such as publications, professional dues, meals, driving, purchases of supplies or equipment, etc.

You and your employer can *both* benefit by converting salary to reimbursements. You'll then pay your expenses with pretax rather than after-tax dollars—plus your employer will not owe employment taxes on the reimbursement amounts as it does on salary.

5. Flexible spending accounts, or FSAs, for medical and dependent-care expenses let you avoid owing tax on a portion of your pay that you set aside to cover these expenses. If your employer offers FSAs through a "cafeteria" benefit plan, make full use of them.

6. Children's salaries paid by a family business effectively let the business take a portion of its income tax free. The business gets to deduct the salary payments at its high tax rate, while a child can earn up to $4,750 *tax free* in 2003 ($4,850 in 2004)—plus another $7,000 ($7,150 in 2004) taxable at only 10%, and additional income over $7,000 to $28,400 in 2003 ($7,150 to $29,050 in 2004) taxable at only 15%.

When a child under age 18 is paid by a parent's unincorporated business, the payments are also free of Social Security and Medicare taxes. And the Tax Court has allowed deductions for reasonable wages paid to children as young as seven.

7. More Social Security benefits may be taken tax free if you invest in appreciating assets, Series EE and I savings bonds, and cash-value life insurance. The increase in the value of such investments adds to your wealth but is excluded from your current income until cashed in—so it won't push your income over the threshold that makes Social Security taxable.

8. Gain on the sale of a home is tax free up to $250,000 ($500,000 on a joint return) when you have used the home as your main residence for at least two of the prior five years. You can make such a tax-free sale once every two years.

If you own other residences (such as vacation or investment properties) in addition to your principal residence, you can move into them for two years at a time to take tax-free gain on them, too, when selling them.

9. Life insurance proceeds are tax free to the beneficiary. They also escape estate tax when the insured individual does not retain "incidents of ownership" in the policy. Achieve this by having the policy owned by another party or a life insurance trust.

Tactic: Instead of leaving taxable bequests of other assets, consider using tax-free life insurance to fund bequests.

10. Borrowed funds are tax free—even if you do not have to repay them during your lifetime. *Examples...*

• Borrowing against the appreciating cash value of a life insurance policy, with the loan to be repaid ultimately from the policy proceeds.

• A "reverse mortgage" on a house that provides the home owner with a stream of income, which ultimately will be repaid from his/her estate.

11. Frequent-flier miles remain untaxed by the IRS—and the IRS has stated that it will not try to tax them in the future without giving advance warning to the public.

12. Capital gain property held until death becomes income tax free to heirs. Currently, at death, the tax basis in the property is stepped up to market value—making all appreciation in the property's value up to that date tax free to those who inherit it.

13. Like-kind exchanges allow you to trade an appreciated property for a similar property —for example, one real estate property for another—while deferring the realization of taxable gain until the second property is sold.

But that property, too, can be disposed of through another like-kind exchange, and so on, deferring taxation on gain indefinitely.

14. Parking paid for by an employer is tax free up to $190 per month in 2003 ($195 in 2004). So is up to $100 per month for transit passes or expenses incurred for carpooling.

15. Tuition reimbursement for as much as $5,250 per year can be provided tax free by an employer to an employee under an educational assistance program.

16. Interest-free loans can be a source of cash at no tax cost to either lender or borrower, up to certain limits. Loans of up to $10,000 have no adverse tax consequences.

Loans greater than $10,000 and as much as $100,000 are treated as if interest is paid on them (interest is "imputed," so taxable interest income results to the lender) but this is only to the extent that the borrower has accrued investment income.

Thus, interest-free loans are tax free if the borrower has no investment income.

17. Long-term health care insurance provides proceeds that are tax free. In addition, premiums on these policies are deductible in an amount that varies by age (from $250 at age 40 or younger to $3,130 at age 71 or older in 2003). These figures increase to $260 and $3,250 respectively in 2004. Premiums paid for by an employer may be a tax-free benefit.

18. All government bonds are tax favored. State and municipal bonds are generally free of federal income tax, and may be free of state tax as well, providing totally tax-free income. Federal bonds are exempt from state taxes.

19. Coverdell education savings accounts, previously referred to as "education IRAs," let investment returns earned in them be used tax free to pay not only college costs but also elementary and high school costs, as well as for books, supplies, after-school programs, tuition, tutoring and even home computers.

20. Section 529 college savings plans let investment earnings be used tax free for education expenses. In contrast to the Coverdell accounts, much more can be contributed to a 529 plan, but 529 funds can be used only for college costs.

21. Scholarship and fellowship grants are tax free when used to pay for tuition and course-related fees, books, equipment and supplies.

22. Accelerated death benefits (viatical settlements) paid on a life insurance policy to a terminally ill insured individual before he/she dies are tax free.

23. Adoption expenses. Employers can provide employees who are adopting children with up to $10,160 in tax-free assistance in 2003 ($10,390 for 2004) to help cover adoption expenses.

24. Employer-provided insurance, such as health and accident, and as much as $50,000 in group term life insurance, can be provided tax free to employees while being deducted by the employer who provides it.

Your Money

More from Janice Johnson...

How to Get Maximum Tax Benefit From Your Home

The family home is the biggest tax shelter most taxpayers have. But few families take full advantage of the tax breaks home ownership entitles them to.

Here's how to do better...

- **Be wary of prepaying your mortgage.** Some people like to prepay their home mortgages because it makes them feel more secure financially. But doing this reduces the best form of low-cost financing you can find these days. And if you prepay your mortgage, you may give up your ability to use tax-favored mortgage financing later, should you need it.

Why: Mortgage interest is deductible only on borrowing used to *acquire* a home—and not on subsequent financing. You can deduct interest on up to $100,000 of home-equity lending, but even borrowing to this maximum may not be enough to tap all your equity in your home if you prepay your principal mortgage significantly.

Example: You have a home that's worth $350,000 and pay your mortgage down to $250,000 through normal payments. You can use a $100,000 home-equity loan to borrow against the home's full value if need be (assuming the lender will give a 100% home-equity loan, instead of the usual 75% limit).

But if you also make prepayments of an additional $75,000 (reducing the mortgage balance to $175,000), even maximum home-equity borrowing ($100,000) will enable you to borrow against only $275,000 of your home's value with deductible interest—$75,000 of its value will be beyond the limit for deductible borrowing.

Best: Pay down other borrowing first—credit card loans, car loans, etc. If you still have additional funds to save, put them in an investment account. By not prepaying your mortgage, you will maximize your tax savings *and* your financial flexibility.

- **Use serial tax exclusions.** When you've used a home as your primary residence for at least two out of five years, up to $500,000 of gain from it is totally tax free on a joint return ($250,000 on a single return).

Opportunity: You can use this break every two years. Say you own a vacation home or residence that you've held as an investment property, and it has appreciated in value. You can sell your first home to take a tax-free gain of up to $500,000, then move into the other home and sell it after another two years to take another gain of up to $500,000.

Planning: If you own a home for only two years, it's unlikely to appreciate greatly in that time. But you can plan ahead. Buy a house or apartment and then use it as a vacation home or investment property for a few years. Move into it full-time after it's gone up in value, then sell it after you live there for two years.

- **Use the second-home mortgage deduction.** Mortgage interest is deductible on your primary residence and on one additional residence. If you own more than one "second" home, you can choose to take the deduction each year for the one that will produce the most tax savings.

Opportunity: Use the mortgage interest deduction to subsidize ownership of a second home that doubles as an investment, or reduces family costs in another manner.

Example: A child is going away to college. Instead of paying for college housing, consider buying an apartment for the child. Use your mortgage interest deduction to help subsidize the cost. The child's housing costs will stay in the family, while the apartment appreciates in value.

- **Use boat and recreational vehicle (RV) interest deductions.** A boat or RV can qualify as a residence if it has living facilities, including a kitchen, a bedroom and a bathroom.

This means that a boat or an RV can qualify as a second home, enabling you to claim the mortgage interest deduction for interest paid on a loan that you use to buy one.

If a boat or an RV is your primary residence because you live in it most of the time, you can claim the mortgage interest deduction for each, if you have both—your primary residence and your "second home."

Tax Guide

●**Use the home-office deduction.** More and more people are working at home these days. If you do, you may be able to deduct a home office.

Requirement: A portion of your home must be used *exclusively* as...

●The primary place where you conduct a business, or...

●A place where you deal with customers or clients on a regular basis, or...

●A place where you perform necessary record keeping for your business when you have no office elsewhere.

Benefits: A qualified home office enables you to deduct otherwise nondeductible home-ownership expenses. These include insurance, maintenance and utility costs allocable to the office. You can also deduct depreciation—a "no cash cost" expense that provides a cash-saving tax deduction.

A qualified home office may also enable you to deduct travel between home and other work locations—turning otherwise nondeductible commuting into deductible travel between two work sites. *But beware of these traps...*

●A home office can be an audit red flag likely to draw IRS scrutiny. That's no reason not to deduct one, but be ready to prove you meet deduction requirements. *Example:* You must be able to prove that you used the office exclusively for work. But an audit notice may not arrive for as long as two years *after* the year for which you deducted the office. That can make it nearly impossible to prove the way you used the office.

As a precaution, photograph or videotape the office to *show* the IRS how you used it, even years later.

●A home office is business property, not residential property. Depreciation deductions taken on the home will be recaptured as taxable income when you sell the home at a gain. The recaptured depreciation is taxable at a tax-favored 25% top rate.

●No home-office deduction is allowed if it exceeds income from the business activity conducted in your home. However, to the extent you create a loss, you can carry the deduction forward to be used in future, higher income, years.

●**Beware of state tax traps.** Do you own real property in more than one state—such as a home in one state and a vacation home in another? When you die, *both* states may tax your estate, resulting in double taxation.

In fact, because each state has its own rules to determine residency, it's possible that each state may deem you to be a resident and assess full state death or estate taxes against you.

Result: True, full double taxation, which is an extremely costly trap.

Self-defense: If you own property in more than one state, consider the consequences under state law with a state tax expert when drawing up your estate plan.

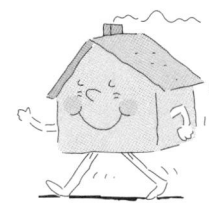

It's Now Easier To Use the Home-Sale Exclusion

Robert B. Coplan, Esq., national director, Center for Family Wealth Planning, Ernst & Young LLP, 1225 Connecticut Ave. NW, Washington, DC 20036.

Home owners enjoy one giant tax break—they don't have to pay tax on up to $250,000 of gain from the sale of their homes (up to $500,000 on a joint return).

The recent pro-taxpayer Treasury regulations, intended to account for the "realities of life," make it a little easier to qualify for this "home-sale exclusion." They clarify when, and to what extent, the exclusion can be taken by various categories of home owner.

THE FULL EXCLUSION

●**Easier to establish "main home."** The full exclusion applies only to the sale of a principal residence. When a taxpayer owns more than one residence, the main home is generally defined as the home in which more time is spent during the year.

However, the new regulations make it clear that this is not an exclusive test. *Other factors that can be taken into account...*

●Where you work.

●Where family members live.

■ *Your Money* ■ ■

- The address that is listed on your federal and state tax returns, driver's license, automobile registration and voter registration.
- The mailing address you use for bills and correspondence.
- The location of any clubs or religious institutions you belong to.

- **The exclusion now can be used for a vacant lot.** In today's hot real estate market, home owners may want to subdivide their property and sell a lot separately from the parcel containing the home.

Gain from the sale of the vacant lot qualifies for the exclusion as long as the sale occurs within two years of the sale of the house. But only one home-sale exclusion amount can be taken between the two properties.

- **Home offices qualify for the exclusion.** If you use a portion of your principal residence as a home office, the regulations provide you with a key tax break when you sell the home. Gain from the sale of the home-office portion can qualify for the full exclusion. No allocation of the exclusion is now necessary when the personal and business portions of the property are within the same dwelling.

Impact: Home owners no longer need fear taking the home-office deduction out of concern that it might taint the exclusion for a future sale.

Legal note: Upon sale, depreciation you've taken on the home office after May 6, 1997, must still be reported as income. It is subject to a 25% capital gains rate. (The exclusion cannot offset this income.)

- **Intricacies of trust ownership clarified.** If a home is owned by a trust—of which the home dweller is treated under tax rules as the trust's owner (so-called grantor trust)—the person residing in the home can use the home-sale exclusion. This new rule also applies to single-owner entities.

Example: If a home is owned by a one-member limited liability company (LLC) and that person lives in the home, the exclusion is not lost. Since the LLC is treated as a "disregarded entity," so that the home owner reports income and expenses on Schedule C of his/her Form 1040, the exclusion can be claimed on the sale.

- **Help for unmarried joint owners and surviving spouses.** Married couples can claim a $500,000 exclusion, even if one spouse holds title to the home (as long as each satisfies the two-year use requirement). But if two or more unmarried people own the home, each owner is eligible for a $250,000 exclusion on his share of the gain (assuming the use test is satisfied).

In the case of a surviving spouse, the exclusion of $500,000 can only be claimed in the year of the deceased spouse's death on a joint return. If the sale takes place after the year of death, the surviving spouse will be limited to a $250,000 exclusion.

A PARTIAL EXCLUSION

If a home owner sells the property before satisfying the two-year use test, the exclusion can be allocated for the portion of the time of ownership, in certain circumstances. *These circumstances include...*

- **Sale for employment reasons.** If a change in jobs forces a taxpayer to sell his home, he may be eligible for a partial exclusion.

Safe harbor: If the distance test used for the moving expense deduction is met, the move is *automatically* treated as a change in the place of employment for purposes of the partial home-sale exclusion.

Required: The distance between the new job location and the former home must be at least 50 miles greater than the distance between the old job location and the former home.

If this test isn't satisfied, a taxpayer can still show that the sale was motivated by a change of the place of employment through facts and circumstances (though the rules don't explain what these are).

Important: A change of job for the home owner's spouse, co-owner of the residence or a person whose principal residence is the taxpayer's home (each of whom is called a *qualified individual*) can also make a sale eligible for the exclusion.

- **Sale for health reasons.** If a home owner sells his home for health reasons affecting him or a qualified individual, the partial exclusion applies. A doctor-recommended change is considered a health reason, as is a move to obtain medical or personal care for illness or injury. A move that is merely beneficial for one's health is not a health reason that qualifies the sale for a partial exclusion.

•**Sale due to unforeseen circumstances.** If a home owner is forced to sell for certain reasons that are outside of his control, the partial exclusion can be claimed. *The new rules enumerate certain unforeseen circumstances...*

•Destruction of the home, including destruction through acts of war or terrorism.

•The home owner or someone in his household dies or goes on unemployment.

•The home owner becomes unable to pay for the housing costs and basic living expenses because of a change in his employment or self-employment status.

•Divorce or legal separation under a decree of divorce or separate maintenance.

•Couple has multiple births resulting from the same pregnancy.

This list of unforeseen circumstances is not exhaustive. If a home owner doesn't fit within any of the circumstances described above, he can still argue that his sale was motivated by unforeseen circumstances.

FINAL WORD

A home owner is not *required* to use the exclusion—an election can be made not to use it for a particular residence. This step might be advisable if he is anticipating the sale of another home within a year or two and the other home has a greater gain eligible for exclusion. Electing not to take the exclusion preserves the right to use it for the other gain.

Again, the regulations allow this election to be made for sales on or after May 7, 1997 (in open tax years). The election is made simply by reporting the gain on the tax return for the year of the sale.

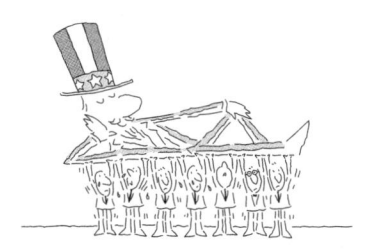

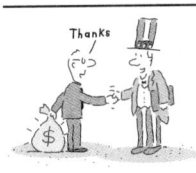

Tax-Free Home-Sale Loophole

To qualify to take tax-free gain on a home sale of up to $250,000 on an individual return ($500,000 on a joint return), you must use the home as your principal residence for two of the five years before you sell it.

Loophole: You do not have to own the home during the years that you use it as your primary residence.

Example: You live for several years in a home that you rent. Then you buy it and move out, renting it to someone else. Before three more years pass, you sell the home. You qualify to take tax-free gain on your sale because you resided in the home for more than two of the five years before you sold it—even though you didn't own it while living there.

Connie Lorz, EA, president, California Society of Enrolled Agents, Lodi.

More from Connie Lorz...

File Even If You Can't Afford to Pay Your Tax Bill

The penalty for not filing a tax return is 20 times that for not paying tax. So, file on April 15 even if you can't afford to pay your tax bill.

Key: The nonfiling penalty is 5% of the tax owed per month, up to a maximum of 25%. If you file on time, the late-payment penalty on any tax you owe is only 0.5% per month—reduced to 0.25% if you pay the IRS through an installment agreement. Automatic installment payments are available for tax bills of up to $10,000.

Details: Go to the IRS Web site, *www.irs.gov,* and search for "An Installment Plan for Your Taxes," then click on "Interactive Installment Payment Process."

■ *Your Money* ■ ■

Uncle Sam Will Help Pay Your Medical Bills

Sidney Kess, New York City–based attorney and CPA. Mr. Kess is coauthor of *1040 Preparation, 2004 Edition* (CCH). Over the years, he has taught tax law to more than 700,000 tax professionals.

When tax season arrives, few of us take the time to maximize our medical deductions. That's unfortunate because many people can significantly reduce their tax bills—if they know which medical services and treatments are deductible.

Anyone who itemizes deductions is eligible to deduct medical expenses. The only requirement is that your total medical expenses not covered by insurance or reimbursed by an employer must exceed 7.5% of your adjusted gross income (AGI).

Example: If your AGI is $100,000, the first $7,500 in deductible medical expenses does *not* count.

You can deduct medical expenses for yourself, your spouse and dependents. If you pay for a child's, parent's or grandparent's medical expenses—insurance premiums, prescription drugs and/or copayments for doctors' visits—you may add these payments to your medical expenses even if they aren't your dependent. You must simply pay for more than half of your relative's annual support.

There are two strategies to help taxpayers reach the 7.5% floor more quickly...

• **Bunch your medical deductions.** This may include accelerating or deferring elective surgery or treatments, such as dental implants or laser eye surgery. For example, if you think you'll be shy of the required percentage in 2004, wait until 2005 to order new eyeglasses, get orthotics for your shoes or incur other deductible expenses not covered by insurance.

Important: Cosmetic surgery and skin treatments are deductible only if they are used to correct a medical condition. Botox injections used to alleviate wrinkles are *not* deductible.

• **Lower your AGI.** If you lower your AGI, you'll reach the 7.5% floor more quickly. You can often accomplish this simply by taking deductions for IRAs, tuition payments, moving expenses, alimony, etc. This is part of general tax planning, so talk with your tax adviser.

DEDUCTIBLE MEDICAL EXPENSES

In addition to health care services that are provided by physicians, nurses and other practitioners, the following medical expenses can be deducted...

• **Prescription drugs and medical aids.** This includes eyeglasses, wheelchairs, blood pressure measuring devices, hearing aids, a seeing-eye dog and its care, etc.

Even drugs, such as *sildenafil* (Viagra), are deductible provided they are prescribed for a medical condition.

• **Weight-loss programs.** This encompasses behavioral and nutritional counseling, prescription medication and surgery prescribed by a physician to treat obesity. It can also include home exercise equipment. Weight-loss programs for general good health or to just shape up are *not* deductible.

• **Stop-smoking programs.** Many smoking-cessation programs, such as Smokenders, are deductible. Over-the-counter treatments, such as nicotine gums and patches, are *not* deductible.

• **Alternative treatments.** Massages, Reiki, reflexology and other alternative treatments are deductible if they're prescribed by a doctor or another licensed health care practitioner. Ask him/her to write a letter describing the medical necessity of the treatment. Keep this note with your tax records.

• **Household care.** It must be required for medical purposes. This includes a health care aide to take care of an elderly person. A person to clean your home would *not* be allowable.

• **Health insurance premiums.** This includes Medicare Part B withheld from Social Security benefits and long-term-care insurance. The amount allowable for long-term-care insurance depends on your age at year-end.

Example: In 2003, people of age 40 or younger have a $250 limit on deductions for long-term-care insurance premiums. Individuals who are age 70 or older have a $3,130 limit on deductible premiums. These figures rise to $260 and $3,250 respectively in 2004.

Tax Guide

- **Nursing home expenses.** The stay must be deemed medically necessary.

Hint: A portion of costs for assisted-living facilities (residence arrangements not primarily for medical care) can be treated as a medical expense. Be sure that the entrance and monthly fees are allocated to show the portion covering medical expenses.

- **Medical travel.** This includes travel to and from doctors, pharmacies, Alcoholics Anonymous meetings, etc. You can deduct your car use at 12¢ per mile in 2003 (14¢ per mile in 2004).

If you must stay overnight at a hotel/motel at or near a health care facility for a consultation or treatment, you can deduct $50 each per night for the patient and a companion.

Travel costs and admission to medical conferences are deductible if the main subject of the conference is an illness or condition that affects you, your spouse or dependent. Lodging and meals are *not* deductible.

- **Home improvements.** Renovations done for a medical reason are deductible to the extent that they do *not* add to the value of your home.

Example: If a doctor prescribes swimming as a medical treatment for a back condition, only the cost of the pool that doesn't add value to the home is deductible. Assume that your swimming pool costs $25,000 and adds $15,000 to the value of your house—$10,000 is a deductible medical expense. An independent appraiser determines how much value the expense adds to your home.

The addition of ramps, widening doorways for wheelchair accessibility and lowering light switches typically are fully deductible because they don't add to the value of the home.

- **Medically related education.** This includes classes and seminars to learn Braille, lip reading or sign language, attendance at schools for the mentally retarded and even clarinet lessons recommended by an orthodontist to treat teeth defects.

To deduct medical costs, save related insurance statements, receipts and canceled checks.

For a listing of additional deductible expenses, go to *www.irs.gov* and type in "IRS Publication 502," or call 800-829-3676.

More from Sidney Kess...

Checking for the AMT

If your income exceeds $58,000 on a joint return or $40,250 on a single return and you reduce the tax you owe by using items such as the deduction for state and local taxes, accelerated depreciation, medical deductions and the tax deferral for gain on incentive stock options, you might owe the alternative minimum tax (AMT). In addition, you could incur a tax bill larger than that calculated under normal rules.

The AMT affects more people each year because it is not indexed for inflation like regular income tax. There's no way to know for sure if you will owe AMT without first working through all the numbers. Be sure to check your AMT exposure while there is still time to counter it.

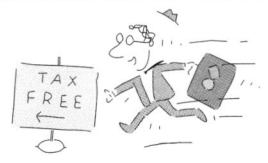

Vacation Tax Breaks

Joseph W. Walloch, CPA, president, Walloch Accountancy Corporation, 290 N. D St., Suite 310, San Bernadino, CA 92401. He is also professor of advanced accounting and taxation at the University of California in Riverside.

With a little ingenuity, you can get the IRS to subsidize your vacation fun. *Here are some tried-and-true ways...*

TRAVEL WITH A PURPOSE

As a general rule, personal expenses, including vacation costs, are not deductible. *But if the main purpose of your trip is business, charity or medical need, you can deduct some or even all of your costs...*

- **Continuing business education.** If your trade or business requires you to take continuing education courses, consider courses that are offered in vacation-like locations. *Deductible business-education costs...*

    - Tuition and registration fees.

    - Travel expenses to and from the location of the school-away-from-home.

- Lodging and 50% of meals while at the destination.
- Local transportation, such as cab rides to and from the airport.

Helpful: The IRS won't disallow your deductions merely because you could have taken a similar course closer to home.

If your spouse or a friend accompanies you, his/her travel expenses are nondeductible. Of course, if you drive, there is no additional cost for having a companion on the trip. Also, a business airline ticket may allow you a free ticket for a companion. And room accommodations may permit your spouse to stay free—the only additional cost for you would be his meals and entertainment.

- **Business trips.** Travel costs within the US are deductible as a business expense if the trip's primary purpose is business. There's no fixed test—all you need is a valid business reason for the trip. Lodging and half your meal costs are deductible for the business portion of your trip.

Example: You travel from Boston to Las Vegas to visit a vendor. Your meetings last three days. You stay for two extra days to catch the shows. Because the primary purpose of your trip is business, your airfare will be fully deductible. Your lodging and meals (subject to the 50% limit) are deductible for the business portion of your stay. The cost of your extended stay is not deductible.

If you extend your stay to get a reduced airfare, your extra lodging and meal costs are considered a business expense. This is the case even if you spend the extra time on personal pursuits.

Caution: Different rules apply to foreign travel. Consult your tax adviser before making foreign business travel plans.

If you're an employee, your unreimbursed business expenses are deductible only to the extent that your total miscellaneous itemized deductions exceed 2% of your adjusted gross income (AGI).

- **Travel for charity.** Travel expenses are deductible if the purpose of your trip is to help a charitable organization.

Example: A trip to work with Habitat for Humanity. Accommodations won't be four-star, but the location might be outstanding.

- **Weight loss.** If a doctor has diagnosed you or your spouse with obesity or a medical condition that would improve from weight loss (such as high blood pressure), you may wish to spend time at a health spa.

For the spouse with the medical condition, the cost of travel to and from the spa and his cost of being there are deductible as medical expenses. The expenses of the other spouse are nondeductible.

Note: Medical expenses are deductible only to the extent they exceed 7.5% of AGI.

VACATION HOMES

Your personal vacation plans can merge with your investment objectives when you buy a vacation home...

- **Interest on acquisition indebtedness up to $1 million to buy a second home is deductible.** If you take a home-equity loan on your main home to buy a vacation home, interest is deductible on up to $100,000 of the home-equity debt.

- **Real estate taxes on a vacation home are fully deductible**—there is no limitation.

Boats and RVs will qualify as a residence as long as they have sleeping, cooking and bathroom facilities.

If you rent out your vacation home for the time you don't use it, you can receive additional tax breaks...

- If the rental period during the year is less than 15 days, rental income is tax free regardless of personal usage. You cannot, however, deduct any related expenses (other than mortgage interest and real estate taxes).

- If your personal use of the vacation home (including use by family members) exceeds 14 days or 10% of the number of days the home is rented during the year (whichever is greater), you must report the income.

But you can offset that income with deductions for interest and taxes, maintenance costs and depreciation (to the extent of rental income).

- If your personal use of the vacation home is less than the greater of 14 days or 10% of the rental days, rental expenses are not necessarily limited to rental income. In this instance, income and expenses are governed by the passive activity loss rules.

In effect, your annual losses in excess of passive activity income are limited to $25,000. You can claim the full $25,000 only if your AGI is $100,000 or less. You can deduct a lesser amount if your AGI is between $100,000 and $150,000, but nothing if your AGI exceeds $150,000.

Keep More Gambling Winnings

Laurence I. Foster, CPA/PFS, former partner and currently consultant at Eisner LLP, 750 Third Ave., New York City 10017.

If you engage in recreational wagering—at casinos, racetracks, state lotteries or even at church raffles—be prepared in case you win big. If you are not sufficiently prepared, taxes will reduce your winnings by much more than they need to.

TAX PLANNING FOR GAMBLERS

The basic tax rule of gambling is that winnings are fully taxable but losses are deductible only *up to the amount of winnings*. Excess losses are not deductible. *But it's not so easy to deduct gambling losses...*

• **You must file an itemized tax return.** Gambling losses are claimed as a miscellaneous expense among your itemized deductions, so you can't deduct them unless you file an itemized return.

Gambling losses are exempt from the rule that miscellaneous expenses are deductible only to the extent that they exceed 2% of adjusted gross income (AGI). All losses can be deducted, up to the amount of gambling income.

However, gambling losses are included in the itemized deductions that are reduced by 3% of the amount by which AGI exceeds $139,500 ($69,750 if married filing separately) in 2003. These figures rise to $142,700 and $71,350 respectively in 2004.

• **You must have proof of all your gambling losses.**

Trap: Many people don't expect to win any big amounts from gambling during the year, so they don't bother documenting their losses. Then, if late in the year they hit a jackpot-type prize, they have no records of the losses they could have used to shelter it from tax.

What to do: Keep a record, such as a diary, of your gambling expenditures year-round—include everything from any money spent on church and school raffles and lottery tickets to casino visits. They can all be offset against any jackpot that you win.

Also, keep proof of expenditures to back up those records. Losing lottery or racetrack tickets aren't convincing because you can get them anywhere, even pick them up off the ground.

Better: Pay for your wagers using a check or credit card, and then retain your canceled check or credit card receipt, just as you would for other deductible expenses.

Also, if you are a regular at a casino, it may keep a record of your wagers for its own purposes—such as to provide "comps" (free meals, show tickets, etc.) to regular customers. For instance, you may play slot machines using a card that keeps track of how much you've played. If a casino does have a record, ask for a copy of it to document how much you have played and lost.

RETURNS AND WITHHOLDING

Your large winning wagers may be subject to income tax withholding and information return filing...

• **Gambling withholding** applies at a 25% rate to winnings of more than $5,000 coming from...

• Sweepstakes.
• Wagering pools.
• Lotteries.
• Other wagering transactions if the winnings are at least 300 times the amount wagered.

Regular gambling withholding doesn't apply to winnings that come from bingo, keno and slot machines.

Noncash payments: A noncash prize, such as a car, that exceeds $5,000 in value, is subject to withholding, even though there's no cash involved to be withheld. In some cases, you

■ *Your Money* ■ ■

may have the option of taking cash instead of the prize. The payer of the prize may require you to provide the cash needed to cover the 25% withholding tax.

• **Reporting.** Gambling winnings are generally reportable to the IRS by the payer, on form W-2G, when winnings are $600 or more and at least 300 times the wager.

But different rules apply to winnings from bingo, keno and slot machines. *Gambling winnings for these games are reportable if...*

• Winnings (reduced by the wager) are $1,500 or more from a keno game.

• Winnings (not reduced by the wager) are $1,200 or greater from a game of bingo or slot machine.

Note: If a Social Security number or Taxpayer Identification Number isn't provided to the payer for use on a W-2G, then winning wagers over the amounts listed here are subject to backup withholding at a rate of 28%, even though they would not otherwise be.

How to handle withholding and reporting: If you win a wager in a casino or at the racetrack that is subject to reporting, you probably will be provided with your copy of the W-2G form right then.

Keep that form to use when preparing your tax return. Don't expect to receive another in the mail in January when you receive your other W-2s and 1099s. If you do not report your winnings, your taxes may be underpaid—and the IRS will know because of computer matching with its copy of the form.

If taxes are withheld from a winning wager or prize, remember that the withholding is only an estimate of the tax you owe, not the actual amount. If your tax bracket is higher than 27%, you may owe more tax. Or, if you have offsetting gambling losses (or other tax-saving items on your return), you may owe less than the tax withheld.

You don't have to wait until the end of the year to even things out. If you recognize that the gambling withholding will result in your taxes being overpaid or underpaid, you can compensate for it right away by adjusting your wage withholding or quarterly estimated tax payments in the other direction.

Some Divorce Costs Are Deductible

The portion of legal fees that relates to tax advice or production of income is deductible. You must get documentation from your divorce lawyer showing what portion of his/her fees relates to tax or income advice.

Also: If you pay your spouse's legal fees, you can't deduct them unless they are classified as alimony, which makes them deductible to you, but income to your spouse.

Randy Gardner, CPA, associate professor of accountancy, University of Missouri–Kansas City and coauthor of *101 Tax Saving Ideas* (Wealth Builders).

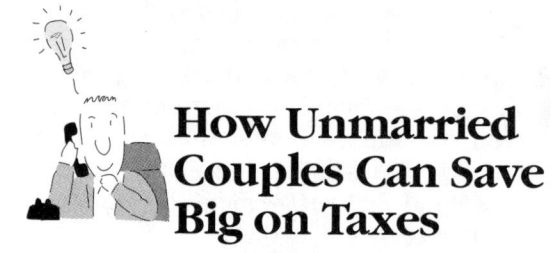

How Unmarried Couples Can Save Big on Taxes

Edward Mendlowitz, CPA, partner, Mendlowitz Weitsen, LLP, CPAs, K2 Brier Hill Ct., East Brunswick, NJ 08816.

Unmarried couples need to plan out their joint finances just as carefully as married couples. There's a bonus—paying close attention to financial planning can create substantial tax savings. *Consider these loopholes...*

***Loophole:* Claim your partner as your dependent.** Unlike married couples, unmarried couples can't file joint tax returns. So they don't get to use the favorable joint-filing tax rates. But one partner may be able to claim a dependency exemption for the other. *Requirements...*

• **Your partner must live with you for the entire year.**

• **You must furnish more than 50% of his/her support.**

• **Your partner cannot have earned more than $3,050 in 2003 ($3,100 in 2004).**

• **Your relationship can't violate state law.**

Example: In some states, living together while unmarried is considered against the law —even if it isn't enforced—therefore, the IRS would not allow a dependency exemption for your partner.

Municipal bond income and other nontaxable income—such as life insurance or certain disability insurance proceeds—are not counted in calculating whether your partner's earnings exceed the income limit.

Note that dependency exemptions on a single return begin to suffer a reduction when adjusted gross income (AGI) exceeds $139,500 in 2003 ($142,700 in 2004). You forfeit the exemptions entirely when your AGI exceeds $262,000 in 2003 ($265,200 in 2004).

***Loophole:* Name your partner beneficiary of your pension plan.** A beneficiary does not have to be a spouse or a relative. Money paid to beneficiaries of qualified plans passes outside your will directly to the people you name as beneficiaries.

The IRS requires you to begin making minimum withdrawals from qualified plans starting no later than April 1 of the year after you turn 70½, or in the year you stop working, if later.

These withdrawals are based on your life expectancy. Withdrawals by your beneficiary after you die generally are based on your beneficiary's life expectancy.

***Loophole:* Hire your partner to work in your business.** As long as your partner's salary is reasonable in relation to the work he does, you can deduct the salary as a business expense. But the company must pay the employer's share of Social Security and Medicare taxes on your partner's wages.

Tax breaks: If your companion's gross income was less than $7,800 in 2003 ($7,950 in 2004), he will not have to file a tax return. The filing threshold is higher for people age 65 or older. And if his taxable income stays under $28,400 in 2003 ($29,050 in 2004), the salary will not be taxed at rates exceeding the 15% federal income tax rate.

***Loophole:* Deduct your dependent partner's medical expenses on your tax return.** When you pay medical expenses for a person you support, you can deduct this person's medical expenses on your tax return even if the person earns more than the income limit of $3,050 in 2003 ($3,100 in 2004).

***Loophole:* Transfer money to your partner free of gift tax.** An individual can give up to $11,000 in 2003 and 2004 each to any number of persons, including his partner, without owing any gift tax on the transfer.

In addition, individuals can give away during their lifetimes up to $1 million free of gift taxes.

Caution: Your estate tax exemption amount ($1 million in 2003, $1.5 million in 2004 and increasing to $3.5 million by 2009) is reduced by any exemption used on lifetime gifts.

Besides all the amounts mentioned above, payments made directly to a school or college to finance an individual's education are not subject to gift tax. The same is true of payments made directly to a health facility for the purpose of paying medical expenses.

You can pay an unlimited amount free of gift tax for the education or medical expenses of your live-in partner—or his children—if you write checks directly to the institution.

***Loophole:* Use trusts to transfer assets to your companion at substantially reduced transfer tax rates.** *The best options...*

•**Grantor retained annuity trust (GRAT).** You place securities, real estate, shares in a business or other assets in a GRAT and retain the right to receive payments of income each year. After the trust term, the assets pass to your companion as beneficiary of the trust.

Example: You transfer $500,000 worth of assets to a 15-year GRAT, keeping the right to receive $35,000 per year. You might incur a taxable gift of only about $200,000, even though your companion will receive $500,000 in assets.

The higher the payout and/or the longer the trust term, the smaller the taxable gift.

Trap: If you (the grantor) die before the trust term expires, trust assets are taxed in your estate.

•**Qualified personal residence trust, or QPRT.** You can transfer a personal residence or a vacation home to a QPRT. After the trust term, the house will pass to the trust beneficiary—your companion. You retain the right to use the house for the trust term. You can keep using the house after the trust terminates, if you pay a fair market rent to the new owner.

■ *Your Money* ■ ■

Key: Deferral reduces the gift tax cost. The longer the term of the trust, the smaller your taxable gift.

Loophole: **Provide for your companion with an irrevocable life insurance trust.** When making annual cash gifts to the trust to cover the premium payments, obtain a "Crummey letter" giving your companion the right of withdrawal. Then the gift is treated as a present interest gift and qualifies for the $11,000 gift tax exclusion. Any proceeds from the irrevocable life insurance trust will be exempt from both income and estate taxes.

Another way: Use excess cash built up in your business to purchase split-dollar life insurance. (With a split-dollar insurance policy, the owner and the company together use company funds to take out a policy on the owner's life.)

How to proceed: On behalf of your companion, set up an irrevocable life insurance trust that will own the policy's death benefit, minus the premiums paid. Upon your death, your company recoups what it paid for the policy and your partner receives death benefits free of estate and income taxes.

Note: There may be current tax to you.

Loophole: **Name your partner as an executor of your will.** Executors collect fees for their services in administering estates. The fees, which are fixed by state statutes, are deducted from the value of the taxable estate, reducing the estate tax owed.

More from Edward Mendlowitz...

Big Loopholes in Preparing Your Tax Return

Two big new tax acts, new regulations and rulings and new court cases are all bound to help you cut taxes on your next return. *Do not overlook all these new tax-saving opportunities...*

EDUCATION LOOPHOLES

• **Annual contributions to the Coverdell education savings accounts were raised** to $2,000 per beneficiary. Contributions for 2003 can be made up to the due date of your tax return, generally April 15, 2004.

This contribution limit is cut back for those joint filers whose adjusted gross income (AGI) exceeds $190,000. It is not available to joint filers with AGI above $220,000.

Even better: Coverdell contributions are now available to cover qualified education expenses —kindergarten through grade 12.

• **Distributions from qualified tuition programs are tax free** if the money is used to pay qualified higher education expenses. You can make contributions to a qualified tuition program and a Coverdell account for the same beneficiary in the same year.

• **More people can now deduct up to $2,500 of interest paid on student loans.** The phaseout range for this deduction has now been increased to AGIs of $100,000 to $130,000 (from $60,000 to $75,000) on joint returns and to AGIs of $50,000 to $65,000 (from $40,000 to $55,000) for single and head-of-household returns.

• **You can deduct up to $3,000 of qualified tuition and school expenses** paid for your higher education or that of your spouse or dependents in 2003. You become ineligible for the deduction when your modified AGI exceeds $130,000 (for joint filers) or $65,000 (for single and head-of-household filers). The deduction increases in 2004.

Limit: You can't take both the tuition deduction and the education credit in the same year for the same student. In addition, the same expenses can't be used to claim the tuition deduction and tax-free withdrawals from qualified tuition programs and Coverdell accounts.

DEDUCTION LOOPHOLES

• **Teachers and other "eligible educators" can deduct up to $250** of the money they spend on classroom books, supplies and computer equipment. Who qualifies? Teachers from kindergarten through grade 12, instructors, counselors, principals or aides who work at least 900 hours during a school year. This deduction only applies through 2003, unless Congress extends it.

• **If you bought a hybrid car, you can deduct up to $2,000** of the purchase price. Vehicles that qualify are the Toyota Prius, Honda Insight and Honda Civic Hybrid.

- **Obesity now qualifies as a disease as far as the IRS is concerned.** This means that overweight individuals now can deduct the cost of weight-loss programs and even home exercise equipment recommended by a doctor as treatment for obesity.

Limits: Medical expenses are deductible only to the extent they exceed 7.5% of your AGI.

Caution: The expense of special diet foods cannot be deducted.

ADOPTION LOOPHOLES

- **The maximum adoption credit is $10,160 in 2003 ($10,390 in 2004)** for each eligible child you adopt, including children who have special needs. Keep in mind that a tax credit, which is a dollar-for-dollar offset against the taxes you owe, is worth more than a tax deduction.

You don't begin to lose some of the credit until your modified AGI exceeds $150,000. Formerly, the figure was $75,000.

RETIREMENT PLAN LOOPHOLES

- **The maximum contribution to traditional IRAs and Roth IRAs for year 2003 and 2004 is $3,000.** Taxpayers age 50 or older by year-end can make additional catch-up contributions of up to $500.

- **The maximum deduction for contributions to a simplified employee pension (SEP) plan is 25%.** The compensation base on which the percentage applies is $200,000 for 2003 ($205,000 in 2004).

- **The maximum permitted elective deferral for SIMPLE-IRA contributions is $8,000 in 2003 ($9,000 in 2004).** Individuals age 50 or older at year-end are allowed an additional catch-up contribution of $1,000 in 2003 ($1,500 in 2004).

- **Premature IRA annuitized distributions can be reduced** by switching to the "required minimum distribution method" for calculating "substantially equal payments."

You can now make a one-time switch to the required minimum distribution method. The change will not be treated as a payment modification that triggers the 10% penalty.

- **The IRS can make "hardship exceptions" to the 60-day rollover rule** for distributions from retirement plans. Generally, a 10% penalty applies to money that is withdrawn from retirement accounts unless the money is returned to the account within 60 days. The IRS may waive the 60-day rollover period in cases of disaster or other events that are beyond the reasonable control of the taxpayer.

MISCELLANEOUS LOOPHOLES

- **New tax breaks for stock options transferred during a divorce.** The IRS ruled that the "assignment of income" doctrine does not apply to transfers of nonqualified stock options and rights to nonqualified deferred compensation as part of a divorce agreement.

Instead, these transfers are free of tax. The receiving spouse recognizes the income when the options are exercised or the deferred compensation is received.

- **Small businesses can use the cash method of accounting.** The IRS issued final rules in 2002, allowing certain small businesses with annual gross receipts of $10 million or less to automatically convert from the accrual to the cash method of accounting.

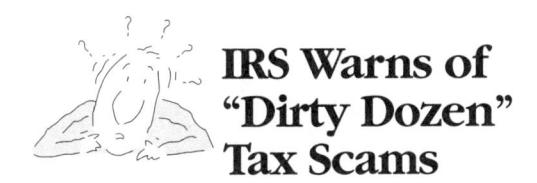

IRS Warns of "Dirty Dozen" Tax Scams

IRS News Release IR-2002-12.

The IRS warns taxpayers to be aware of these common tax scams during the tax-filing season. If you encounter one of these or some other suspected tax fraud, report it to the IRS by calling 800-829-0433. The "dirty dozen"...

- **African-Americans get a special tax refund as reparation for slavery.** There is no such refund, so don't pay anyone to tell you how to claim it.

- **Taxes need not be withheld from your wages, provided you know the secret.** There is no secret.

- **"I don't pay taxes—why should you?"** Con artists who do pay taxes falsely claim they don't, and offer to sell you their secret.

■ *Your Money* ■ ■

- **"You've won a prize that you will get after you pay us the tax on it."** If you win a prize, you will pay any tax on it *to the IRS,* nobody else.
- **"Untax yourself for $49.95."** This old scam is now being sold on the Internet. It claims to teach you that taxes are "voluntary." Many sellers of these packages have been criminally convicted—but more are still out there.
- **Social Security "refund" scam.** For an up-front fee, someone offers to help you prepare a claim for a refund of Social Security taxes—a refund that the law does not allow.
- **"I can get you a *big* refund...for a fee!"** The scam artist charges an up-front fee to get you a refund—and may actually get one by using a false W-2 or Social Security number.

Snag: IRS computers will catch the false filing and you'll have to pay back the refund with penalties after the scam artist is gone.

- **Share dependents to get earned income credits.** Unscrupulous tax preparers use one family's children on another family's tax return to get tax credits. But the IRS prosecutes the preparers and penalizes the taxpayers involved.
- **An IRS agent comes unannounced to your house to collect tax.** Real IRS agents give notice of their visits in advance, carry photo ID and don't collect taxes in person. Report impostors by calling a special hotline number, 800-366-4484.
- **"Put your money in a trust and never pay taxes again."** Promoters charge thousands of dollars to set up trust schemes that are fraudulent. They leave you controlling the assets you supposedly put "in trust," so this income is taxable.
- **Improper home-based business.** Promoters exaggerate the tax savings of a home office while not revealing the rules you must meet to have a real tax-qualified one.
- **Disabled access tax credit for pay telephones.** The con artist claims you can get a $5,000 tax credit for installing a pay telephone with volume controls. But the real disabled access credit applies only to bona fide businesses that comply with the technical legal requirements.

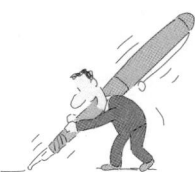

Don't Make Mistakes with Your Social Security Number

A wrong Social Security number makes a tax return "not processable." The IRS says that even if a tax return reports a correct taxpayer identification number (TIN) for an individual, an incorrect Social Security number on the Form W-2 accompanying the return will result in the return being "not a processible form," one that is frozen for refund purposes. Moreover, interest will not run on any refundable amount. The refund (without interest) will not be paid until the IRS obtains the correct Social Security number.

IRS Service Center Advice 200233003.

Simple Ways to Avoid Underpayment Penalties

Larry Torella, CPA, tax partner, Eisner LLP, 750 Third Ave., New York City 10017. He is author of his firm's annual year-end tax-planning guide.

Our tax system is a pay-as-you-go system. Your taxes for the current year are paid throughout the year by withholding and estimated tax payments.

The combined total of these payments must be at least 90% of the tax you ultimately owe, or you'll pay a penalty for underpayment of estimated taxes.

THE EASY WAY

But you can avoid the penalty if you base your estimated taxes for this year on one of the following two "safe harbors"...

- **Pay in at least 90% of this year's tax liability.**
- **Pay in 100% of last year's tax liability.**

If you do that, you'll avoid penalty no matter how high your current bill turns out to be.

Tax Guide

Important exception: If your adjusted gross income last year was greater than $150,000 (or $75,000 if married filing separately), you cannot use the 100%-of-the-prior-year's-tax safe harbor. Your safe harbor is 110% of last year's tax. You must pay in this amount to avoid underpayment penalties or rely on the 90% rule.

Problem with safe harbors: While reliance on a safe harbor helps you to avoid an underpayment penalty, it may cause you to overpay your taxes.

THE ANNUALIZED METHOD

To match your tax payments more closely with the time when income is earned, you can figure out your estimated taxes utilizing the "annualized" method. This method is helpful to taxpayers who earn most of their income late in the year. They don't have to make estimated tax payments before the income is received. The tax payment is tied to cash flow.

Self-employed professionals in particular—who work for clients throughout the year but only collect for it late in the year—should be sure to look at the annualized method.

Disadvantage: When using the annualized method, you must complete IRS Form 2210, *Underpayment of Estimated Tax by Individuals, Estates, and Trusts*. This form is very complicated—therefore, it's best to consult a tax professional about it.

YEAR-END ADJUSTMENTS

To more closely figure estimated tax payments, you might try to adjust your income tax withholding near the end of the year to make up for any projected shortfalls in estimated payments.

Example: An employee who receives a year-end bonus can apply all of it toward his estimated taxes. Under the Tax Code, withholding from wages and other compensation is treated as if it had been made throughout the year—even if actually made on December 31.

You can also boost your wage withholding at year-end to cover tax on items such as gains from property sales and year-end mutual fund distributions and other income from which tax is not withheld.

If one spouse has wages subject to withholding while the other does not (the other spouse is self-employed, for example), then the employed spouse can adjust his/her withholding to cover the estimated tax obligations of the couple.

FINDING THE CASH TO PAY

The best way to meet estimated tax payments is to put aside a set amount each week into a money market account or another short-term instrument. That way, the funds will be available to you on the estimated tax due dates, which are January 18, April 15, June 15 and September 15.

If you lack the discipline to set aside funds for estimated tax payments, you can have withholding on…

• **Social Security benefits** (at the rate of 7% for taxpayers in any of the lowest three individual rates—10%, 15% and 25%). Complete Form W-4V, *Voluntary Withholding Request,* by selecting the withholding rate you want. Submit the form to your local Social Security office.

• **Unemployment benefits** (at the rate of 10%).

• **Pensions and IRAs.** Withholding on periodic pension distributions (such as monthly benefits) is just like withholding on wages—it's based on the withholding allowances you claim.

Withholding on required minimum distributions from IRAs and qualified plans is made at the rate of 10%. In both cases, you can opt out of withholding entirely or increase the withholding amount. Distributions from qualified plans eligible for rollover treatment that are not transferred directly to an IRA or other plan are subject to *mandatory* 20% withholding.

The nonpayment option: The penalty for underpayment of estimated taxes is really just an interest rate—currently 4% (which is adjusted quarterly). For anyone short of the cash needed to pay estimated taxes, the penalty is not so burdensome. For example, if you don't pay your January payment until April, you'll owe the penalty for just three months. For more information, see IRS Publication 505, *Tax Withholding and Estimated Tax.*

■ *Your Money* ■ ■

Tax Cost of Settling A Debt

If you settle a debt for less than you owe, the amount forgiven will represent taxable income to you as long as you remain solvent. The creditor is supposed to send Form 1099C for that amount to you and the IRS.

Caution: Even if you do not receive the form, the creditor may have informed the IRS. You may be required to report the amount forgiven as miscellaneous income and pay any tax that results.

Mike Kidwell, vice president, Myvesta.org, a financial management organization in Rockville, MD.

Avoid Underreporting Penalties

If your tax returns underreport the tax you owe, a 20% "accuracy-related penalty" may apply. But the penalty can be avoided by making "sufficient disclosure" on the return concerning the deductions and other items that caused the underreporting of tax.

Useful: The IRS has published rules regarding what constitutes adequate disclosure so taxpayers can avoid the penalty regarding specific items, such as charitable contributions, medical expenses, interest expense and so on.

Backup: If you will be taking "aggressive" positions on your return, look up the disclosure rules to learn how to minimize risk.

Details: Revenue Procedure 2002-66, IRB 2002-42, 724.

Randy Bruce Blaustein, Esq., senior tax partner, R.B. Blaustein & Co., 155 E. 31 St., New York City 10016.

More from Randy Bruce Blaustein...

Should You Pay Taxes With a Credit Card?

When paying taxes with a credit card the processing charge is 2.49% of what you owe—and you are charged interest if you fail to pay the credit card company immediately.

When it might make sense: If you use a card that gives frequent-flier miles or rebates worth more than the processing fee.

To pay by credit card: Contact Official Payments Corp. (888-272-9829 or *www.officialpayments.com*)...or LINK2GOV Corp. (888-729-1040 or *www.pay1040.com*).

Alternative: Reduce the processing fee to 2.25% by using Intuit's *TurboTax* software filing package and paying with a Discover card.

Also from Randy Bruce Blaustein...

How to Give a Collectible To Charity

Giving a collectible to charity may allow you to take a tax deduction for its current full value—even if you paid much less for the item years ago.

To get this deduction: You must have owned the object for more than one year and must donate it to a public charity or nonprofit group, not a private foundation. It must be appraised by a qualified unrelated party. For the full write-off, you must donate to a group that doesn't sell the item but keeps and uses it in its exempt purpose.

Example: A museum that will display a piece of sculpture.

When You Can't Pay On Time

If you can't pay your taxes by the deadline, ask the IRS about its installment plan. This lets you spread out your tax payments over three years. You'll be charged a setup fee of about $43 plus interest and a penalty per month on your unpaid balance.

Cost: Typically less than taking out a loan or using your credit card.

You can use this strategy if you owe less than $10,000 in taxes and haven't previously defaulted on IRS payments. If you owe more, consult a tax adviser.

Steve Rhode, president and cofounder of Myvesta.org, a financial management organization in Rockville, MD.

Electronic Refund Trap

The IRS won't replace an electronic refund that was stolen by fraud.

Facts: An individual filed a tax return with the help of a volunteer return preparer at a clinic. The individual asked for an electronic refund, and provided the routing information for his bank account. But the return preparer substituted information for another account and absconded with the refund after it arrived.

IRS position: The original refund was correctly sent to the bank account listed on the return, so the IRS cannot send a replacement refund to the taxpayer.

IRS Legal Memorandum 200236025.

Has Your Refund Check Been Intercepted?

If you owe state taxes, your federal tax refund check might never arrive. Under a new program, the IRS and state tax authorities share information. When a federal tax refund is due to a person who owes back state taxes, the IRS will send the check to the state instead. So far, 24 states have joined the growing program.

Harley Duncan, executive director, Federation of Tax Administrators, Washington, DC.

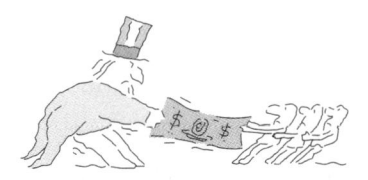

Even Honest People Get in Trouble with The IRS—What to Do If You're Accused

Donald W. MacPherson, Esq., specialist in criminal and tax law and head attorney, MacPherson Group, PC, 3404 W. Cheryl Dr., Phoenix 85051, *www.beatirs.com.* He is author of *Tax Fraud and Evasion: The War Stories* (MacPherson & Sons).

An angry employee or ex-spouse makes charges against you to the IRS. A business partner or an associate engages in wrongdoing that you weren't aware of—but the IRS thinks you were. An investment adviser misleads you into making an offshore investment that turns out to be a tax-evasion scheme.

It's bad enough to owe the IRS back taxes—but facing criminal tax charges is a nightmare. It can happen to you even if you have done nothing "criminal" at all.

In a civil case, all the IRS wants is money. You can end the case easily and quickly by paying up, or you can go to the IRS Appeals Division to try to reach a compromise with an appeals officer.

It is critical, however, to recognize the signs of a criminal investigation and demonstrate your innocence *before* IRS investigators put in so much effort that they become personally committed to pursuing your case. Officials are likely to believe they are right—and demand penalties greater than a tax payment. In criminal cases, the IRS seeks jail time, fines and restitution.

WARNING SIGNS

•**An IRS "special agent" gets involved.** IRS *revenue agents* handle civil audits...*revenue officers* deal with collection matters.

Special agents, however, are criminal investigators. If one contacts you about your taxes or asks questions of others about you, you are under criminal investigation.

•**A special agent signs paperwork related to your case.** Sometimes, special agents don't contact you up-front because they don't want to tip you off to a criminal investigation. However, they will sign paperwork that you might see.

■ *Your Money* ■ ■

Example: The IRS issues a summons for your bank records that is signed by a special agent. Depending on the case, the bank may —or may not—notify you.

•**Tax audit or collection efforts suddenly stop.** When a special agent takes over a case, he/she often puts a "hold" on everything that IRS revenue agents or officers have done on that case.

Example: During the course of a long-running tax dispute, the IRS starts taking steps to seize your property—and then suddenly stops without explanation.

What to do: Ask for a "specific" transcript of your tax account to find out why the IRS stopped what it was doing. You can request it from your regional IRS Disclosure Office. Your tax adviser can read the codes to determine whether a special agent ordered a hold on further action. *Code 914* means a criminal investigation is underway, while a *Code 912* means that an investigation is closed.

IF YOU ARE BEING INVESTIGATED

•**Obtain legal counsel immediately.** If a special agent shows up at your door or you learn in some other way that special agents are involved in your case, consult a lawyer who is experienced in handling criminal tax matters. Do not simply turn to your tax preparer or a CPA—he is not qualified to deal with criminal law. You will have time to find an attorney since the average investigation lasts four years.

Ask a local lawyer for a referral, but be sure to ask the prospective attorney how much experience he has in this specific area.

•**Be silent.** An agent can use whatever is said in court. Don't say anything to the special agent. Caution family members and business associates that they might be contacted and to stay silent. This may not be easy— agents are trained to get people to talk.

Example: A team of special agents may appear at your door at dawn before you are awake and thinking clearly...or after 7 pm, while you are relaxing with family or friends.

Self-defense: Know your rights. You don't have to say anything to a special agent who visits unexpectedly. You do not even have to open your door to an IRS special agent if he doesn't have a warrant. Instead, politely ask the agent to identify himself and request his business card. Agents are required to show photo identification and badges and give their employee identification numbers.

Then say no more. If he insists on talking to you, ask him to call back later to make an appointment for an office meeting with you, during which you will be accompanied by legal counsel.

To learn more about IRS criminal enforcement practices and specific dangers that can lead to criminal tax prosecution, visit the IRS's criminal investigation Web page at *www.ustreas.gov/irs/ci*. It offers data on criminal tax prosecutions and convictions as well as a list of prevalent "tax scams."

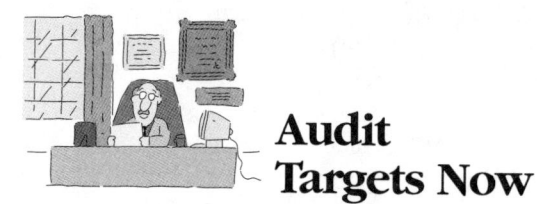

Audit Targets Now

Irving L. Blackman, CPA, founding partner, Blackman Kallick Bartelstein, LLP, 300 S. Riverside Plaza, Chicago 60606, *www.taxsecretsofthewealthy.com*.

Today's IRS may be "kinder and gentler," but beware. *There are three subjects about which it is on the warpath...*

•**Auto donation programs.** Many of the programs that purportedly donate vehicles to charity are scams. The IRS is checking them. *Warning signs...*

  •A claim is made that you can get a deduction worth more than you could get by selling the car. *Reality:* Your deduction can't be worth more than what you could get by selling it, times your tax bracket rate.

  •You hear you can claim a deduction even if you don't file an itemized return. You can't.

  •You deduct full blue book value when the car is worth less.

Caution: Those who donate the cars are the targets of the audit.

•**Sham trusts.** There are dozens of programs out there—offered in seminars, over the Internet and by referral—that promise to show how to use trusts to (1) protect assets from creditors, and (2) escape income and estate taxes. Many of these trusts are offshore.

Reality: A trust may help you achieve asset protection. But any trust program that promises to help you avoid income or estate taxes is a phony—stay away from it. These trusts are another red flag to the IRS.

• **"Secrets" of tax avoidance.** Scam artists are always coming up with new ideas that they say you can use to avoid taxes. They claim their secrets will let you deduct your personal living expenses as business costs or some other bogus claim. But they always ask for your money first.

Reality: There are no secrets in the tax law. If you're unsure about something, tell the person making the offer you'll check it with an expert. If he tells you the experts don't know about this yet, forget it—you are dealing with a scam artist.

More from Irving Blackman...

Tax Breaks Can Help You Buy Long-Term-Care Insurance

Long-term-care policies that meet specific conditions are deemed "tax qualified." Benefits paid by these are tax free...people who get a qualified policy on their own can deduct part of the cost as a medical expense (from $250 at age 40 to $3,130 if age 71 or older in 2003 and from $260 at age 40 to $3,250 if age 71 or older in 2004)...self-employed people can deduct 100% of their cost from gross income. Businesses can provide long-term-care insurance as a tax-free benefit they can deduct.

Some policies return the full premium cost to the insured's heirs at death, making the insurance "free" in dollar terms.

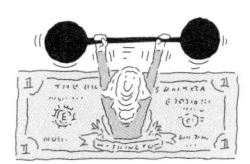

Tax Guide

What the IRS Doesn't Want You to Know About Its Audit Process

Martin S. Kaplan, CPA, PC, 11 Penn Plaza, New York City 10001. He is author of *What the IRS Doesn't Want You to Know* (Wiley).

The IRS is now in the midst of a near-total reorganization, so its processes are in disarray. *What this means to taxpayers...*

• **The IRS audit rate is at an all-time low.** The rate for personal returns fell to 0.49% during the fiscal year ended September 30, 2001. That's down from a historical range of 1.5% to 2.3%.

About half of all IRS audits now are done as "correspondence audits," in which the IRS sends a letter asking for documentation—such as a receipt for a charity deduction.

The audit rates for businesses have also dropped. The audit rate for corporations with assets of $1 million to under $5 million declined to 2% from 7.78% in 1997—a decrease of nearly 75%.

• **Audits are now more common for low-income individuals** than for high-income individuals. Because of the high error rate on low-income tax returns claiming the earned-income credit, the IRS says Congress wants it to pay closer attention to them.

Taxpayers with incomes of less than $25,000 had an audit rate of 0.4%. Those with incomes of $50,000 to below $100,000 had an audit rate of only 0.23%.

Among taxpayers who reported business income on Schedule C, the audit rate was 2.7% for those with gross receipts below $25,000, versus only 1.2% for those with gross receipts above $100,000.

Don't be complacent: The IRS still conducts 600,000 audits each year. IRS computers score returns to target those most likely to contain errors or discrepancies. Also, the IRS computers "examine" every return and match the figures on information returns, such as W-2s and 1099s. In September 2002, the IRS started up a new "super audit program" that involves line-by-line audits.

Your Money

AUDIT BATTLE PLAN

Do not overestimate what the IRS auditor knows. He/she knows almost *nothing* about you that is not on your tax return. The IRS's record-keeping system is archaic—with information spread over several largely obsolete computer systems that don't communicate with each other. Any information the auditor gets to use against you will come *from you. Dos and don'ts...*

•***Don't* volunteer anything.** Consult your tax preparer before answering any questions. Be concise, and say nothing more. When an auditor asks for additional records, ask him to put his request in writing. Ask for at least one month to retrieve records from your files. Produce only what was requested.

•***Don't* make friends with the auditor.** Small talk about family, business, vacations, hobbies, etc. will only provide the auditor with more subjects to investigate. In fact, the IRS manual instructs auditors to encourage small talk for this reason—and even to create awkward silences to encourage taxpayers to volunteer something to "break the ice."

Self-defense: Instead of attending the audit yourself, hire a tax professional to represent you. Your tax preparer may not have experience handling IRS audits. CPAs and lawyers are generally more experienced, but they charge $200 to $300 hourly. Unless your return is very complex, an enrolled agent—a federally authorized tax practitioner—is a good choice at somewhat lower rates.

•***Do* arm yourself with the auditor's handbook.** More than 50 auditing guides for IRS agents are available at no cost to taxpayers. Go to the "Businesses" section at *www.irs.gov* or call the Government Printing Office, 866-512-1800.

CORRESPONDENCE AUDITS

IRS personnel who handle correspondence audits are *not* trained tax examiners. These workers are required only to have graduated from high school.

To minimize exposure to a correspondence audit, promptly provide whatever is requested in the first letter you receive. This is *especially* true if you can't fully meet the request.

Example: You receive an IRS letter asking for records supporting a $1,500 charity deduction. You have canceled checks and required acknowledgments from recipients for only $1,000. If you promptly send the records you have, the clerks handling the audit will credit you for the $1,000 and bill you for the tax on the difference—and that will be *the end of it*.

If you delay your response, make an unconvincing excuse for your missing records or try to argue, you risk having your case "passed up" to trained IRS auditors who may examine your entire return. At that point, you may be asked to come into the local IRS office to continue the audit.

HOW TO APPEAL YOUR CASE

First, take your case to the IRS Appeals Division. For less than $25,000 of taxes, you probably won't need professional representation. You may get a chance to settle. Appeals officers, unlike auditors, have the authority to accept compromise settlements.

Information: The IRS offers free help for appeals at *www.irs.gov*. Also, see IRS Publication #5, *Appeal Rights and Preparation of Protests for Unagreed Cases*.

If you can't reach an agreement at the appeal, the Tax Court's Small Case Division now hears cases involving as much as $50,000 of disputed taxes. You don't need a lawyer, but you must file within 90 days of receiving a deficiency notice. Obtain forms from Clerk of the Court, US Tax Court, 400 Second St. NW, Washington, DC 20217...or at *www.ustaxcourt.gov*.

Key: You get another chance to negotiate with the IRS when you file a case in the Tax Court. Ninety-eight percent of cases filed are settled before trial.

More from Martin Kaplan...

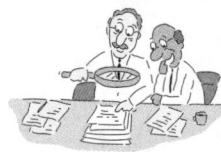

Is Your Tax Professional Doing a Good Job? How to Tell...

You'll have to place a lot of trust in any tax professional you hire to prepare your tax return. But how do you know if the professional is doing a good job? You can't tell by just looking at your tax return—if you could, you'd be able to prepare it yourself.

Here are the main things to look for and questions to ask when evaluating a professional tax adviser or seeking a new one…

FOUR CATEGORIES

You want to employ the kind of tax professional that best meets your needs. *There are four kinds…*

•**Certified public accountants (CPAs)** must pass rigorous professional examinations and keep their accounting skills up to date with annual continuing education.

•**Tax attorneys** also are professionally educated and certified, with expertise lying more in the areas of litigation and dispute management than tax accounting.

•**Enrolled agents** are tax specialists who qualify to practice before the IRS either by having worked for the IRS for at least five years or by having passed a challenging IRS-administered examination.

•**Seasonal tax return preparers** work for firms such as H&R Block, Jackson Hewitt or smaller firms (or themselves). The firms train the preparers.

There's no one "best" kind of tax professional. Within each category, different individuals have different specialties. The "best" for you depends on your particular needs. *Examples…*

•A CPA may be best if your return includes complex business or accounting issues.

•An attorney should be consulted if you anticipate possible litigation with the IRS, or if any issue of fraud exists regarding past returns.

•An enrolled agent who worked inside a particular division of the IRS may have insight that could be helpful in your specific situation.

•Seasonal preparers have the least professional expertise, but may provide the best value for a straightforward tax return with little examination risk.

AUDIT SERVICES

One of your most important rights as a taxpayer is the right to be represented by a professional in your dealings with the IRS. You don't even have to personally attend an audit in most cases, but can send your professional on your behalf.

This not only can save you aggravation, but also prevent you from making costly revelations or procedural mistakes when personally dealing with an auditor.

You can be represented before the IRS at an audit or IRS Appeals proceeding by a CPA, attorney or enrolled agent—but not by a seasonal preparer (another reason to use seasonal preparers only for low-audit-risk returns).

The policies of particular tax professionals regarding representing clients to the IRS may differ. Be sure you understand the extent of representation you can expect from your professional during an audit dispute, and its cost, before any dispute arises.

PLANNING SERVICES

With luck you'll never be audited, and so never need to be represented during an audit. Key to minimizing your audit risk is the quality of the service you receive from your tax professional in tax *planning,* as well as return preparation.

Planning ahead is vital. If you just give a box of records to your professional after year-end to use in preparing your tax return—and your professional routinely accepts this practice—neither of you is doing a good job at minimizing your taxes.

One good measure of the quality of service you are getting from your tax professional is the amount of advance planning you do with him/her to reduce your taxes on a looking-forward basis.

Does your professional…

•**Give you face-to-face meeting time** to discuss your situation and plan the coming year's tax strategies, after reviewing the results on the past year's tax return?

•**Send you tax-planning and record-keeping materials** at the beginning of every year, or coordinate with you on software you can use to keep records throughout the year?

•**Keep you informed throughout the year** about changes in the Tax Code and in IRS rulings, regulations and procedures that could affect your situation?

■ *Your Money* ■ ■

Remember, after year-end, when you collect your final records for the year, it is too late to use most potential tax-saving strategies—the year is done.

If you aren't getting such advance planning help now, then ask for it. If the response you receive is inadequate, look for another adviser.

RETURN PREPARATION

Of course, preparing the tax return itself is a key task for any tax professional. *To verify the quality of the job that will be done, ask...*

• **Will your return be prepared personally** by the professional you meet and plan with, or will the task be delegated to a subordinate?

• **How many meetings will be required** to prepare and review your return? The average taxpayer will require one or two, while the average small business two to four.

• **What procedures are there to double-check your return** after it is completed?

• **Is up-to-date technology used by the professional to prepare returns?** Good tax software greatly reduces the error rate in complex tax calculations—as well as reducing the billable hours that must be spent on a return.

Best: UltraTax from Creative Solutions and *ProSystems fx Tax* by CCH.

• **Can you communicate with your professional by fax, E-mail or through a firm's Web site?** During the crush of the tax-filing season, electronic communication can be very useful in avoiding the delays involved in sending documents or information personally, by mail or even by express delivery.

BEYOND THE RETURN

Taxes are just a part of your total financial position. CPAs, attorneys and enrolled agents who understand your situation can also give valuable advice about larger related issues such as business organization, pension and estate planning. Plus, they may be able to provide valuable referrals to professionals in related fields—such as investment planning, insurance planning, Medicare planning, etc.

The more your tax professional does to help you minimize your taxes on a looking-forward basis, integrating tax strategies with planning for your larger financial concerns, the better service you are receiving.

Also from Martin Kaplan...

Smart Reasons to File an Amended Tax Return

There are a variety of new reasons to file amended returns. In one case, you even get more time to file than the standard three years.

Don't worry: The risk of being selected for audit as a result of filing an amended return is slight. Amending a return does *not* give the IRS extra time to audit that year's return.

• **New business incentives.** *The Job Creation and Worker Assistance Act of 2002* became law *after* some taxpayers had already filed their 2001 returns. Changes they may have been entitled to claim can be claimed on amended returns filed before April 15, 2005, in most cases. *They include...*

• Bonus depreciation, which applies to property bought and placed in service on or after September 11, 2001.

• Increased depreciation limit for cars due to the addition of bonus depreciation to the first-year amount.

• **Deductions for "lost" assets.** You can deduct securities that have become worthless and debts you are owed but that you can't collect. You must do so in the year in which they became worthless.

Trap: You may not know exactly when an asset became worthless, especially if litigation or bankruptcy was involved.

Solution: If you *now* know the year in which you *should* have taken the deduction, file an amended return. You can do so up to *seven* years back—currently, back to 1996.

• **Casualty loss deductions.** If you suffered a casualty loss due to a storm, flood or other disaster in a place designated a disaster area by the president, you may deduct this loss on your tax return for the year, or amend the prior year's return and deduct the loss in that year.

• **Tax-free gains on home sales.**

Tax Guide

Old rules: If you own and live in a home for two of the five years before selling it, you can take $250,000 of the gain tax-free if you file a single return…$500,000 with a joint return.

New rules: Even if you do not meet the "two-year test," you can take a tax-free gain if you sell the home for any of these reasons—a job change, medical reasons or "unforeseen circumstances," such as divorce or separation.

New rules also apply if part of your home, such as a home office, was used for business. If you sold a house before the rules were announced in December 2002, you can file an amended return to claim more of the tax-free gain. The new rules, which are retroactive to May 7, 1997, are available at *www.irs.gov*. Search the site for "Home Sale Exclusion Rules."

•**Overlooked income.** If you made an error on a prior year's tax return that resulted in underpayment of taxes, correct it with an amended return. This will minimize interest and penalties if the IRS finds your mistake.

Common examples: You forgot to include income from an IRS Form 1099 when you prepared your return, or the 1099 arrived after you filed your taxes.

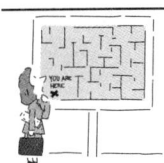

Inside the IRS

In the following articles, Ms. X, Esq., a former IRS agent who is still well connected, reveals inside secrets from the IRS…

PLANNING BEFORE AN AUDIT

If you have been notified of a tax audit, plan your defense carefully. Try to anticipate the questions you will be asked, and be prepared with the answers. The better prepared you are, the more credible you will appear. Once an audit target's credibility has been firmly established, IRS auditors tend to limit the scope of their inquiry. They often close the case without pursuing every issue they originally planned to review.

Example: To support a deduction you claimed for charitable contributions, staple each canceled check to the appropriate receipt and present all your documents in an organized folder. Any deduction claimed for a contribution for which you have no receipt should be listed on a separate page in the folder with a complete explanation of the circumstances surrounding the contribution.

IRS AGENTS AND YOUR PRIVACY

IRS management has decided that revenue agents may drive by an individual's home to determine whether there exists some "reasonable indication of the likelihood of unreported income." Management says this does not violate a provision of a 1998 law that restricts agents from using "specific financial status audit techniques," which include in-depth questioning about lifestyle to find unreported income. Revenue agents may also use commercial databases to search public records relating to purchases of real estate.

Inside information: Unreported income is usually discovered by IRS agents when money is used to buy cars, boats, vacation homes and insured jewelry and artwork.

WHEN INFORMATION OVERLOAD ACTUALLY HELPS

One of my general rules is never volunteer information to the IRS during a tax audit…and answer only the question that was asked.

Exception: By providing an IRS agent with voluminous records which contain information that won't help their case or hurt your case, the audit may be completed much faster than you expected. Few IRS agents have the time to spend hours reviewing piles of documents.

Strategy: Summarize the information you give the agent, presenting conclusions in the light most favorable to your position.

WHAT IF YOUR TAX PREPARER SUGGESTS SOMETHING THAT RESULTS IN A PENALTY?

IRS guidelines (Section 10.34(b) of Circular 230) require attorneys, CPAs and certain other tax practitioners to inform their clients of the penalties reasonably likely to be applied with respect to a tax return position advised, prepared or reported by the practitioner.

How this can help you: If your tax preparer suggests a strategy or position that sounds too good to be true, demand a written explanation

■ *Your Money* ■ ■

from the preparer. Make sure he/she explains the penalties you will be liable for if his advice is ignored by the IRS. This written statement may help you to avoid IRS penalties by helping establish that you relied on the advice of an independent tax professional as to the tax treatment of an item.

TAKING THE IRS TO COURT

Most disputes with the IRS are resolved in the US Tax Court. There are good reasons for this. You can go to Tax Court without first paying the tax the IRS claims you owe. Also, a Tax Court proceeding is held before a judge with no jury. The judges are well versed in tax matters.

Alternative: Pay the tax first, file a refund claim and then take your case to a US District Court. In District Court, the case can be heard by a jury, which has little or no knowledge about the tax law. This could very well be to your advantage.

THE IRS's NEW SECRET WEAPON AGAINST TAX SCAMS

The IRS now has a new way to deal with tax scams.

Old way: Focus only on taxpayers who pursue the phony tax-saving schemes. Audit their returns to recover the lost tax.

New way: Go to court and get injunctions against unsavory return preparers and scam promoters. The injunction prevents a preparer from completing a tax return that claims a "slavery reparations tax credit" or a promoter from selling a "common law trust" that, supposedly, is not required to pay tax. Failure to comply with the terms of the injunction amounts to being in contempt of court, with the expectation that a prison sentence will be imposed.

SOMETHING FREE IS USUALLY TAXABLE

Winners of contests and prizes are generally surprised to learn that the fair market value of the product or service they won must be included in their income for tax purposes.

Here's another situation: Recently, a US District Court, in *Townsend Industries, Inc.* (DC SD Iowa, No. 4:01-cv-10176), determined that the costs of a company's annual employee fishing trip were taxable wages to the employees.

Caution: Before you accept anything of value, consider the tax consequences. It may turn out to be cheaper to reject the freebie than to pay tax on it.

HOW TO DEDUCT YOUR SPOUSE'S EXPENSES ON A BUSINESS TRIP

A favorite audit target for revenue agents is personal travel costs, generally for a spouse who tags along on a business trip. Proving that your spouse had a legitimate business purpose in making a trip is usually difficult. But some of the costs of traveling with your spouse can be deducted. Those are costs that would be incurred whether you traveled alone or with your spouse. The cost of a rental car, for example, would be fully deductible. So would the cost of many hotel rooms. You could also pay for one airline ticket (fully deductible) and your spouse could use frequent-flier miles. Also, identify meals to which business associates invite their spouses, and deduct the cost of those meals for both you and your spouse.

WHAT'S AN ABUSIVE TAX SCHEME?

As a starting point, the IRS has created four categories of abuse…(1) Frivolous returns— such as claiming that income is not subject to tax…(2) frivolous refund claims (such as slavery reparations)…(3) abusive domestic trusts (such as deducting personal living expenses)…and (4) offshore schemes (such as hiding income and assets). Look for the IRS to pressure the Justice Department to bring more criminal cases against offenders to put an end to the billion-dollar revenue drain each year.

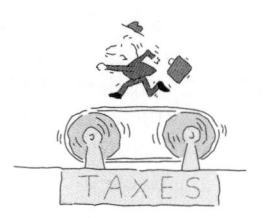

■■ Your Money ■

10 Better Investing

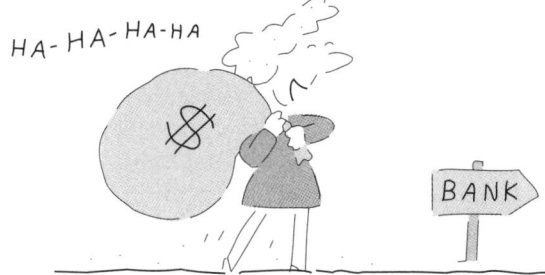

10 Principles for a Tricky Market

I have developed a game plan, a plan that will help today's investor survive and even succeed in this tricky market environment. *My plan is based on 10 principles that should guide all investors now...*

THE 10 PRINCIPLES

1. Protect your principal. More than anything else, after three years of a down market, you don't want to lose the capital that you have now.

2. Be your own benchmark. There are a lot of reasons not to compare your portfolio's performance with the S&P 500. Among other things, you will have bonds and cash as well as stocks.

Better: Compare how your investments are doing with how much you need to achieve your goals.

3. Buy and adapt. This is my way of saying that you need to have a dynamic, not rigid, approach. There are instances when buy and hold simply doesn't make very good sense... and this is one of them. Stubbornness in the face of a constantly changing investment environment is not smart.

4. No matter what your age, have an offensive plan *and* a defensive strategy. Even for young investors, it's a mistake to take on too much risk because the early money grows the most. Compounded over, say, 25 years, even 6% will turn into a large amount. Conversely, even an 80-year-old needs some risk (equities) in his/her portfolio—if only to overcome the effects of inflation.

5. Plan short term for the long term. Most planners force people to focus on the long term. This strategy can create paralysis in the short term.

Vern Hayden, CFP, president, Hayden Financial Planning Group LLC, Westport, CT 06880. He is author of *Getting an Investing Game Plan: Creating It, Working It, Winning It* (Wiley).

Best: Plan in three- to five-year segments that provide a guide as to what you should be doing now.

6. Look at the risk as well as returns. If you ask people if they would rather have a 50% chance of earning $10 or an 80% chance of earning $8, most people would wisely choose the latter. But that's not how they invest! Look at the risk undertaken by the dot-com mutual funds making 100% or more in the 1990s. At that time, the fear was missing out on those big returns.

7. Hit the books or the Internet to educate yourself about the basics of investing. For example, learn to tell the difference between sound advice and a sales pitch.

8. Avoid investing in sectors—unless you're immune to the high risks, and you crave the adrenaline rush. Sectors tend to go in and out of favor without much warning.

9. Keep score. Your mutual fund statements should clearly show how you're doing. Unfortunately, you may have to do the work yourself to monitor how your initial investment is growing…or not. Above all, do not just fork over your money and forget about it.

10. Act like a professional…or get the help of one. If you have the time, talent and temperament to manage your own money alone, go for it. Otherwise, find a professional financial planner who can work with your goals, your resources and your value system.

THE RIGHT MIND-SET

To have a successful game plan, investors need to have three Cs…

• **Commitment** to stay with the plan.

• **Consistency**—so as to resist getting off track with every shift in market sentiment.

• **Courage** to resist the latest hot investment trend.

You must pay attention to risk. Everybody pays lip service to risk these days, but I find that there is generally a big gap between the actual risk in someone's portfolio and his/her individual risk tolerance. Many investors are simply unaware of the risks inherent in their mutual funds. And risk levels fluctuate from time to time. They're not constant.

Most critical: The gap between how much you *think* you can afford to lose and the actual, emotional reaction when your portfolio drops by even 10%.

Problem: Most financial planners cite the numbers from investment research firm Ibbotson Associates in which large-cap stocks are said to average an 11% annual return since 1926. What these average figures don't explain is that the market has fluctuated between a loss of 43% and a gain of 54% in any one given year. I make it a policy to tell investors that they could face a big loss on a short-term basis.

We cannot control the market. We can only control the risk they're assuming. When people are extremely upset over losses, I'm quick to pull the plug and get them out as smoothly as possible. They will probably miss the first 10%, 15%, even 20% when the market finally turns up, but they can sleep at night.

Manage Investments Monthly

Talk with your financial advisers monthly about your investments. It's fine for busy people to hire financial advisers to manage their money and even make investments for them. But your money is still yours. Checking in regularly helps make that point—and keeps you involved in your investments, even if you do not manage them on a day-to-day basis.

Ellen Hoffman, Washington, DC, Business Week Online columnist specializing in retirement issues and author of The Retirement Catch-Up Guide *(Newmarket), www.retirementcatchup.com.*

More from Ellen Hoffman…

Read All Investment Statements

Monthly and annual statements can be a chore to read and understand. But people and computers make mistakes. It's your money—you need to keep a close watch on it. Even if you use a financial adviser, talk with him/her regularly—and keep track of your own investments.

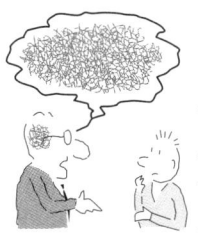

When to Hire an Investment Adviser

Investment advisers can be worth the cost if they prevent you from trading too frequently. A recent study showed that investors without advisers redeemed their mutual fund shares at a higher rate than investors with advisers—and ended up with significantly lower returns. On average, investors made 20% less money if they traded on their own than if they had advisers preventing them from trading too frequently.

Gavin Quill, senior vice president and director of research, Financial Research Corp., Boston, and leader of a study of fund investors' performance from 1996 through March 2000, conducted for Phoenix Investment Partners, Ltd., Hartford.

Find Investment Analysts With the Best Records

Investment analysts are under fire for giving careless advice and engaging in conflicts of interest. But some have provided much more accurate analysis and forecasts than others, and a new Web site identifies them. StarMine Investor identifies the most accurate forecaster for each of more than 4,000 stocks, as well as the most accurate forecasters for stock picking and earnings projections. It also identifies "bold" earnings estimates—forecasts by analysts with top-rated records that differ from the consensus.

More: Visit *www.starmine.com.*

How to Profit from Today's Headlines

Peter Navarro, PhD, associate professor of economics and public policy, Graduate School of Management at University of California, Irvine. He is author of If It's Raining in Brazil, Buy Starbucks: The Investor's Guide to Profiting from News and Other Market-Moving Events *(McGraw-Hill).*

Most investors haven't a clue about how to read stock market cycles or identify the next hot industry sector. But they can learn by practicing what I call *macrowave investing.* That means tracking and interpreting the broad economic developments shaping the stock market.

Once you know how to read the trends, you'll know which sectors are likely to thrive ...and which are likely to wilt. The tools you need are already at your fingertips—in newspapers and magazines and on radio, cable TV and the Internet.

SPOTTING MARKET TRENDS

Macrowave events are those that are important enough to influence the stock market. *They are...*

•**Economic news.** Some of the most important items are consumer confidence, monthly purchasing managers reports, employment, retail sales and worker productivity. Slightly less significant are gross domestic product, housing starts, industrial production, producer prices and US trade.

Example: High consumer confidence in 2001 signaled unexpected strength in consumer-driven sectors, such as housing and automobiles. Similarly, strong productivity helped the technology sector thrive in the 1990s. The wave of interest rate hikes by the Federal Reserve, several oil price shocks and broader inflationary fears led to the recession after March 2000.

•**Corporate news.** Earnings reports flag sectors in which profits are growing or lagging. Watch sector-leading companies for crucial indications of a sector's fortunes.

Example: If sector leader Intel warns of weak sales in semiconductors, as it did in late August 2002, then all the other semiconductor

■ *Your Money* ■ ■

manufacturers are likely to indicate declining profits. This trend will then expand to the makers of semiconductor-manufacturing equipment and—in a sector this large—eventually will be felt in the broad economy.

- **Government news.** The two key US government economic tools are monetary policy, which manages interest rates and the money supply…and fiscal policy, which determines taxation and government spending. Changes in these areas can move the market.

Example: In 2000, higher interest rates from the Fed contributed to popping the technology bubble, which pushed the economy into recession. Aggressive rate cuts in 2001 helped to moderate the recession while they simultaneously triggered large gains in economically sensitive sectors, such as autos and housing.

- **External shocks.** These include unpredictable events, including OPEC production cuts, the September 11 terrorist attacks and corporate financial scandals. These events can dramatically affect the entire market as well as individual sectors.

While these events are unpredictable, their impact is fairly easy to estimate. The September 11 attacks were a total shock—yet it was obvious that such sectors as hotels, airlines and insurance would suffer. It was equally obvious that sectors to benefit would include defense and alternatives to travel, such as teleconferencing.

The corporate accounting scandals, which began with Enron and spread to such companies as Global Crossing, Tyco and WorldCom, cast a pall over the entire stock market for many months.

TRACKING TRENDS

Publications, broadcasts and Web sites allow anyone to track trends. *My favorites…*

- **Active Trader.** The best magazine for investors and traders using macrowave theory.

Cost: $59.40*/yr. 800-341-9384 or *www.activetradermag.com*.

- **Barron's.** Weekend reading for a look back and forward at economic and market news.

Cost: $145/yr. 800-544-0422 or *www.barrons.com*.

*All prices subject to change.

- **Bloomberg News Service.** The Web site of this financial news service is one of the most useful for interpreting how economic events influence the markets. *www.bloomberg.com*.
- **Bloomberg TV.** Offers the most balanced global coverage.
- **Economy.com's Dismal Scientist Web page.** The best economic statistics on the Web.

Cost: $29.95*/month…$295/yr. *www.economy.com/dismal*.

- **Investor's Business Daily.** Read it daily, particularly the "Big Picture" column.

Cost: $295/yr. 800-831-2525 or *www.investors.com*.

SECTOR INVESTING

Exchange Traded Funds (ETFs) are important tools when investing in sectors. They are essentially sector-specific mutual funds that trade like stocks on the American Stock Exchange. You can invest in almost any sector using iShares, which track an entire industry sector…or HOLDRS, an ETF-like instrument that is a subset of about 20 of the sector's leading stocks.

By looking up their prices, earnings and volume histories, you can see which sectors are hot, which are turning hot and which are losing momentum. Quotes are listed in the financial sections of most newspapers.

Examples: Semiconductors (SMH), biotech (BBH) and oil services (OIH) are likely to suffer in a recession. Health care (IYH) and pharmaceuticals (PPH) should suffer less.

Information on ETFs—including stocks or indexes in each—is available on the American Stock Exchange Web site at *www.amex.com*.

The downside to ETFs is they include some stocks that are not a sector's strongest. I prefer to use ETFs to track a sector and also buy the three or so strongest stocks in the sector.

*All prices subject to change.

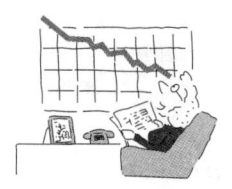

Stick with What You Have

If you are unsure about which stocks to buy in an erratic stock market, sticking with what you have is often the best strategy. If you bought and held gold through the 1970s and Japanese stocks through the 1980s, you would have beaten 99% of all investors. Similarly, investors who bought a representative sampling of US stocks at the start of the 1990s and sat tight for the next 10 years would have seen their money grow by 1,100% over the decade.

Bill Bonner, founder and chief executive, Agora Inc., publishers of financial and investment materials, Baltimore, *www.dailyreckoning.com.*

Wall Street Research You Can Trust

Dave Kansas, deputy managing editor of *The Wall Street Journal Online,* a former senior reporter for *The Wall Street Journal* and former editor in chief for *TheStreet.com.* He is author of *TheStreet.com Guide to Smart Investing in the Internet Era* (Doubleday).

In the past, only top clients of Wall Street brokerage houses had access to detailed stock research.

Now, there is much more available to the individual investor. But with some top Wall Street analysts under investigation for conflicts of interest, it is difficult to know which sources you can trust.

Instead of buying a stock based on a tip from a chat room or news program, here are the best resources and strategies you can use to do your own research…

•**Focus on the main valuation measurements.** *Stock screens allow you to sift through…*

•Price-to-earnings ratios (P/Es). Use P/E to compare any stock to its competitors, an industry average or the stock market.

•Price-to-book ratio. This tells you how the price of the stock compares to its *book value*—the amount you would get if you sold all the company's assets minus its liabilities. This measure is especially useful for companies that have a lot of "hard" assets, such as heavy equipment or financial stocks, for which the assets include loans and cash.

•Price-to-cash-flow ratio. This ratio measures how much cash a company is generating above its day-to-day business expenses. It is important because earnings can be finagled but cash is much harder to falsify. Excess cash flow lets a company raise dividends, make acquisitions, buy back its own stock and ride out problems. Useful when comparing businesses, the lower the price-to-cash-flow ratio, the more appealing the stock.

•**Watch the economy.** Gauge its effect on potential holdings.

Example: An RV manufacturer may have a great balance sheet and reasonable valuation, but because of the economy, fewer people will be buying recreational vehicles.

BEST STOCK SCREENS

My favorite free ones…

•**MSN Money** offers preset screens, including ones for small-caps with high momentum …cheapest stocks of large, growing companies…and highest-yielding stocks in the S&P 500 index. *http://moneycentral.msn.com.* Click on "Investing," "Stocks," then "Stock Screener."

•**Quicken.com.** This user-friendly stock screen will let you plug in up to 41 variables. *www.quicken.com.* Click on "Brokerage," then "Quotes & Research, then "Stock Screener," which is under "Additional Stock Research."

•**Zacks.com.** This site's screening tools let you slice and dice analyst earnings estimates as well as earnings surprises/disappointments in ways that are not possible anywhere else. *http://my.zacks.com.*

To use a stock screen: Type in the stock's ticker symbol or use the site's ticker-symbol lookup feature. Pick out the screen you want from the menu, and specify a time period.

DATABASES

•**EDGAR.** Public companies are required to file forms, such as quarterly reports and notices when insiders sell stock, with the Securities and Exchange Commission. These reports provide invaluable information.

■ *Your Money* ■ ■

Cost: Free at *www.sec.gov*...or for a monthly fee at *www.edgar-online.com,* which provides search capabilities for the EDGAR database.

•**Hoovers Online.** Comprehensive data on more than 12 million companies and 300 industries. Basic information is free of charge. *www.hoovers.com.*

THOUGHTFUL EXPERTS

•**James J. Cramer.** A former hedge fund manager and full-time market pundit. Writes daily market commentaries for *RealMoney,* the subscription arm of *TheStreet.com.*

Cost: $24.95/month...$229.95/yr. *www.thestreet.com/realmoney.*

•**Robert Green.** He reports from tech conferences and interviews CEOs to help you find stocks with a competitive edge.

Cost: $9.95/month and up. *www.briefing.com.*

•**Jon Markman.** His weekly column highlights companies with great long-term potential. *http://moneycentral.msn.com.* Click on "Investing," "Insight," then "SuperModels." Free.

•**Gary B. Smith.** A stock trader who uses technical analysis. He is a columnist for *RealMoney* and a commentator on Fox cable television's *Bulls & Bears.*

Cost: $24.95/month...$299.95/yr. *www.thestreet.com/realmoney.*

*All prices subject to change.

How to Protect Yourself from Bad Broker Advice

If you lost money as a direct result of a broker's advice, you may be able to recover some of it through arbitration. But you must be able to prove you bought the stock based directly and solely on the broker's flawed recommendation. Write a letter of complaint to the firm. If the matter is not resolved to your satisfaction within two months, file an arbitration claim quickly. Investors recover about half of their money more than half the time in securities arbitration.

To file a claim: The National Association of Securities Dealers' Dispute Resolution Forum (212-858-4400 or *www.nasdadr.com*) provides rules and filing costs for NASDAQ and AMEX claims. For NYSE filings, call 212-656-2772 or go to *www.nyse.com/arbitration.*

David E. Robbins, Esq., Kaufmann, Feiner, Yamin, Gilden & Robbins, LLP, and author of the Securities Arbitration Procedure Manual *(Lexis Law).*

Self-Defense Against Increasing Brokerage Fees

Investors are being charged more as brokerage firms try to increase revenues to make up for a sharp decline in trading. Some firms now charge order-handling fees...others are raising prices for everyone except frequent traders and people with substantial balances.

Self-defense: Combine all your accounts at one firm if that helps you meet requirements for lower fees. If family members also have accounts at the firm, ask your broker to consider the total of all accounts together for fee purposes. Get rid of small positions in mutual funds if the fund company charges a fee for small balances.

John Markese, PhD, president, American Association of Individual Investors, 625 N. Michigan Ave., Chicago 60611, www.aaii.com.

More from John Markese...

High-Net-Worth Services Now Available to More People

High-net-worth services are now available to more investors as banks and brokerages redefine what it means to be wealthy. It used to take $1 million or more to qualify for the special services, such as asset-allocation guidance and help with your tax and estate planning. Charles Schwab now provides private-client accounts to people who have $500,000 or more invested... Fidelity offers special services for those investing $300,000 or more...E*Trade has a $100,000 minimum for special services.

Caution: These accounts can carry annual fees. Know all the costs before opening one.

Easy Way to Find High-Dividend Stocks

Nancy Dunnan, financial adviser and author in New York City. Her latest book is *How to Invest $50–$5,000* (HarperCollins).

With the cut in the tax rate on dividends to 15% (5% for those in the 10% or 15% tax bracket), investors are hunting for dividends.

To locate high-dividend stocks, check out the "Summary & Index" section of *Value Line Investment Survey*. It's available at many public libraries and most brokerage offices. This weekly publication analyzes approximately 1,700 stocks. The Summary & Index (also known as Part I) has a page entitled "Highest Dividend Yielding Stocks." It gives the recent price, P/E ratio, yield and industry group, along with the stock's ranking (1 to 5) for "Timeliness and Safety." The stocks are arranged by yield, starting with the highest-yielding one in the *Value Line* universe. You can also find the 10 highest-yielding stocks, updated daily, at *www.dogsofthedow.com*.

Don't choose a stock *only* because it has a high dividend or because you expect dividends to become totally tax free—they may not. Be sure the company can cover its dividend with its earnings and not have to reduce or eliminate its payout during tough times. Its "fundamentals" need to be solid—it should have increasing revenues, and it should not be burdened by too much debt.

Also, with many companies you can choose not to receive the dividend check but instead have it automatically reinvested in additional shares of the company's stock.

Brokerage Statement Reminder

Julie Jason, JD, LLM, managing director, Jackson Grant & Co., investment advisers, 1177 High Ridge Rd., Stamford, CT 06905, *www.juliejason.com*.

Always open brokerage statements even if you fear bad news about your holdings. You could miss serious problems in your account such as unauthorized purchases, sales or incorrect wire transfers that must be corrected within 60 days.

Red flag: If you receive a so-called "happiness letter" that says, "We appreciate your business and hope you are happy with the service you receive...Please sign and return this letter..." it means that the branch manager has some reason to be concerned about your broker's handling of your account. He may suspect churning, unsuitable purchases or simply going against your investment objectives. Never just sign and return the letter. That might signify your approval.

Instead: Write to the branch manager and ask for a written response explaining his concern in detail.

Smarter Investing with Dollar Cost Averaging

Stick with dollar cost averaging—investing the same amount in the same investment at regular intervals, whether the market goes up or declines—even if the market stays in the doldrums. It can be upsetting to contribute money every month and see statement totals continue to decline. But that means you are buying more stock each month with the same amount of money. When the market turns up —as it always has in the past—you will have accumulated more shares and will be better positioned to benefit.

Dennis M. Gurtz, CPA, CFP, senior financial planner, American Express Financial Advisors Inc., Bethesda, MD.

■ *Your Money* ■ ■

How to Profit from Insider Trading Legally

Jonathan Moreland, New York City–based director of research, *InsiderInsights.com,* an independent on-line analysis newsletter.

Practically everyone knows that insider trading is illegal—except in circumstances when it isn't.

Government regulators are now preparing to increase penalties for improper profiteering following scandals at Enron, ImClone, WorldCom, etc.

Legal trading by insiders—exceptionally well-informed company executives and directors—will continue. So long as these trades are not based on specific, nonpublic information and are reported to the Securities and Exchange Commission (SEC), they are legitimate.

Although there is a time lag of as much as 40 days between the date of an insider trade and when the public sees it, academic studies have proven that the information can be used profitably.

HOW OUTSIDERS CAN PEEK

Insiders must file SEC Form 4 to disclose changes in their holdings of company stock. By tracking Form 4s, anyone can see what insiders are doing.

Look up these forms at no charge on the SEC's Web site, *www.sec.gov/edgar.shtml*...at Yahoo! Finance, *http://finance.yahoo.com*...or with Quicken, *www.quicken.com. Look for...*

•**Clusters of disclosure activity.** A single insider can be wrong.

•**Stock trades of a significant value—** $50,000 or more.

•**Relatively large percentage changes in holdings.** A vice president selling $100,000 in stock may be much more significant than the chairman unloading $500,000 if the former has decreased his/her position by a larger percentage than the chairman.

Several services collect and analyze all Form 4 activity—so you don't have to search company by company.

Some of these services include my own at *www.insiderinsights.com*...Washington Service (*www.washserv.com*)...and Vickers Stock Research (*www.vickers-stock.com*). Subscriptions may be tailored to include trading alerts, stock rankings and track records of trades by the insiders themselves.

Cost: $75* to $350 per month.

Investors should use the Form 4 information only as a beginning point. Growth in revenue and earnings is the key to stock appreciation. Stock prices generally do not fluctuate just because of insider trades.

Recent scandals are likely to raise requirements for reporting of insider trades. Proposed SEC changes would reduce filing time for insider trades that are larger than $100,000 to just two days.

*All prices subject to change.

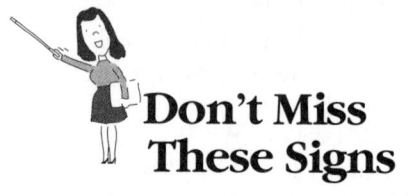

Don't Miss These Signs

Be on the lookout for the following warning signs of troubled firms...

•**Extensive use of *gain on sale* accounting,** which lets a company book profits based on estimated future profitability.

•**Below-average return on capital.**

•**A large amount of stock selling** by company executives and other insiders.

•**Projections about market potential** that run against broad market research.

•**Customer service problems** as well as bad press.

•**Abrupt resignation of senior executives in the company.**

You can find out about such things by searching the quarterly filings public companies are required to make to the Securities and Exchange Commission at *www.sec.gov/edgar.shtml*.

A. Larry Elliott, president and CEO, EDA, Inc., executive search firm, Vienna, VA, and coauthor of *How Companies Lie: Why Enron Is Just the Tip of the Iceberg* (Crown Business).

What Mutual Funds Won't Tell You

Larry E. Swedroe, director of research and a principal at Buckingham Asset Management, Inc., St. Louis. The firm manages more than $500 million for individuals and institutions. He is the author of *What Wall Street Doesn't Want You to Know* (St. Martin's) and *Rational Investing in Irrational Times* (Truman Talley).

Lean times are likely to make fund marketers more aggressive—and sneakier—than ever. *Here are five things you're not likely to hear from a mutual fund company...*

•**Our ads are misleading.** In advertisements and prospectuses, funds are required by the Securities and Exchange Commission to post their one-year, five-year, 10-year and/or since-inception returns through the end of the most recent quarter. But many fund families still make misleading claims.

Most common: Promoting the company's best one-year performer and implying that all of its funds are equally successful...or claiming to beat an inappropriate benchmark.

Example: A mid-cap fund should compare itself to the S&P 400 index, not the S&P 500 index, which represents the largest American companies. In the three years that ended December 31, 2002, the average mid-cap blend fund beat the S&P 500 by more than 10 percentage points but lagged the S&P 400.

•**Index funds are more profitable than managed funds** even in a down market. In bull markets, passively managed funds with low expenses and virtually 100% of assets invested in stocks are hard to beat.

In bear markets, active managers theoretically should have the upper hand because they can lighten up on equities before prices drop or short-sell stocks by betting that they will go down.

The facts speak otherwise. During the bear market—over the three years ending December 31, 2002—54% of large-cap funds, 72% of small-cap funds and 77% of mid-cap funds failed to beat their benchmarks, according to Standard & Poor's.

Fund managers were unable to call the start of the bear market in time to avoid major losses...or were suckered into bear-market rallies before the real bottom came.

A few managers will outperform in both bull and bear markets over the next decade. But trying to find those rare individuals is a form of gambling, not investing.

If you insist on active management, find a fund whose performance doesn't depend on a star manager. Look for low expenses...low turnover...and a consistent style.

•**Sector funds—except for real estate funds—are too risky.** Most sector funds, such as technology, telecommunications and health care, aren't for investors. They're for speculators. They typically have high expenses and are purchased and sold like hot stocks, which makes their performances volatile.

Real estate, on the other hand, is an effective diversifier of risk because it isn't highly correlated to other US equity asset classes and is a good hedge against inflation.

To gain broad real estate exposure, buy a mutual fund that invests in real estate investment trusts (REITs), which are publicly traded real estate companies. Over the long term, REITs have moved out of sync with the S&P 500 index, smoothing returns in choppy markets. From 1975 to 2002, REITs produced an average annual rate of return of 15%, versus 13.3% for the S&P 500, according to Ibbotson Associates.

Be sure to hold REIT funds in tax-deferred retirement accounts because they pay big dividends, which are taxed at a higher rate than capital gains.

For information on REITs: National Association of Real Estate Investment Trusts (800-362-7348 or *www.nareit.com*).

•**You need more diversification than just our S&P 500 index fund** can provide. Investors have flocked to index funds that track the S&P 500. But its makeup—the bigger the market capitalization of a company, the greater percentage it occupies in the index—means that megacap growth stocks dominate.

In fact, the biggest 50 stocks make up about 60% of the S&P index. At certain times, the two

■ *Your Money* ■ ■

largest, General Electric and Microsoft, each have accounted for 5% of the entire index.

Better: Invest among global asset classes. Put 70% in US index funds, (20% large-cap value, 20% small-cap value, 10% large-cap blend, 10% small-cap blend, 10% REITs) and 30% in international index funds.

•**Long-term bonds are risky.** Investors have not been compensated for the extra risk associated with bonds whose maturities are longer than three years. Over the period from 1975 to 2002, holding one-month US Treasury bills has provided a risk-free rate of return of 6.5%, according to Ibbotson Associates. Extending the maturity to one year increases the rate of return by about one percentage point. However, pushing the maturity to five years adds only an additional 0.3%...and extending it to 20 years actually causes returns to fall by almost 0.5%.

Best: Limit the maturity of your fixed-income holdings to between one and three years. Buy only US government bonds or municipal bonds rated AA or AAA. Or use a Vanguard short-term bond fund, and buy short-term Treasury bonds directly from the US Treasury Web site at *www.treasurydirect.gov.*

For tax-deferred accounts, I advise Treasury inflation-protection securities (TIPS), for which the principal and interest are adjusted for inflation. For more information, go to *www.publicdebt.treas.gov/com/comnewmk.htm.*

For taxable accounts, I like the Series I bonds. For information, go to *www.savingsbonds.gov.*

Use Expense Erosion

Expense erosion is better than expense ratio for deciding whether a mutual fund is too expensive to own. It relates cost to returns—a more expensive fund with substantially higher returns may be a good choice.

To calculate expense erosion: From a fund's five-year annualized gross return before expenses, calculate what percentage was lost to annual expenses.

Example: A fund with an annualized gross return of 5% and 1% expenses has 20% erosion.

C. Meyrick Payne, senior partner, Management Practice, market-focused strategic consultants, Stamford, CT.

Corporate Bond Warning

Don't invest in corporate bonds when looking for a safe place for money. The safest ones pay little more than US Treasuries—but are subject to state and local taxes, which Treasuries are not. Treasuries can be bought without commission...are easier than corporate bonds to resell before maturity...and cannot be called before maturity. There are some higher-rate corporate bonds that may seem attractive compared with Treasuries—but those rates come with significantly higher risk.

The bottom line: When buying bonds for safety, stick with Treasury issues or insured/pre-refunded munis.

Andrew Tobias, Miami, FL–based author of *The Only Investment Guide You'll Ever Need* (Harvest).

Better Way to Buy Bonds

Buying savings bonds with certain credit cards can boost the return from a bond purchase. Bonds are available for purchase at *www.savingsbonds.gov.* If you buy them with a credit card that offers cash back, you are effectively buying the bonds at a discount—which raises your net return. Even if you sell the bonds within the first five years and pay a penalty of three months' interest, you may still net more with a cash-back credit card than the bonds officially pay.

Daniel J. Pederson, president of The Savings Bond Informer, Detroit, and author of *Savings Bonds: When to Hold, When to Fold and Everything In-Between* (TSBI).

Better Investing

Don't Hang on to These Savings Bonds

Americans own more than $9.4 billion of savings bonds that have stopped paying interest, forfeiting more than $350 million in interest annually.

If you own old savings bonds, learn what they are worth and whether they are still paying interest. Just click on "Have Your Bonds Stopped Earning Interest?" at *www.savingsbonds.gov.*

Barbara Weltman, attorney in Millwood, NY, www.bwideas.com. She is author of many books, including Bottom Line's Very Shrewd Money Book *(Bottom Line Books).*

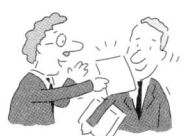

Smart CD Buying

Buy certificates of deposit (CDs) and annuities on-line to get the best interest rates. Look for sites that evaluate and compare these products, such as *www.bankcd.com...www.annuityratewatch.com...*and *www.bankrate.com.* Once you find the product and the rate you want there, go to the site of the firm offering that product.

Jim Bruene, founder and editor of the Online Banking Report, *Seattle.*

Second Homes Are Seldom Good Investments

There are some financial advantages to owning a second home—mortgage-interest tax deduction...and depreciation and expense deductions if you rent out the house for more than 15 days. But second homes can be expensive to maintain, and the insurance costs can be high. Consider purchasing a second home only if you want to use it for your own vacations. Homes that are located on oceanfront property have the greatest appreciation potential.

Michael Abelson, PhD, real estate consultant and associate professor of management, Texas A&M University, College Station.

Investment Real Estate Can Supercharge Your Portfolio

William G. Brennan, CPA/PFS, CFP, Capital Management Group, LLC, Washington, DC 20036.

With savings yields at historically low levels and the future of the stock market uncertain, investors are looking for alternatives.

One possibility: Real estate.

The forecast for investment property looks encouraging...

•**Demand for commercial and residential space will grow** as the economy rebounds.

•**Supply is reasonable** because the real estate sector did *not* experience overbuilding in the 1990s' economic boom.

Incentive: Tax advantages can help boost returns from direct real estate investments.

Potential problem: Owning an investment property can be a very time-consuming proposition. Do not underestimate the effort that will be involved.

FIRST THINGS FIRST

Tax breaks won't turn a bad real estate investment into a good one. So, selecting a promising property remains a prime concern. *In addition to location, look for...*

•**Stage of development.** There's certainly more risk—and more growth potential—in buying a to-be-built property, rather than one that's already fully rented.

•**Condition.** If you're considering the purchase of an existing building, first find out if it needs repairs.

Your Money

- **Price.** Don't pay more than other buyers are paying for similar properties. Your accountant can help you evaluate the investment value of a property based on net operating cash income and estimated annual appreciation.
- **Legal entanglements.** A savvy lawyer can ensure that you will hold clear title and avoid costly environmental headaches, such as soil contamination.

LIMITED LIABILITY

Increasingly, the owners of investment real estate are creating limited liability companies (LLCs) to hold each property. *This strategy offers key advantages...*

- **LLCs are taxed like partnerships,** so corporate income tax is avoided. Losses flow through to the owners, known as members.
- **LLCs confer limited liability.** Any claims arising from operating the property won't jeopardize your other assets. Conversely, if you are personally subject to a creditor's claims, real estate held in an LLC may be protected.
- **Most states permit one-member LLCs.**

LEVERAGE

Among the tax breaks available to real estate investors are interest deductions. If you use a mortgage to buy property, you can write off the interest.

Example: You buy investment property for $1 million, paying $200,000 down and taking out an $800,000 interest-only mortgage. With an 8% interest rate, you'll owe $64,000 a year in interest, which you can deduct.

Most real estate investors want the property to pay out enough net income from operations to cover mortgage payments. Otherwise, they'll have to go into their own pockets to make these payments.

DEPRECIATION DEDUCTIONS

In addition, real estate investors benefit from depreciation deductions, which represent a non-cash expense.

In general, commercial real estate and improvements must be depreciated over 39 years. For residential properties, the scheduled depreciation is 27.5 years.

But not every penny invested in real estate needs to be depreciated over such a long time period. Items such as carpeting and furniture can be classified as personal property, depreciable over seven years. Parking lots and landscaping may be classified as land improvements, depreciable over 15 years. However, the land itself is *not* depreciable.

Hire a professional appraiser or valuation expert to help you classify various components of your real estate investment for speedier depreciation deductions.

SHELTERED CASH FLOW

Suppose that you buy a $1 million property with an $800,000, 8% mortgage, as described earlier. Your net operating income (NOI) is $100,000, while your depreciation deduction is about $36,000.

From your $100,000 NOI, you'll pay (and deduct) $64,000 in interest, which leaves you with $36,000 in cash—an 18% return on your $200,000 down payment. Your $36,000 depreciation deduction will leave you at breakeven, on paper.

Result: Even though you pocket $36,000, you'll owe no income tax.

Instead, suppose the depreciation deduction actually caused a tax loss. Can you deduct that loss? *It depends on various circumstances, thanks to the passive activity rules...*

- **If you have passive income,** perhaps from another real estate investment, the loss can offset this income.
- **If you're classified as a real estate professional,** it may be easier for you to deduct this loss.
- **For most people,** passive losses up to $25,000 per year are deductible if adjusted gross income (AGI) is less than $100,000.
- **If your AGI is above $100,000,** your ability to deduct passive losses will gradually fade to zero, at an AGI of $150,000.

Examples: Suppose you have a $24,000 loss. With AGI of $102,000 or less, you could deduct the entire amount. At $125,000 in AGI, halfway through the phaseout range, you can deduct $12,500 worth of passive losses.

The other $11,500 ($24,000 minus $12,500) is a suspended loss, and suspended losses can be deducted against any future passive income.

Otherwise, all suspended losses are deductible when you dispose of the property.

THE ENDGAME

Depreciation deductions, as described earlier, reduce your annual tax obligation *and* reduce your basis in the property.

Trap: When you dispose of your property, you'll owe tax on the depreciation you've taken, at a 25% rate.

Example: Over 10 years, your $1 million investment has appreciated to $1.4 million. However, you have taken $360,000 worth of depreciation deductions. That $360,000 will be taxed at 25% on a sale, for a tax obligation of $90,000. In addition, your $400,000 appreciation will be taxed at 18%, for a tax of $72,000.

Result: On a property sale, you will owe $162,000 in tax. State and local taxes may add to the amount you'll owe.

Strategy: Instead of selling, you might refinance the property.

Example: With a property that's worth $1.4 million and an 80% mortgage loan, you can borrow $1,120,000. Repaying the original $800,000 loan leaves you with $320,000 in cash. That $320,000 in cash will be tax free. No sale has been made, so no tax is triggered.

Caution: You now have a larger debt to service, so this strategy will only make sense if the property's NOI has increased over the years, providing more cash to cover the additional debt service.

Refinancing your property isn't the only alternative to a sale. If you're moving to another part of the country, or if you want to own a different type of property, a like-kind exchange under Tax Code Section 1031 may be appropriate.

You can trade for any other type of real estate investment property. Typically, you'll sell your property first, have an intermediary hold those proceeds, then direct the intermediary to purchase a replacement property. As long as you receive neither cash nor debt reduction, no tax will be due.

Depending upon future tax law, if you die while holding your original investment property or replacement property, your heirs may inherit it with a step-up in basis.

With a basis step-up, all the gains and depreciation deductions taken during your lifetime may avoid income tax.

MAKING IT A HOME

Another exit strategy may be viable if you own a modest investment property—exchange that property for a house or a condo of comparable value.

How: Rent this house or condo for at least enough time to file a tax return, treating it as rental property. Then, move into it yourself.

Under current law, no tax will be triggered on the exchange. You will retain the basis you had in the property as investment real estate.

After making this house your principal residence for at least two years, you can sell it and exclude up to $250,000 worth of taxable gain from your income. If you're married, the exclusion from tax goes up to $500,000.

---

10 Top Tax Strategies for a Shrunken Portfolio

Arthur M. Seltzer, CPA, Brown Smith Wallace, LLC in St. Louis. He writes on tax matters and is a regular guest on a local radio station's financial information program. He gives presentations on estate planning and other tax-related issues to lay and professional groups.

The eyes of the world are on Wall Street these days. While much of the gains of the past decade have been wiped out, stock prices are improving once again.

US stocks have rebounded from depressions, World Wars and other catastrophes of the past 100 years, and they're bouncing back from the recent chaos, too. The following savvy moves can help you cut taxes and position yourself to better cash in on the market upswing.

Here's what to do...

•**Double up on loss positions.** If you're holding stocks that are down, this is an ideal time to take losses, particularly if you can do so without affecting your investment position. Net capital losses of up to $3,000 per year, in excess of gains, may be deducted.

■ *Your Money* ■ ■

Problem: You can't take a capital loss if you buy the identical security within 30 days before or after the sale, which is known as the "wash-sale rule."

Tactic: Buy an equal amount of the security you wish to sell. After waiting for 31 days, you can sell the original lot and avoid the wash-sale rule. You can also sell first and wait 31 days to repurchase the stock, but then you lose out if the stock goes up in the interim.

Example: In 1998, you bought 100 shares of ABC stock at $50. In November 2003, ABC sells at $20, and you believe the company is undervalued. On November 1, 2003, you buy another 100 shares, paying $20 per share. On December 2, 2003, with the trading price at $30, you sell the original lot that you bought at $50.

You can take a $2,000 capital loss on the sale of ABC. You have cash of $1,000, less commissions, and you still own the stock.

An alternative would be to sell ABC and buy XYZ, which is in the same industry and is also down. You don't have to wait 31 days or come up with additional cash.

• **Buy stocks "on sale."** This can be an excellent time to buy depressed stocks. If they move up quickly, you can sell at a profit.

Trap: Gains taken on securities held for a year or less are short-term capital gains and are taxed at ordinary rates, up to 35% this year.

Losses you realize on your existing holdings can completely offset such gains, delivering tax-free profits. You may be able to take enough losses to zero out any gains, in which case there is no reason to wait out the year before cashing in your profits.

• **Give family members stocks you expect to appreciate in value.** The annual gift tax exclusion is $11,000 per recipient ($22,000 for gifts given by a married couple).

This means you can give up to $11,000/$22,000 worth of stock to each child, grandchild, friend or relative free of all gift tax. At lower stock market levels, more shares can be given away without exceeding the exclusion amounts.

If the shares you give rise in price, that appreciation will be out of your taxable estate.

Tactic: If the stocks are worth less than your cost, you can sell them, realize a capital loss and then give away the cash from the sale.

• **Fund Section 529 plans and Coverdell education savings accounts.** In recent years, Congress has developed some wonderful tax-saving opportunities to accumulate funds for educating your children and grandchildren. Investment earnings inside Coverdell education savings accounts (formerly education IRAs) and Section 529 plans can be withdrawn tax free if used for specified education expenses.

When the stock market is below its previous high, you can buy more with the dollars you invest. The future growth is taken from your estate, but you can retain a degree of control over the accounts.

The increased potential for tax-free growth from a market rebound makes this an especially good time to create and fund these vehicles.

• **Fund your IRAs and Roth IRAs now.** For 2003 and 2004, a working taxpayer can contribute up to $3,000 to an IRA. For one-income couples, the nonworking spouse also can make a $3,000 contribution.

As an alternative, you can contribute $3,000 to a Roth IRA. Those contributions are not deductible, but subsequent withdrawals will be tax free if you follow the rules. Your modified adjusted gross income (MAGI) must be less than $95,000 (single return) or $150,000 (joint return) to make full Roth IRA contributions. At slightly higher MAGI levels, partial contributions are permitted.

You don't have to make your 2003 IRA contribution until April 15, 2004, but if you contribute now you'll enjoy tax-free appreciation inside the account if stocks rise.

• **Make catch-up IRA, Roth IRA and 401(k) contributions.** If you're 50 or older this year, you can contribute an extra $500 to an IRA or Roth IRA and an extra $2,000 in 2003 and $3,000 in 2004 to your 401(k). Again, you might as well put this money in now, to buy low. By April, your investment might buy a lot less than it does now.

• **Fund other retirement plans.** If you're self-employed or a business owner, you may be able to sponsor a SEP or some other qualified retirement plan. Chances are you expect to make a contribution sometime in 2004 and take a deduction on your 2003 return.

You may be able to make contributions as late as October 15, 2004, if you get a filing extension, and still take a 2003 tax deduction. But it's best to contribute now to lock in a tax deduction.

You also may be able to make tax-deductible contributions now to shelter taxable income from freelancing or a sideline business.

●**Convert an IRA to a Roth IRA.** You can move some of the depressed stocks from your IRA into a Roth if you qualify and are willing to pay taxes on the current value of the stock… which may not be much.

Example: Converting an IRA that was worth $30,000 in 2003 would have generated $30,000 in taxable income. If that IRA is currently worth only $20,000, additional taxes are reduced by one-third.

Even better, you can pick and choose which securities to convert, selecting stocks that maximize potential growth and limiting the tax cost to the amount you are willing to pay. You can pick the time to convert specific investments.

Fallback position: If your guess is wrong and the stocks go down more, you may be able to "recharacterize" the Roth back to a regular IRA and avoid paying the tax.

Roth payoff: After five years and once you reach age 59½, all Roth IRA withdrawals are tax free.

Note: You aren't eligible to convert a regular IRA to a Roth if your AGI exceeds $100,000.

●**Take required minimum distributions in depressed stock.** If you are age 70½ or older, you must take minimum distributions from your IRA. You may also have to take distributions from other tax-deferred retirement plans.

If your IRA now includes stocks that are depressed, but that you expect to recover, think about taking the distribution in stock rather than in cash.

Example: Say you must take at least a $30,000 distribution from your IRA this year. Instead of cash, you can take out $30,000 worth of stocks that are reduced from their highest prices.

You will owe tax on the distribution, of course, but subsequent appreciation in the stock will be taxed when you sell it—at favorable capital gains rates, which can be as low as 5%. If you hold the stock for the rest of your life, the potential taxable gain will disappear at your death.

Getting the stock out of the IRA will reduce the distributions required in the future.

●**Remove depressed stocks from your IRA.** Your income may be too high for you to be eligible for a Roth IRA conversion. In this case, you still can get some of the same advantages by moving depressed issues from your IRA to a taxable brokerage account.

You'll owe tax on the withdrawal, but lower stock prices will hold down your tax bill. As long as you're at least age 59½, you'll avoid the 10% early withdrawal penalty.

Once stocks are out of the IRA, subsequent appreciation will qualify for favorable long-term capital gains rates and a basis step-up at death.

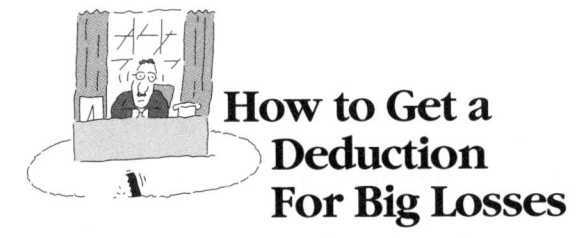

How to Get a Deduction For Big Losses

Janice M. Johnson, JD, CPA, financial consultant, 301 E. 52 St., New York City 10022. She was previously with American Express.

Active stock traders can get a full loss deduction for big losses in their portfolios, instead of only a capital loss deduction, which is limited to the amount of net capital gain plus $3,000 a year.

How: File a Section 475(f) "mark to market" election. This causes gains and losses to be taxed at year-end even if not realized, and makes losses incurred during the year or at year-end deductible against ordinary income.

Requirement: You must be a stock "trader." You should trade frequently, hold most shares one year or less to profit from short-term price swings and expend a significant effort in managing your trading.

■ *Your Money* ■ ■

A 475(f) election for 2004 must be filed by April 15, 2004. It makes *gains* taxable at ordinary rates, too—but you can save tax-favored long-term gains for other investments by segregating them from your trading account. Consult a tax professional.

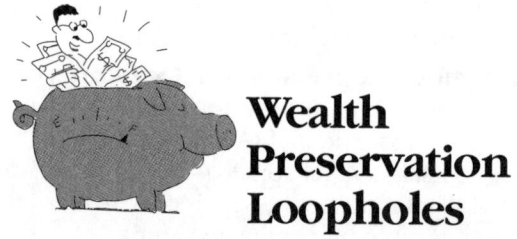

Wealth Preservation Loopholes

Edward Mendlowitz, CPA, partner, Mendlowitz Weitsen, LLP, CPAs, K2 Brier Hill Ct., East Brunswick, NJ 08816.

To hang on to your hard-earned money, it is important to understand the tax consequences of major financial decisions before you make them.

Loophole: **Begin this learning process by reviewing your tax returns for the past three years.** Line by line, look for items that have changed and made a difference in your taxes. Watch for those items in the future. If you typically have large capital gains income, for example, consider offsetting it by selling securities on which you have losses.

Loophole: **Exercise some of your incentive stock options (ISOs) each year.** Often, that's better than waiting until just before the expiration date to exercise them all.

Reason: When you exercise ISOs, the difference between the fair market value of the stock and the exercise price is a "tax preference" item. This is included in the alternative minimum tax (AMT) calculation if the stock is not sold in the year acquired. Avoid the AMT by exercising small amounts of ISOs each year, just below the amount that would put you into an AMT position.

Loophole: **Shelter part-time business income with a tax-deferred retirement plan.** In 2003, you can contribute up to $40,000 to a defined-contribution plan ($41,000 in 2004).

Strategy 1: When net income from a part-time business is less than $9,000 in 2004, you may be better off with a SIMPLE plan, to which you can contribute up to $9,000 a year. To take deductions for 2004, you must set up a plan by October 1, 2004.

If your net business income exceeds $9,000, you might be better off with a 401(k) plan, to which you can contribute up to $13,000 per year. If your income is more than $13,000, you might be better off with a combined 401(k) and defined-contribution plan where you can contribute 25% of income plus up to $13,000. For example, if your net income is $20,000, you can contribute $18,000 ($5,000 plus $13,000).

In addition, people age 50 or older by year-end can add $3,000 more to the 401(k) in 2004.

Strategy 2: People over age 50 should consider setting up a *defined-benefit* retirement plan. It may permit much larger deductible contributions than under a defined-contribution plan. You have until December 31 to create a qualified plan for 2004.

Loophole: **Have shares of stock in your employer's company that are held in a 401(k) plan distributed directly to you** rather than rolled over to an IRA. Employees who receive shares of corporate stock that have been contributed to their 401(k) accounts have two choices when taking shares out. *They are...*

•**Roll over the shares into an IRA** and pay no tax.

•**Have the shares distributed to them and pay taxes...**and possibly owe an early withdrawal penalty.

When you roll over company stock into an IRA, you or your IRA beneficiaries will pay tax on the full value of the shares when they are withdrawn from the account. IRA distributions are taxed at ordinary income rates—up to 35%.

Better: Have all the company stock in the 401(k) distributed directly to you and pay tax at the time of distribution. If the stock is greatly appreciated, consider paying tax on the cost of the stock to the company when it was contributed to the plan, not its fair market value.

When you then hold the shares for more than one year and sell them, the proceeds will be taxed at favorable long-term capital gains rates.

Loophole: **Analyze a mutual fund's capital gains exposure before you buy shares.** While funds must distribute their dividends and interest to their shareholders every year, nothing prevents them from building up long-term gains in their portfolios. So two funds that look identical may produce very different after-tax returns when they sell the shares they own.

Example: Because of appreciation, the value of a fund may include as much as 50% of capital gains appreciation. If a fund manager sold stock, shareholders would receive their proportionate share of long-term capital gains. Another fund's value might comprise only 10% of unrealized capital gains, and the tax bite to shareholders would be much lower.

Call the fund or look for the capital gains exposure in analyses prepared by Morningstar, Lipper or other fund data providers.

Loophole: **Consider using family limited partnerships for gifts of closely held stock.** When making gifts of closely held shares to a family limited partnership, you can retain the general partnership interest and give children the limited partnership units over time. The general partner has complete control over the partnership.

Tax impact: Gifts of family limited partnership units can be discounted—that is, reduced in value—to take into account minority interests and lack of control and marketability. This reduces the gift tax owed on the interests.

Gifts of family limited partnership interests also remove future appreciation in shares transferred from the estate of the original owner.

Loophole: **Instead of cash, donate appreciated long-term stock to favorite charities.** When you do this, you can deduct the full fair market value of the shares and owe no capital gains tax on the stock's buildup in value since you bought it.

Example: You own 100 shares of stock, bought 10 years ago for $15 per share. When you donate the shares, now worth $50, you deduct the full $5,000 fair market value—not your $1,500 cost. You also avoid paying capital gains tax on the $3,500 of appreciation in the shares.

More from Edward Mendlowitz...

How to Avoid Taxes When Buying And Selling Mutual Funds

Even if you lost money in the bear market, you may still owe hefty taxes on your mutual funds. *Use these techniques to avoid or at least lessen them...*

• **Use *specific identification accounting* when selling shares.** The IRS generally calculates gains and losses on fund shares with "first-in, first-out" (FIFO) accounting, which means using the price that you paid for the shares you have held the longest.

Specific identification accounting allows you to sell select shares to get the best tax result.

Example: You bought shares of the same fund first for $10, then $30 and then $60. They are worth $40 now. If you sell a portion of the shares, under FIFO accounting rules you will be deemed to sell the $10 shares first—for a $30 taxable gain.

Specific identification rules, on the other hand, let you select the shares you sell. You can sell the $60 shares to produce a deductible capital loss. If you want to report a gain, select the $10 or $30 shares.

This method for accounting can create a specific amount of gain that can be matched against an offsetting loss.

Specific identification accounting requires more paperwork than FIFO. You must keep records showing purchase prices and dates for all fund shares. Your sell order must specify the specific shares to be sold on the sale confirmations. Your broker or fund firm may not track these records—you must do it.

• **Buy tax-efficient funds.** Investors incur two types of tax on mutual funds—tax on the sale of fund shares and tax on gains earned inside the fund. Gains earned inside the fund are distributed to shareholders annually as taxable dividends.

Trap I: Tax bills from an actively managed fund often include more short-term capital gains, which are taxed at a higher rate than long-term capital gains. This lowers your total after-tax return.

■ *Your Money* ■ ■

Trap II: The actively managed funds have higher fees and expenses than most index funds, which are not actively managed. Compare fees on similar funds.

These factors can significantly reduce mutual fund returns. To protect yourself, look for index funds or actively managed mutual funds that are tax efficient. Funds state in their prospectuses if they manage trades to minimize taxes. You also can find this information on fund Web sites or at *www.morningstar.com*.

•**Track reinvested dividends.** When dividends from a fund are reinvested, they become, in effect, the cost of new shares.

Add the dividends to the cost basis of your holdings when you sell your shares. If you don't, you risk overstating your taxable gain or understating your loss.

Example: You purchase fund shares for $5,000 and receive $100 in dividends, which you reinvest in additional shares. Your basis in the shares is now $5,100.

•**Check a fund's capital gains exposure.** Even tax-efficient funds can incur large capital gains when they sell to finance shareholder redemptions. That means you might owe a gains tax even as the fund value declines. Go to *www.morningstar.com* to find out how much of a fund's value is preexisting appreciation on investments. If you are comparing two similar funds and one's value is based more on appreciation, the other fund may be the better investment.

•**Time purchases and sales around the dividend date.** Every mutual fund has an annual dividend date on which it distributes internal gains—and the tax liability on them. If you buy a fund just before the dividend date, which typically is close to the end of the year, you will pay a price that already has been factored into the dividend—but you will owe tax on it. If you wait until after the distribution, you will pay the same price and avoid the tax.

Also sell fund shares just before the dividend distribution.

•**Avoid wash sales.** If your fund shares have declined in value but are still an attractive investment, you might want to sell them for a tax-deductible loss and repurchase them later.

Wait 31 days to repurchase shares. The wash-sale rule bars deductions for losses incurred on securities sold and repurchased within 30 days.

If you do not want to reduce your stock market investments at that time, use money from the sale to purchase shares of a different fund that has a similar objective and track record or an index fund.

Silver Lining to the Bear Market

Many excellent established funds have big losses on their books. They can carry these losses forward and avoid distributing capital gains for years. Investors in these funds do not have to pay any tax on the funds' gains until the retained losses are used up.

Steve Savage, editor, No-Load Fund Analyst, *Orinda, CA 94563.*

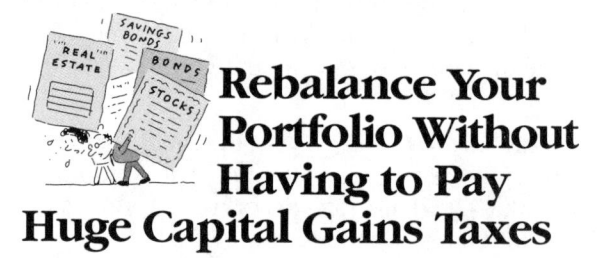

Rebalance Your Portfolio Without Having to Pay Huge Capital Gains Taxes

Glenn E. Frank, CPA/PFS, CFP, principal, Tanager Financial Services Inc., 800 South St., Waltham, MA 02453.

A sophisticated asset allocation divides up your portfolio between stocks and bonds, growth and value stocks, large- and small-company stocks, etc.

Rebalancing is a technique for bringing the portfolio back into line after some assets have grown and others have shrunk. The rocky markets of the past few years highlight the importance of rebalancing, which may require the advice of a tax professional.

Example: During the late 1990s, the large-company growth stocks (especially technology issues) experienced tremendous returns. For many investors, that portion of their portfolios grew while others dwindled.

Investors who rebalanced at the peak of the market would have trimmed large-capitalization growth stocks and put the proceeds into bonds, value stocks and small-cap stocks. Such tactics would have limited the investor's exposure to the bear market of 2000–2002, which hurt large-cap growth stocks badly.

Morningstar reports that large-cap growth funds lost 14.1% in 2000, 22.6% in 2001 and another 28% in 2002. At the same time, bond funds had three excellent years while small-cap value funds returned 19% in 2000 and 17.2% in 2001—during a bear market! Small-cap value funds did, however, have a negative 9% return in 2002, but they still outperformed large-cap growth funds significantly.

TAXES AND REBALANCING

On paper, rebalancing makes perfect sense. You sell what is high and buy what is low. Although there are no guarantees, investment cycles generally recur over time, meaning that today's losers may be in the winner's circle tomorrow. *But investors face two problems with this strategy…*

- **Emotions.** Many investors find it difficult to sell what has been hot and invest in what's been cold. They fear losing future profits.

- **Taxes.** Rebalancing your portfolio means selling those assets that have gained a great deal. If this rebalancing is done in a taxable account—rather than in an IRA or a 401(k)—taxes will be due.

Taken together, these two concerns keep many investors from rebalancing their portfolios. Although it may be difficult to overcome the emotional hurdle, the tax pitfall can be cleared by dividing your portfolio.

THE INSIDE STRATEGY

Consider using a variable annuity to facilitate rebalancing.

How it works: You buy a variable annuity from a financial firm, investing the money in a lump sum or in a series of payments. The money you invest can be directed among several subaccounts, which may resemble mutual funds. Indeed, mutual fund portfolio managers manage many variable annuity subaccounts.

This strategy makes sense if you have only a relatively small amount in your self-directed retirement plan. If you have a large IRA, for example, it is not necessary to purchase a variable annuity as a rebalancing tool.

Tax advantages: Inside a variable annuity, any investment income or capital gain remains untaxed. Switching among subaccounts won't generate a tax bill.

Disadvantages: Variable annuities generally have higher costs than mutual funds. Also, all income is taxed at ordinary rates when you take withdrawals, so you cannot benefit from favorable long-term capital gains rates.

TAX-DEFERRED REBALANCING

If you divide your portfolio between a regular taxable account and a variable annuity, you'll be able to rebalance without owing taxes.

When rebalancing means taking gains, you would take them inside the deferred annuity, avoiding taxes. New money going into the taxable account can keep your financial portfolio in balance.

Example: You have a $500,000 taxable portfolio. With half of that money, you purchase a variable annuity.

If you're going to liquidate investments to buy a variable annuity, choose assets that will produce a tax loss or a small gain upon sale.

Once you invest in a variable annuity, certain asset classes are best held there, rather than in a taxable account.

Example: If your asset allocation calls for you to hold real estate investment trusts (REITs) and/or junk bonds, they should be held inside the annuity. These assets tend to produce a great deal of dividends or interest each year, the tax on which is deferred inside the annuity.

If your investment mix includes tax-exempt municipal bonds or municipal bond funds, they should be held *outside* the variable annuity.

Otherwise, your asset classes should be divided fairly evenly between your taxable account and the variable annuity. When it's time to rebalance, you take your gains inside the annuity.

Example: Your asset allocation calls for you to hold 10% of your portfolio in small-cap value stocks. According to your plan, you would rebalance if that allocation tops 15%.

Say your small-cap value stocks now are worth $80,000 (16% of your $500,000 portfolio). You need to sell $30,000 worth of those value stocks to get down to $50,000 (the 10% target).

Selling $30,000 worth of small-cap value stocks in a taxable account would trigger a sizable gain.

But if you hold half ($40,000) of your small-cap value stocks in a variable annuity subaccount, you can sell $30,000 of those stocks and incur no taxable gain. That $30,000 can go into large-cap growth stocks, international stocks or other depressed asset classes, bringing your allocation back to desired levels.

What if you have only $20,000 worth of small-cap value stocks inside the annuity? You could sell them all, reducing your total holdings to $60,000 (12%).

Eventually, new money you're investing in your taxable account could go to other asset classes, reducing the small-cap value portion.

HELP WITH HARVESTING

Using a variable annuity as a mirror portfolio can help with another problem you'll face when you rebalance—harvesting tax losses.

Good tax planning calls for you to take capital losses when securities decline because those losses can be deducted or used to offset capital gains.

Trap: Taking losses means selling the losers, which is exactly the opposite intention of a rebalancing strategy.

Example: In 2003, you might have taken losses on international stocks. That would have reduced your allocation to those stocks even further, at a time when rebalancing called for cutting small-cap value and adding international equities.

Solution: With this mirror-portfolio approach, you could have taken losses on international stocks in your taxable account. By buying international stocks inside your variable annuity, you could maintain or increase your overall commitment to that asset class.

COMPREHENSIVE PLANNING

Look at your taxable accounts and your variable annuities as separate components of your overall portfolio.

Don't forget to include your holdings inside an IRA, 401(k) or another tax-deferred retirement plan.

Example: If you have $250,000 in taxable accounts, $250,000 in a variable annuity and $50,000 in a 401(k), your asset allocation should be based on a total portfolio of $550,000. A 10% small-cap value allocation would mean holding $55,000 in small-cap value stocks, counting all of your holdings.

Bottom line: Base your rebalancing on your overall portfolio. For the best tax results, take losses in your taxable account and gains within your tax-deferred variable annuity or your tax-deferred retirement account.

TIME AND MONEY

Keep three points in mind when you shop for a variable annuity...

• **Breadth.** You'll want a variable annuity with enough subaccounts to include the asset classes in your portfolio.

• **Cost.** A variable annuity probably will have higher expenses than a portfolio of mutual funds. Nevertheless, there are variations among variable annuities, so look for one with relatively low costs.

• **Holding period.** Do not buy a variable annuity if you expect to bail out soon—you'll owe surrender fees plus a 10% penalty before age 59½.

However, if you hold on to it for 10 years or longer, the tax advantages likely will outweigh the extra expenses you'll incur as well as the lost tax benefit of long-term capital gains.

Tax-Deductible Investment Expenses

Tax-deductible investment expenses include fees paid to accountants, financial planners and lawyers for tax and investment advice... custodial and trustee fees paid to brokerages and mutual fund companies...phone and postal expenses for managing accounts...annual cost of a safe-deposit box to hold investments...

and subscriptions to investment publications. These miscellaneous itemized deductions are deductible to the extent that they exceed 2% of your adjusted gross income.

Caution: If you are subject to alternative minimum tax—as more people are every year—you will lose some or all of these deductions.

The New Rules of Personal Investing by financial correspondents of *The New York Times* (Times).

Don't Make Costly Tax Return Mistakes

Jerry Wade, CFP, CFS, and Ryan Berg, CPA/PFS. Mr. Wade is president and Mr. Berg is manager, Tax Planning Services, Wade Financial Group, Inc., 5500 Wayzata Blvd., Minneapolis 55416.

When you put together your return, you'll want to take every legitimate tax deduction that you can. Unfortunately, some investors make expensive errors and omissions. *Here are their biggest mistakes...*

CARRYFORWARDS

Only $3,000 worth of net capital losses can be deducted against ordinary income every year. Any excess can be carried forward.

Strategy: Check prior tax returns for loss carryforwards. If you have net capital gains in 2003, those carried-over losses can offset them.

Other types of carryforwards from investments may be valuable now.

Example: You were in an old tax shelter that wound up last year or you sold rental property. Suspended passive losses now can be deducted against gains from that venture.

Similarly, if you rent investment property, including a vacation home, you may have suspended passive losses you were unable to deduct. If that property generated taxable income last year, old losses may wipe out your tax obligation.

ITEMIZED DEDUCTIONS

Miscellaneous itemized deductions in excess of 2% of your adjusted gross income (AGI) can be deducted. *Investment expenses that fall into this category include...*

- **Subscriptions to publications** you rely on for investment advice.
- **Books** related to your investments.
- **Depreciation on a home computer** to the extent you used it for tracking investments, asset allocations, and tax gains and losses.
- **Computer software** and on-line services used to track your investments.
- **Legal, accounting or advisory fees** that are related to your investments.
- **Rent on a safe-deposit box** that's used to store income-producing securities and related documents.
- **IRA trustees' fees,** if they are billed and paid separately.
- **Travel expenses** (such as trips to your financial adviser) related to your investments. If you own rental property out of town, trips to the property may be deductible.

Caution: The costs of traveling to or attending investment seminars are not deductible.

UNDERVALUING YOUR BASIS

As mentioned, miscellaneous deductions are only deductible to the extent they exceed 2% of your AGI, so investment expenses may not be deductible, especially for high-income investors.

Trap: Even if the 2%-of-AGI hurdle is cleared, your deduction effectively will be pared if your AGI is more than $139,500 ($69,750 if married and filing separately) or if you are subject to the alternative minimum tax (AMT). These figures are $142,700 and $71,350 respectively in 2004.

In addition, any investment expense you are able to deduct as a miscellaneous itemized deduction may reduce the amount of investment interest expense you can deduct.

Strategy: Instead of piling up nondeductible investment fees or fees that won't save you much in taxes, add those fees to the basis of your securities in order to reduce the tax upon an eventual sale.

Rationale: When you buy a stock, the brokerage commissions you pay are added to the basis of the stock. If that's the case, why not add an investment advisory fee to the basis of your holdings?

■ *Your Money* ■ ■

Example: You had invested $100,000 in mutual funds five years ago. Counting $10,000 in reinvested distributions, you have increased your basis to $110,000.

Last year, you sold those funds for $120,000. At first glance, this would be a $10,000 taxable gain. However, you have paid your investment adviser $5,000 over the years. Your tax pro says that you might be able to justify adding as much as 80% of that amount ($4,000) to your basis, as long as your claim is properly documented.

Result: If $4,000 can be added, your basis would be $114,000 and you would have a $6,000 capital gain, not a $10,000 gain.

TRAPS AND OPPORTUNITIES

This technique falls into a gray area of the tax law, without guidance from the IRS one way or the other. Discuss with your tax preparer.

Whether or not you add investment fees to your basis, be sure to track reinvested dividends and reinvested capital gains. If you sold securities last year, increase your basis by the amounts you previously reinvested—you have already paid tax on this income.

Trap: If you don't increase your basis, you will be paying tax twice on those reinvestments.

INTEREST EXPENSE

Investment interest expense outlays are *not* considered miscellaneous itemized deductions. Consequently, they are not subject to the 2%-of-AGI rule. Thus, interest you paid on money you borrowed to buy or hold investments may be fully deductible.

Trap: Such interest is only deductible against taxable net investment income—your taxable investment income (generally exclusive of long-term capital gains and dividends) minus any deductible investment expenses.

Example: You had $10,000 in investment interest last year and $8,000 in net investment income. You can deduct $8,000 worth of your investment interest expense on your 2003 return, but you must carry forward the other $2,000 of excess investment interest expense.

Strategy: As above, check the prior years' returns for carryforwards of investment interest expense. If you have one, it can be deducted if you report sufficient net investment income for 2003.

CRUNCH THE NUMBERS

In some cases, handling investment interest expense can be tricky.

Key: Your net investment income includes taxable interest and short-term capital gains. You also can include long-term gains and dividends if you choose to forgo favorable tax rates on this income.

If you do include the long-term gains, those gains are taxed as ordinary income. This may pose a difficult problem.

Example: Your investment interest expense in 2003 was $10,000. Your net investment income, excluding long-term gains, was $8,000. As above, you can deduct $8,000 in investment interest expense and carry forward the excess $2,000.

Suppose, though, that you also had $5,000 in long-term capital gains in 2003. You can count $2,000 as investment income. This would permit you to deduct the entire $10,000. However, that $2,000 would be taxed at your ordinary income rate, not the favorable long-term capital gains rate.

Questions: Are you better off with the larger current deduction? Or are you better off paying lower taxes on capital gains and carrying forward the excess $2,000 investment interest expense?

Crunch the numbers with your tax professional to find out what would be better.

MATCHING ALERT

The IRS devotes a tremendous amount of effort to document matching. Whatever investment income is reflected on the Form 1099s you received, make sure that this income is reflected on your tax return.

Key: That includes any dividends you reinvested, too.

Trap: Discrepancies are likely to draw the attention of the IRS. Make sure to account for all reported investment income.

■■ Your Money ■

11

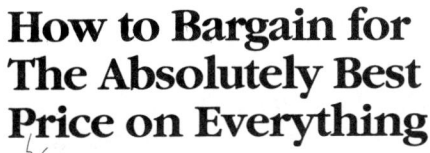

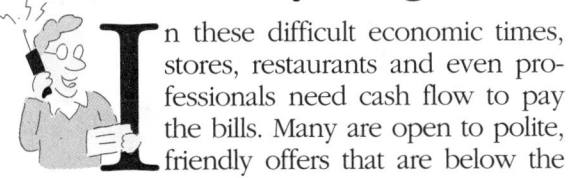

Consumer Confidential

How to Bargain for The Absolutely Best Price on Everything

In these difficult economic times, stores, restaurants and even professionals need cash flow to pay the bills. Many are open to polite, friendly offers that are below the stated price.

A Harris Interactive poll conducted in 2002 found that an average of 14% of people asked their doctors, dentists or pharmacists if they would lower their prices...and almost half of them agreed to do so.

BEST STRATEGIES

The key to getting a better price is to ask for one. You don't have to be pushy or deceptive. Casually say, "Can you do a little bit better?" Many stores—even department stores—are willing to cut their prices, but they don't advertise it.

Talk to the person in charge, but do it out of earshot of other customers. A manager is less likely to make a deal if he/she has to give it to others as well.

Create a relationship. Think of bargaining as a joint effort to resolve a problem rather than just a win-lose situation. *To build trust with the other party...*

•**Chat for a minute or two.** To show interest, ask the seller what he thinks are the best manufacturers and materials, for example. This sets a positive tone, defuses tension and gives you time to decipher the seller's motivations. What would he consider a successful result?

Example: This summer, we went into a home-improvement center to buy deck furniture. The manager was complaining about how much fall and winter inventory kept coming in. From that point on, our bargaining

Rob and Terry Adams, longtime bargain hunters, Box 27309, Bay Point, FL 32411. They are coauthors of *The Bargain Hunter's & Smart Consumer's Field Guide* (Avebury).

angle was to help take excess summer stock off his hands.

- **Focus on what's fair.** Your goal isn't to steal from a seller—it's to pay a price with which you're comfortable.

- **Show respect.** Keep your tone confident —not negative or confrontational. If you criticize an item, do it gently.

Avoid saying, "I'm not paying that much for an outdated computer." Instead, try, "I can see from the package that this computer has been out of the store and repacked. I'm wondering if you can take something off the price."

- **Avoid adversarial body language.** Try to position the item so that you and the seller are looking at it side-by-side, rather than facing each other.

- **Never make the first offer.** It locks you into a price range without finding out how low the seller is willing to drop. It also allows him to control the bargaining and move the price up higher. Instead, ask him about bargains or sales. Follow up by asking for the best price.

- **Wait before counteroffering.** If you counteroffer immediately, the seller will feel that you didn't take his original proposal seriously. Wait a moment, then repeat his price to show that you're listening. Say, "So you want $400 for this item. Let me think about it for a minute." Speak slowly and deliberately.

Make sure you give your reasons for paying less before you counteroffer. Say, "That's more than I can afford." If you mention a price first, the other party won't pay attention to the rest of what you say.

- **Invoke a higher authority.** Say, "I love this car and want to buy it. But my wife will never agree to the price." This lets you bargain for a lower amount without sounding unreasonable. Use a series of higher authorities to ratchet down the price.

Example: Your mechanic (authority number two) says the car needs $1,200 in work, and your accountant (authority number three) says that now isn't a good time for you to buy a car.

Smart: If the "higher authority" tactic is used on you, stick to your original position.

Example: A large-screen TV is listed at $995. You want to pay $800. The salesman will sell it for $900 if his manager approves. Typically, the manager will say, "I'm told that you're offering $900. If you come up to $925, it's yours." Tell him, "You're mistaken. Your *salesman* offered $900. I'm offering $800." If the manager is in a position to bargain, he'll say, "Let me see what I can do" and look up the price and inventory status.

- **Use the power of silence.** After making your counteroffer, say nothing and wait for a response. Talking too much drains the potency of your rejection. Many people offer a number, then raise it before the seller even reacts.

- **Be honest**—but don't reveal everything right away. Dumping a lot of information on the seller at once reduces your ability to make strategic choices as the haggling goes forward.

Example: If you notice a defect in the item, keep it to yourself until you negotiate the best possible price. Then, when the deal nears completion, point out the defect and bargain down the price even more.

- **Avoid ultimatums.** Take-it-or-leave-it offers rarely work because they put the seller on the defensive and challenge him.

Better: Ask, don't demand. Say, "I would like this painting as a gift for my sister. We're at the end of our vacation, and we don't have that much money to spend. Would you take $50 for it?"

- **Think outside the box.** We often come up with creative solutions by listening closely to what the seller is saying.

Example: The owner of a lawn-mowing service gave us a price and wouldn't bargain. As we spoke, he complained about how long it took to load his equipment after each job and drive around town. *Solution:* We got six neighbors to use the service, and the owner gave us all a lower price.

- **Don't be afraid to return if you walk away.** An impasse isn't a failure as long as you end positively. Say, "I'm sorry we could not come to terms. But I enjoyed talking to you. Maybe we can work something out in the future."

When you do complete a deal, make sure that the next time you see the seller, you tell him how much you enjoy the item and appreciate his help. Sellers rarely get positive reinforcement and will be more likely to make deals with you in the future. We did this with our home-improvement store manager after we bought the deck furniture. Now, he actually calls us whenever he has items that are steeply discounted.

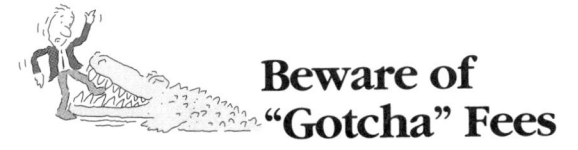

Beware of "Gotcha" Fees

Mary Hunt, editor, *Cheapskate Monthly* in Paramount, CA, www.cheapskatemonthly.com. She is author of *Debt-Proof Living* (Broadman & Holman).
Barbara Rollin, consumer advocate in San Diego and author of *Ask! The Revolutionary New Guide for Getting Total Customer Satisfaction* (Griffin Trade). Her Web site is www.askexchange.com.

Thoroughly fed up with his bank, a friend recently decided to terminate all of his accounts.

Final insult: The teller said he could do it for free if he took his money, $6,000, as cash. A check would cost $10.

"Gotcha" fees like these are mounting. *Some of the worst offenders...*

- **Banks.** Besides ATM fees, some banks may impose minimum-balance penalties, charges for overdraft protection, fees for copies of checks.
- **Phone companies.** Cellular-service bills are rife with surprises, such as charges for calls that go unanswered for more than 30 seconds.
- **Car rentals.** Surcharges may include fees for extra drivers, highway maintenance, airport access, airport recovery and vehicle license fee recovery.
- **Airlines.** Expect new or higher charges for excess baggage, ticket changes, paper tickets.
- **Hotels.** Some assess electricity surcharges, resort fees, Internet fees—even if you don't use the services.

To win at the "gotcha" game, we must all become better players. Read your opponent's playbook—the fine print that you receive in the mail—so you don't miss notices about new or increased fees. Be suspicious. Ask questions. Then summon the courage to say "no."

Timing is critical in getting fees waived.

Example: Travelers have more power when making advance reservations than at check-in. When reserving your room, inquire what fees, if any, you will be expected to pay during your stay. Ask if they can be waived. If not, ask for other compensation—such as a room upgrade.

Attitude is critical for getting what you want. Remember the old adage—honey will catch more flies than vinegar. Ask nicely.

More from Mary Hunt...

Cheaper Diamonds

Diamond jewelry can be bought for less than $100 at Wal-Mart, Kmart and other discount stores as well as through home-shopping channels. Many of the diamonds—called Indian diamonds because they are cut and polished almost exclusively in India—come from smaller, less-perfect stones that never used to be brought to market.

Penny-Pincher's Guide to Saving Money

Clark Howard, self-made millionaire and author of *Get Clark Smart: The Ultimate Guide to Getting Rich from America's Money-Saving Expert* (Hyperion). He also hosts *The Clark Howard Show*, a nationally syndicated radio program on consumer advice.

A lot of people think I am the cheapest person they know—but my philosophy is more about finding value than depriving myself of life's pleasures.

No matter what your income, if you spend less than you make—and do everything you can to avoid debt—you will get much more guilt-free pleasure out of occasional splurges. *Here are my favorite ways to save...*

■ *Your Money* ■ ■

- **Travel to a city on sale.** Instead of choosing the destination and then shopping for the best fare, look for cheap airfares first. You have to be flexible, but there's a great payoff. From Atlanta, I have traveled to San Francisco for $79, to Salt Lake City for $110, to Tucson for $99 and even to Honolulu for $182, all round-trip.

  To find deals, register for free weekly E-mail notification of fare sales at all the airline Web sites. Also, check *www.travelzoo.com…www. orbitz.com…www.expedia.com…*and *www. travelocity.com.* Comparison shop.

  The best hotel deals can be found on *www. hotwire.com* and *http://travel.priceline.com.*

  If you do not have a computer, find great prices through a travel agent. Ask several agents to plan the same trip, and compare their prices.

- **Buy a used auto.** Two- or three-year-old cars cost about 40% less than the new vehicles. Despite this fact, used-car sales were down in 2002, while new-car sales had their fourth-best year ever. Look for reliable models at *www.consumerreports.org.* To figure out how much a car is worth, go to *www.edmunds.com* or *www. kbb.com.* Expect to pay somewhere between the average trade-in price and the average retail price, adjusting up or down for extras and mileage. Pay a mechanic to inspect the car before you buy.

- **Pay less for long distance.** Twenty years ago, a one-minute long-distance call averaged 69 cents. Today, if you have a cell phone, you can get long distance at no extra charge as part of your calling plan. Or purchase prepaid long-distance calling cards at retail stores.

  Cost: Less than 3.5 cents a minute.* If you have a speed-dial feature on your phone, program in the calling card number for inexpensive calls with less hassle.

  If you prefer the convenience of dialing from home without punching in lengthy code numbers, try *www.zoneld.com.*

  Cost: 3.9 cents a minute.

- **Pay off your credit card balance faster.** I hope that you are among the 40% of credit card holders who pay off their balances in full each month.

  *All prices subject to change.

If not, Marc Eisenson, a credit card expert and coauthor of *Invest in Yourself: Six Secrets to a Rich Life* (Wiley), found that you can pay off any balance 75% faster by taking your regular monthly payment, splitting it in half and making half payments every 14 days.

Why this works: The credit card companies calculate interest daily, so getting money to them more quickly reduces the interest you pay on your remaining debt.

To make sure payments aren't late, set up an automatic bill-paying account.

- **Increase the deductibles on insurance policies.** Making small claims raises the risk that your insurer will cancel your homeowner's policy. Instead of having a $500 deductible, raise it to $1,000 or more, and save big on premiums. I raised my homeowner's insurance deductible to $2,500 and saved 38% on my annual premium. The same principle applies to auto insurance.

- **Never buy state-of-the-art technology.** For example, you might pay $1,500 for a computer system with all the newest bells and whistles. I paid $399 for a monitor and computer at a warehouse club. It does everything I need. You also can find such low-cost computers in retail stores and on-line.

- **Do not handcuff yourself to a particular home-security company.** Steer clear of any company that requires you to sign a multiyear contract. The long-term contracts prevent you from shopping for better deals, and you may be charged penalties if you move or decide to change companies.

  Beware of companies offering one-year contracts with rollover provisions that renew automatically. Look for a company that charges no more than $20 per month.

  Important: Make sure your alarm station monitors your home for fire and that it's been approved by Underwriters Laboratories, the product-safety testing organization.

- **Don't buy premium gasoline—unless you must.** Only about 5% of cars require premium gas, but 20% of all gas sold is premium. Premium grade costs about 20 cents a gallon more than regular—for a 15-gallon gas tank, that's $3 more every time you fill up. Using a higher-grade gas doesn't help—and may even damage—the engine. Check the owner's manual for the grade of gas recommended.

The best gas deals can be found at discount stores and warehouse clubs—about 15 cents a gallon less than branded locations. Quality is the same.

•**Skip the fancy bottled water.** Most tap water is clean and tastes good. In blind taste tests I conducted for a TV report four years ago, tap water won, even though most of the testers were avowed bottled-water drinkers.

Expensive bottled waters can cost more than $1. If you prefer bottled water, try one of the less expensive private labels. Wal-Mart's Sam's Choice brand costs about 20 cents for a 20-ounce bottle. If you purchase a one-gallon jug, the price may be less than one-half penny per ounce.

Cheaper still: Attach a filter to your faucet.

More from Clark Howard...

Cost-Cutting Secrets

It's always a good idea to keep your spending under control. Today, with the slower economy and lower stock and bond returns, cutting the cost of living is the hottest topic on my talk show.

Here are some of the best cost-cutting ideas discussed recently...

•**Make the most of today's used-car glut.** With dealers offering 0% financing on new cars and millions of cars coming off lease, the used-car market is flooded with two- and three-year-old vehicles. The price of a new Mazda MPV LX minivan is about $22,825. A used 2001 model can be as low as $15,790, according to CarsDirect.com.

Important: Never buy a used car until a mechanic has checked it. You want a diagnostic mechanic certified by Automotive Service Excellence who is familiar with today's cars. Some AAA affiliates offer referrals to diagnostic mechanics.

•**Have Virgin Mobile USA as your cell phone company.** If you use a cell phone only occasionally, you don't need a calling plan from one of the big national cellular operators offering unlimited minutes, weekend minutes, etc. Instead, look into prepaid cellular phone service from Virgin Mobile USA, the same company that runs the Virgin chain of music stores and Virgin Atlantic Airlines. For information on prices and plans check their Web site at *www.virginmobileusa.com* or call 888-322-1122.

•**Schedule your vacation, then pick the destination.** Travelers used to pick a vacation destination and then decide when to go. Today, it's best to do it the other way around. Schedule your vacation time first. Then, as your departure date approaches, shop among all the travel bargains available for the cheapest package for when you plan to go.

With the global economic slowdown, you can get some fabulous travel bargains—as long as you're flexible about destinations. You may go to Italy this year when Hawaii was on your mind. But eventually, you'll make your way around the world—and at a huge discount.

•**Switch to a discount Internet service provider.** With basic AOL Internet service costing up to $23.90 a month, plenty of smaller competitors now offer dial-up access for $10 a month or less.

United Online—created by the merger of bargain services Juno and NetZero—charges $9.95* a month for basic service and $14.95 a month for SpeedBand, a high-speed Web surfing plan (*www.untd.com*). Joi Internet (*www.joiinternet.com*) charges $6.95 a month for Joi Unlimited and $9.95 a month for Joi Express.

Strategy: Try a discount Internet service provider for one month. If the service proves reliable, sign a one-year contract.

•**Take advantage of super bargains in furniture.** If you haven't gone furniture shopping lately, you may not know that bargain imports from Asia and Eastern Europe are now flooding the market.

The US furniture market is reeling because prices on these import items are just unbelievable. My Chinese-made desk is a reproduction of a piece normally found in designer showrooms for around $1,400. I paid $300 for it.

Another great way to save on furniture is to buy used or repaired furniture at flea markets.

*All prices subject to change.

■ *Your Money* ■ ■

Our dining room table would have cost $10,000 or more new. We got it at a flea market, in excellent condition, for $1,400.

Strategy: Most areas now have a furniture flea market one weekend per month. Don't make a bid until the final two hours Sunday afternoon. Dealers are most willing to bargain then, so they won't have to truck home what they didn't sell.

• **Get your TV from a dish.** Prices of cable service just keep rising—especially if you opt for the new digital cable installations. You can almost always save by getting your TV via a dish from DISH Network at *www.dishnetwork.com* or DIRECTV at *www.directv.com*.

DISH Network has a great deal. For $24.99* a month, the service includes all the typical cable fare. Although you can save a ton with satellite, most end up paying as much as they would with cable because they take more options—but they get more channels.

• **Explore the new generic products.** You could always save money buying a retailer's generic version of *branded* products. But the quality was not always great. Today's story is the rise of branded generics, where the retailer creates and promotes a brand name for its line of generics.

Branded generics cost about 30% less than national brands. That's less than the 50% or so that the old-style generics used to save you, but the quality of today's store-brand generics is excellent.

• **Make your own housecleaning products.** Create cleaning products out of items that are likely to be in your pantry, such as white vinegar, baking soda and ammonia. Go to *http://organizedhome.com* for recipes. You'll be using nontoxic products and will save around 90% of the retail price of household cleaners.

• **When you rent a car, ask for the smallest one available.** Half the time, the rental company will not have the compact car you order and will have to give you a larger model —at the small-car price.

*Price subject to change.

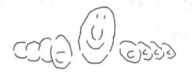

Best Coupon Savings

For coupons offered by everyone from local stores and grocers to more than 200 major retailers, check out *www.ultimatecoupons.com*. Coupons can be printed by your computer for use in stores such as Wal-Mart, Eddie Bauer and Target, or be used electronically at on-line retailers. The site also offers a Web buying guide, free newsletter, links to extensive product reviews and more for the smart bargain hunter.

SmartMoney, 250 W. 55 St., New York City 10019.

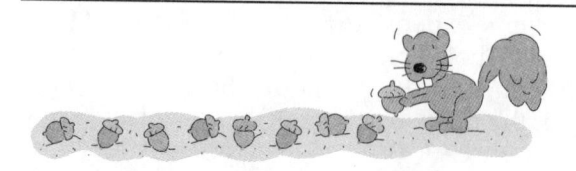

Painless Ways to Save From *Bottom Line* Readers

Warren Cromer, Suzanne Gregg, Steven Halverson, Valerie Kestner, Liz Langston, Bruce Snider, Lindy Spiezer, Marcia Spires and other *Bottom Line* readers who contributed anonymously.

Readers from across the country write in to tell *Bottom Line/Personal* how they avoid needless expenses. *Here are just a few of their suggestions...*

FINANCIAL

• **Pay your regular bills automatically** with a no-fee credit card that offers rewards, such as cash back or free gasoline. Have that card automatically paid off monthly by your bank. You will earn rewards for purchases and avoid late fees...and you won't have to worry about bills while traveling. You also won't need as many checks and stamps.

Examples from Robert McKinley at Cardweb.com: Cash back/no fee—Fleet Cash Dividend Platinum/Titanium Visa, 888-506-1586. *Gas/no fee/rebates*—ExxonMobil MasterCard, 866-427-7322.

• **On nonroutine bills, mark the due date on the lower left corner** of the envelope. Wait until just before that date to mail them so that your money stays in the bank earning interest longer.

• **Use a credit card that offers monthly statements that break down your expenses** into categories. Then you will be able to see where your money is going and start to save in new areas.

• **Buy checks from a mail-order company.** They are half the cost of what some of the banks charge.

Example: *secure.checksinthemail.com* or 877-397-1541.

• **Buy a rubber stamp that bears your return address.** Use address labels only for important correspondence.

SHOPPING

• **Ask for discounts if you pay cash** for major purchases.

• **Use the Internet to find bargains** on everything from merchandise to vacations.

Examples: *http://travel.priceline.com...www.travelocity.com.*

• **Assess whether you need high-speed Internet service.** You can save $20 a month if you're willing to use your phone line and a dial-up service.

• **Buy quality**—cars, appliances, tools, furnishings, etc. Quality items last longer, so they are cheaper in the long run.

TRAVEL

• **Stay at airport hotels.** By staying near the airport the night before your trip, you may be able to save by leaving your car in the hotel garage at a lower rate than the one at the airport.

AUTO

• **Maintain your car.** You can make it last for 100,000 miles. Keeping the tires properly inflated will boost your mileage and reduce tire wear.

• **Change your car's oil yourself.** Buy oil, oil filters and air filters in bulk. Each oil change will save you the fee.

ELECTRICITY

• **Install ceiling fans** to avoid running the air conditioner as often.

• **Replace some regular lightbulbs with fluorescent bulbs.** The initial higher cost will be more than repaid by their longer life and energy efficiency.

EATING

• **Take advantage of early bird specials.**

• **Bring your lunch to work** and a bottle of water to the gym. Pack water or soda on car trips to avoid buying expensive drinks at service stations.

ENTERTAINMENT

• **Get—and use—a library card.** Besides books, libraries often loan videos and music at no cost.

• **Restrict or avoid pay-per-view TV.** You can save about $20 a month if you pass up a movie a week.

Keep Up with Safety Recalls

To stay aware of the latest safety recalls, enter your E-mail address at *www.safetyalerts.com,* and you will receive notice of all recalls in 15 categories, such as food, autos, outdoor items and cosmetics. Or you can specify only the categories that interest you. The service is free.

Kiplinger's Personal Finance, 1729 H St. NW, Washington, DC 20006.

If You Break an Item in a Store...

You don't have to pay for anything you break in a retail store—even if the store posts a sign saying, *You break it, you buy it.* Breakage is covered by a store's insurance or is tax deductible from the store's income. If you want to pay anyway, ask for evidence of the item's cost to the retailer. Pay only that amount —not full retail.

Barbara Weltman, attorney in Millwood, NY, www.bwideas.com. She is author of many books, including Bottom Line's Very Shrewd Money Book *(Bottom Line Books).*

■ *Your Money* ■ ■

On-Line Auctions: The Latest Strategies For Buyers and Sellers

Dennis Prince, Rocklin, CA–based author of four books about on-line auctions, including *AuctionWatch.com's Guide to Online Buying and Selling* and *Starting Your Online Auction Business* (both from Premier). He specializes in buying and selling movie memorabilia and baby boomer toys and games.

When should a seller use the "buy-it-now" option? What's the best way for a buyer to place a last-second bid? *Here's what you need to know now...*

SELLERS

• **Stick with eBay except for certain items.** Although Yahoo! at *http://auctions.shopping.yahoo.com* and Amazon.com at *www.amazon.com* also run general auction sites, both lag far behind eBay's 50 million users. The more buyers there are, the more likely you'll get fair market price or higher.

Several auction sites have significant volume in specific categories. Compare sales prices of items similar to yours at these sites and at eBay. *Use whichever site brings the higher prices...*

• Computers and consumer electronics—*www.ubid.com...www.dellauction.com* for Dell computers.

• Pottery—*www.potteryauction.com.*

• Stamps—*www.stampauction.com.*

• **Use the *buy-it-now* option judiciously.** For a five-cent fee, eBay sellers now can offer buyers the option of preempting the auction by snapping up the item at a buy-it-now price named by the seller.

Downside: If you set the price too high, you might discourage buyers from considering your item. If you set it too low, you might sell below market value.

Typically, the price is set at a slight premium to the amount similar products have fetched in the past.

Choose the buy-it-now option if...

• The category is hot, as Spider-Man comic books and collectibles were when the movie came out.

• A gift-giving holiday is approaching.

• The item is the hardest-to-find component of a set. Buyers might be willing to pay a premium to complete their collections.

• **Schedule the auction's close for a Sunday evening.** Most eBay bids are placed in the final minutes of an auction, so you want to close when the greatest number of buyers are available. In my experience, that is Sunday evening at 9 pm Eastern time, 6 pm Pacific time. Saturday evening is the second-best option.

Helpful: Opt for a seven-day auction starting the previous Sunday evening. This gives people who log on only once a week a chance to see your item. Use a three- or five-day auction only if a gift-giving holiday is rapidly approaching—holiday buyers tend to want things right away.

BUYERS

• **Don't feel pressured to buy.** So many people now sell on-line that even relatively rare items pop up with some frequency. There is never a need to overpay. If you lose one auction, another will come along.

• **Know how to make a last-second bid.** eBay auctions have what is known as a "hard close." When the auction period runs out, no more bids are accepted for that auction. Many smart buyers wait until the final seconds before making their moves, rather than bidding heavily earlier in the process and driving up the price.

A last-minute bid is always a big gamble because you don't know how long you can wait to get your bid in. Sometimes, you're able to get a bid in when no time remains on the auction clock—other times, a bid with five seconds left on the clock is not accepted.

My trick to improve the odds: I keep two windows open on my computer screen—one with my bid ready for submission, the other indicating the status of the auction with the clock ticking down.

When the auction clock doesn't tick off each passing second—for example, when it jumps right from 25 seconds remaining directly to 23 or 22 seconds—it's an indication that eBay's servers are moving slowly. Then I know I had better get my bid in with five to seven seconds to spare if I want it to register before the auction is over.

If the servers are humming along, the clock will tick off each passing second, and I'll put my bid in when there are three seconds left.

Another option: Use a service from eSnipe.com, which makes your last-minute bid for you. You open a free eSnipe account and type in the auction number and amount you wish to bid. If you win the auction, eSnipe.com charges a small fee to your credit card, usually 1% of the purchase price. You can use eSnipe only for bids on eBay.

Yahoo! and Amazon.com both have an auto-extension feature that makes last-second bids less effective. Auctions at these sites end when no bids are made for a period of five minutes. In theory, an auction could go on forever.

• **Search under misspellings.** Savvy buyers have done this for years, but it bears repeating because the bargains can be big. Most shoppers search under the correctly spelled heading. There's less competition in an auction when the item description is misspelled.

Examples: I once found a *Poseidon Adventure* movie poster at a fraction of its usual cost by searching under "Posidon Adventure." The cheapest Beanie Babies often are sold as "Beenie Babies."

Swap Good Deeds

With the "time dollar system," neighbors donate an hour of time to each other, without putting a dollar value on it.

Example: An hour of legal services is worth an hour of baking services. Because the hours are not valued, the IRS does not consider this barter, and there are no tax problems.

Bonus: Trading hours of time cements community relations and can help you get assistance you need in return for doing things you are good at.

More information: The Time Dollar Institute (202-686-5200 or *www.timedollar.org*).

Where to Retire, 1502 Augusta, Houston 77057.

How to Get the Best Prices On-Line

Find the best prices on-line by visiting Web sites that compare costs at multiple retailers.

Examples: *www.mysimon.com* checks dozens of retailers and lists the top 10 sellers in various product categories. *www1.dealtime.com* and *www.pricegrabber.com* offer price comparisons...customer reviews and ratings...and total price, including shipping and tax. *www.pricescan.com* lets you search for the best prices on different items with the same features.

Family Fun, 114 Fifth Ave., New York City 10011.

Keep Your Old Monitor And Save

Cathode-ray-tube (CRT) monitors sold with PCs today are barely improved over ones sold as many as seven years ago. If you buy a new computer from a company that makes computers to order—such as Dell, Gateway or Hewlett-Packard/Compaq—you can omit the monitor and save several hundred dollars. Check with the manufacturers to make sure your current monitor offers 640 x 480 pixels and that it will work with your new computer.

Dana Blankenhorn, Internet consultant and writer at a-clue.com in Atlanta.

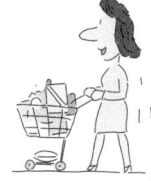

Easier Merchandise Returns

When returning merchandise, if you can't find your receipt and paid with a credit card, bring your monthly statement. Or provide the date and time you bought the item—the store may be able to trace it through its computer system.

■ *Your Money* ■ ■

Caution: Many major retailers are tightening up return policies and now require receipts... refuse returns after a certain number of days... will not give cash refunds in many circumstances...have return penalties, which they frequently call "restocking fees," of up to 15% of the purchase price.

Bottom line: Always ask about the store's return policy before making a purchase.

George Whalin, president and CEO, Retail Management Consultants, San Marcos, CA.

How to Shrink Your Medical Bills By 25% or More

Sue Goldstein, host of *The Diva of Discounts*, a radio program on KAAM-AM 770, Dallas/Fort Worth. She maintains the Web site *www.biggerbetterbargains.com*.

The cost of medical care continues to climb. And even if you do have insurance, it rarely covers everything. *But you can cut costs...*

NEGOTIATE A BETTER DEAL

More patients are negotiating with their doctors for reduced fees. If you would like to try, phone your physician *before* scheduling an appointment. Ask what you can do to lower your bill. Would there be a discount if you paid with cash...or scheduled your appointment for an off-peak time? What if you agreed to come in on short notice when the doctor had a cancellation? You could get 25% off your bill—possibly more.

You might even be able to barter for medical care if you have a skill or service that the medical professional needs. Are you a Web designer, landscaper, architect or accountant? Ask the physician if he/she is interested in trading services.

If a procedure is medically necessary but you have no insurance and money is tight, tell your doctor. Most physicians are willing to bend on price under these circumstances.

COSMETIC SURGERY SAVINGS

Cosmetic surgery is rarely covered by health insurance, so cosmetic surgeons are often open to negotiation. Some board-certified surgeons may offer significant discounts to patients who are flexible about scheduling.

About 13% of all scheduled cosmetic surgeries are postponed. This can leave doctors with open operating-room time. If you're ready to jump in when one of these gaps occurs, the doctor might discount his regular rate by as much as 15%.

Important: Ask the surgeon to show you his portfolio of patients' before-and-after pictures. Get at least three references. Also call your state's medical society—listed in the *Yellow Pages* under "Medical Associations"—to learn about disciplinary actions, license suspensions or other complaints.

GO TO A TEACHING HOSPITAL

Local teaching hospitals, dental schools and chiropractic schools often offer inexpensive medical care. Students lack the experience of older doctors, but they typically are well supervised. If they can't handle something, more experienced doctors are on hand to help. Contact local teaching hospitals or schools for more information.

Resource: The Association of American Medical Colleges (202-828-0400 or *www.aamc.org*).

DISCOUNT HEALTH CARE CLUBS

Discount health care clubs offer big savings on prescription drugs...doctor visits...even eyewear and hearing aids.

The best club I have found is Meds of America (800-388-8284 or *www.medsofamerica.com*). For $8.95* a month, uninsured or underinsured people can purchase prescription medications at discounts of up to 85% off regular rates. Check the Web site to see if the drugs you need are among the more than 3,500 offered.

For $29.95 a month, members have access to the discount pharmacy and also receive price breaks from medical providers. There are more than 275,000 physicians participating nationwide, offering savings of 30% to 50% on average...and over 15,000 dentists offering savings

*All prices subject to change.

of up to 80%. Discounts do vary, so members should ask about prices before making their appointments.

There is also an average savings of up to 30% at a variety of neighborhood pharmacies for those who need prescriptions immediately or who would like to deal with a pharmacist face-to-face.

These discounts are available because the participating doctors, dentists and pharmacies want to build their businesses and don't want insurance company hassles.

FREE MEDICATIONS

Major pharmaceutical companies may provide drugs to certain people at no cost or at steep discounts. There are more than 1,100 drugs available through 78 pharmaceutical company programs.

To be eligible for these discounts, your insurance must not cover the prescription. You also must make enough money that you don't qualify for government health care programs—but not so much that the pharmaceutical company thinks you can afford to pay.

Income requirements vary from company to company, but people making less than $25,000 a year are generally eligible for most programs. Anyone with big prescription drug bills—$300 per month or more—who is making less than $50,000 may also qualify.

These programs are based on income, not assets. Even if you own a nice home, you still could qualify if you are retired or temporarily unemployed.

To find out if you are eligible and if the drug you need is covered, call the drug manufacturer.

You can also purchase a pamphlet listing the drugs covered from The Cost Containment Research Institute, a public interest group.

To order the pamphlet: Institute Fulfillment Center, *Free and Low Cost Prescription Drugs,* Box 210, Dallas, PA 18612 or *www.institutedc.org.*

Cost: $6* (for printed copy); $4.95 (for online copy).

FREE COUPONS

Many pharmaceutical companies run free, week- to month-long trial-offer programs for certain drugs. All that consumers need to do is clip a coupon from a magazine or download one from a Web site and have a doctor write a prescription. Rules vary, but in many cases, you can use the coupon even if it is not your first prescription for the medication.

Don't assume that these coupons always are good deals. The drugmaker might be offering the free trial because a competing drug—perhaps even a cheaper generic version of the drug—is coming to market. The drug company is banking that you won't want to go to the bother of switching medications. Always ask your doctor if there are cheaper or more effective alternatives.

To find out if a coupon is available for a particular drug, check the company's Web site. To find the site, look up the company or drug name on a search engine, such as *www.google.com.*

DISCOUNTS ON ADJUSTABLE BEDS AND NONALLERGENIC MATTRESSES

For people with certain heart conditions or back problems, adjustable beds are medical necessities. For allergy sufferers, nonallergenic mattresses can be a must.

City Mattress Factory (800-834-2473) sells all types of mattresses and adjustable bed frames, typically for half the retail price of brand-name mattresses even after factoring in shipping.

Example: An adjustable double bed at City Mattress costs about $900, rather than the $2,000 you would pay for one that's advertised on television.

IF MONEY IS EXTREMELY TIGHT

If you have no insurance and require medical treatment, one option is to participate in a clinical trial. You receive free complete medical exams, free treatment and may even get paid for your trouble.

Downside: The treatment that you receive might not yet be proven effective—it could even be dangerous, although this is rare. Also, if you participate in a "blind" study, you might be given a placebo instead of the experimental drug.

If you are interested in participating in a clinical trial, contact Research Across America

*All prices subject to change.

■ *Your Money* ■ ■

(972-241-1222 or *www.researchacrossamerica.com*)...or Radiant Research (425-825-5100 or *www.radiantresearch.com*).

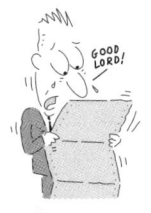

Check Hospital Bills Carefully

Studies show that 90% of all hospital bills have errors—and 75% of those errors are in the hospital's favor. Before you go into the hospital, find out what your health insurance covers and what is excluded. While in the hospital, keep records of major tests, treatments and medications, or have a family member or friend keep them for you.

After your hospital stay, check your insurer's explanation of benefits (EOB) carefully to be sure you understand all charges and know what you are expected to pay. Compare the EOB and your notes with the bill the hospital gave you on discharge to check for errors. If you find mistakes, tell the hospital and your insurance provider.

Charles Inlander, president, People's Medical Society, Box 868, Allentown, PA 18105, and author of *Take This Book to the Hospital with You* (St. Martin's).

More from Charles Inlander...

Work with Your Doctor To Reduce Costs

Patients should tell their physicians which type of health insurance they have.

Reason: Most doctors will try to hold down a patient's out-of-pocket expenses by working with the type of coverage the patient carries.

Examples: Prescribing a medication on the "approved" list instead of equivalent ones that are not...or prescribing a generic drug instead of a brand name to patients who lack drug coverage.

Cheaper Contact Lenses

Buying contact lenses on-line, by mail or at a warehouse club is dramatically cheaper than buying them through your eye doctor. Some optometrists may not want to give you a prescription to use elsewhere. But 28 states have laws that require them to do so at your request or automatically. The remaining states have no such laws on the books.

To find out about your state: Go to *www.1800contacts.com*.

Also: Ask your optometrist to match any lower price you find.

Kiplinger's Personal Finance, 1729 H St. NW, Washington, DC 20006.

How to Save on Prescription Drugs

Robert M. Hayes, Esq., president and general counsel, Medicare Rights Center, a nonprofit advocacy group for consumers, 1460 Broadway, New York City 10036.

During the past few years, HMOs that had offered drug benefits have cut benefits or dropped out of Medicare. Drugs you take may no longer be covered, or the HMO may cover generics only. But, there are ways to cut drug costs.

FINANCIAL ASSISTANCE

•**State assistance.** Over half the states have drug-coverage assistance programs. Income qualifications and coverage vary. For a list of state assistance programs, contact Medicare at 800-633-4227 or *www.medicare.gov*.

•**Veterans Health Administration.** If you are an honorably discharged veteran and use VA facilities, most prescriptions are only $7.*

For information: Department of Veterans Affairs (877-222-8387 or *www.va.gov*).

Editor's note: Some VA facilities have waits of up to six months for new patients.

*All prices subject to change.

Consumer Confidential

DRUG DISCOUNT CARDS

Discounts offered by drug manufacturers and other organizations may be subject to income restrictions. Most discount cards are free. For a complete list of drug-discount programs, contact Medicare Rights Center, *www.medicarerights.org* (click on "Discount Rx Resources"). *Examples...*

- **AARP** (800-424-3410 or *www.aarp.org*). ***Annual fee:*** $12.50.*
- **Costco Ageless Care Programs** (800-869-5494 or *www.agelesscare.com/costco*). ***Annual membership:*** $131.40 to $299.40.
- **LillyAnswers Card** from Eli Lilly & Company (877-795-4559 or *www.lillyanswers.com*). $12 administrative fee for a 30-day drug supply of any Lilly retail-distributed drug.
- **Advance Rx** (800-238-2623 or *www.advancerx.com*).
- **Medco Health** (877-733-6765 or *www.yourplan.com*). ***Annual fee:*** $25 (single) or $40 (family).
- **Pfizer for Living Share Card** (800-717-6005 or *www.pfizerforliving.com*). $15 fee for a 30-day supply of most Pfizer drugs.

MAIL-ORDER/INTERNET PHARMACIES

Some offer up to 75% off prescription drugs. *Examples...*

- **DrugPlace.com** (800-881-6325 or *www.drugplace.com*).
- **Familymeds.com** (888-787-2800 or *www.familymeds.com*).

Note: A list of drug prices from on-line pharmacies is available at *www.destinationrx.com*.

*All prices subject to change.

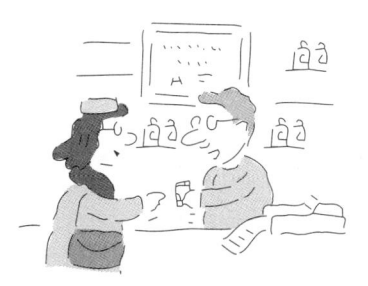

Cutting Medication Costs

To save money on medications, speak to a pharmacist at your insurance company. Find out from him/her what medications your plan covers for your condition and at what payment levels. Take this information to your doctor. Doctors often think of medicines in terms of clinical effectiveness, not cost.

If your insurance doesn't offer a drug benefit or you are uninsured: Tell your doctor cost is important, and ask if there is a less expensive but equally effective drug available.

C. Daniel Mullins, PhD, associate professor of pharmacoeconomics, University of Maryland School of Pharmacy, Baltimore.

More Savings on Drugs

Nancy Dunnan, financial adviser and author in New York City. Her latest book is *How to Invest $50–$5,000* (HarperCollins).

Many pharmaceutical companies will give free or reduced-cost prescription drugs to those who cannot afford them. Most programs are limited to low-income people (less than $12,000 per year), although some expensive drugs—for transplants and cancer, for example—are available to those who have annual family income as high as $60,000.

Each drug company determines eligibility for its program. In general, you cannot have private insurance or qualify for a government or other assistance program. Depending upon the company, you either fill out an application form with the company or go through your doctor. Once your application is approved, you will receive a three-month supply of medication. Some prescriptions are renewed automatically, some are not.

To get started, contact NeedyMeds (215-625-9609 or *www.needymeds.com*), a free information service. Enter the drug name to find out who to contact, the manufacturer's income requirements and how to enroll. Be sure to read the site's frequently asked questions.

■ *Your Money* ■ ■

If you don't find the drug listed here, go to the Pharmaceutical Research and Manufacturers of America (800-762-4636 or *www.phrma.org*).

Finally, if handling the paperwork is overwhelming, The Medicine Program (573-996-7300 or *www.themedicineprogram.com*) will do it for you for a $5* processing fee per prescription drug request.

*Price subject to change.

More from Nancy Dunnan...

If You're Overcharged For a Funeral...

If you think a funeral home is overcharging, begin by getting the full name of the director of the funeral home. Call and ask him/her to send you a detailed, written explanation of all charges within five business days. Follow up your request with a written letter to him and submit one copy to the Better Business Bureau in the city or town where the funeral home is located.

If he doesn't respond or if he does and you still think the bill is unfair, get in touch with the Funeral Consumers Alliance (800-765-0107 or *www.funerals.org*) and the International Cemetery and Funeral Association (800-645-7700 or *www.icfa.org*). The Alliance will answer your request for help within 48 hours. The Association has a free mediation service. Let the director know that you are looking for resolution through both groups. That should motivate him to resolve the issue.

Also from Nancy Dunnan...

How to Buy a Diamond Ring

When looking to buy a diamond ring, you can pick a reliable local jeweler as well as read some excellent consumer information on the Jewelers of America Web site at *www.jewelers.org*. They can also be reached at 800-223-0673. Members of this trade organization must make an annual ethics commitment, which gives you a degree of protection.

Also, be sure to contact your local Better Business Bureau (*www.bbb.org*) to see if complaints have been lodged against a specific store.

Even the Federal Trade Commission (*www.ftc.gov*) has gotten into the act. Its free publication, *All That Glitters—How to Buy Jewelry*, discusses imitation diamonds and lab-created stones, such as cubic zirconia.

Once you've decided on a stone or ring, take it to a gemologist/appraiser. For names, contact the National Association of Jewelry Appraisers (410-897-0889)...or the American Society of Appraisers (703-478-2228 or *www.appraisers.org*).

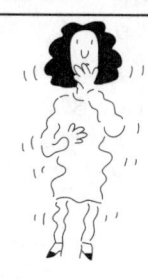

When to Buy a New Mattress

Consider a new mattress if you wake up sore, stiff or unrested. Choose one that yields to your body's contours. Firmer is not necessarily better. Side and stomach sleepers need more give than back sleepers. Women's hips need to sink deeper than men's. Some mattresses are split down the middle, and each side has a different degree of firmness.

When shopping: Buy only from a retailer that lets you return or exchange your purchase within 30 or 60 days.

Stephen Hochschuler, MD, chairman of the Texas Back Institute, Plano, *www.texasback.com,* and coauthor of *Treat Your Back Without Surgery* (Hunter House).

How to Buy Better Sunglasses

Jeffrey Weaver, OD, director of the clinical care group, American Optometric Association, St. Louis.

The price of sunglasses is no indication of quality. But if you buy them from your eye doctor rather than a drugstore, you may have a better chance of exchanging them if you are not satisfied.

184

Criteria for choosing a good pair: The lenses should block 99% of UV radiation, in both the UVA and the more damaging UVB wavelength ranges.

Note: You must depend on the label for this information unless you have a light meter. The label may indicate that the lenses either block or absorb more than 99% of UV or transmit less than 1%.

The glasses also should block 75% to 90% of visible light. Sunglasses that have the American Optometric Association (AOA) seal of acceptance meet all these requirements. Other sunglasses also may meet them. There is no legal requirement to have a label, and there is only a voluntary standard for quality.

For driving: Wear gray (best) or brown lenses, which allow correct color perception.

For active sports and children: Lenses should be impact resistant. Polycarbonate is the best material.

To minimize reflected glare from roads, water or snow: Polarized lenses.

Electronics at a Discount

Refurbished electronic products are available at deep discounts at *www.refurbdepot.com*. You can save from 20% to 80%. The products—mostly store returns—include CD recorders, scanners, digital cameras and more. They carry manufacturers' warranties of between 30 days and two years. Manufacturers test products thoroughly before labeling them refurbished.

SmartMoney, 250 W. 55 St., New York City 10019.

Save on Detergent

Use only half as much detergent as laundry- and dishwasher-detergent makers recommend. You will save money…your clothes and dishes will get just as clean…and you won't end up with excess detergent collecting on washer parts, leading to costly repairs. Detergent makers consistently recommend that consumers use more of their products than is necessary.

Gary Foreman, editor of *The Dollar Stretcher*, Box 14160, Bradenton, FL 34280, and former certified financial planner.

Low-Cost Alternatives to Cleaning Products

To avoid the high cost of cleaning products, try these cheap or no-cost alternatives…

• **All-purpose cleaning.** Lemon juice, at full strength or diluted with water.

• **Toilet bowls.** Chlorine bleach. Pour in half a cup, let it sit for 30 minutes, then scrub any stains away.

• **Drains.** Flush out pipes once a week with three quarts of boiling water.

• **Windows and other glass.** Add one-fourth cup of vinegar or rubbing alcohol to a quart of water.

• **Wood furniture and floors.** Wipe the wood with a cloth or mop dipped in cool tea —then polish.

Terri McGraw, host of the syndicated TV show *Mrs. Fixit Easy Home Repair*. Based in Syracuse, NY, she is author of *Mrs. Fixit Easy Home Repair* (Pocket). Her Web site is *www.mrsfixit.com*.

How to Avoid Carpet-Cleaner Scams

Cut-rate carpet cleaners are almost always bait-and-switch scams. Once in your home, they insist you pay extra for everything—sometimes even for the detergents. Thorough carpet cleaning costs 20 to 60 cents per square foot, depending on the type of carpeting, how dirty it is, if you have allergy concerns and how much furniture must be moved.

■ *Your Money* ■ ■

Carpet cleaners without formal training in chemicals can be dangerous. Find a certified professional at *www.iicrc.org,* and insist on a written estimate. A hot-water extraction cleaning for a home with 500 to 1,000 square feet of carpeting takes about two hours and up to four hours to dry.

Cleaning your home's carpets every six to 12 months extends their life and improves indoor air quality.

Joe Polish, owner of a carpet-cleaning firm and president of Piranha Marketing, which advises more than 3,500 carpet-cleaning companies nationwide, both are in Tempe, AZ.

A Home Energy Audit Can Cut Energy Bills in Half

Mark Ginsberg, member, board of directors, Office of Energy Efficiency and Renewable Energy, US Department of Energy, Washington, DC.

Most home owners can cut their energy bills by 10% to 30% on existing homes, and up to 50% on homes that are being constructed.

Most people have no idea how many "energy leaks" they have in their homes or how much even a small leak may be costing them.

Useful: Have an expert conduct an "energy audit" of your home. The expert will examine your home's construction and your energy bills, and may use equipment such as infrared cameras to detect heat leakage and air blowers to find air leaks.

Leading sources of air leaks in homes: Floors, walls and ceilings, 31%...ducts, 15%...fireplaces, 14%...plumbing, 13%...doors, 11%...windows, 10%...fans and vents, 4%...electric outlets, 2%.

Cost of an audit: $50 to $400—but remember that some utilities help subsidize conservation expenditures. And, there are do-it-yourself kits available.

For more information on energy audits: Call the US Department of Energy at 800-363-3732 or go to *www.eere.energy.gov.*

More Energy Savers

Jon Koomey, PhD, staff scientist and group leader of the energy end-use forecasting group, Lawrence Berkeley National Lab, which does research on energy and environmental issues, Berkeley, CA, *www.lbl.gov.*

Try out some of these helpful strategies for lowering energy expenses around your home...

•**Appliances.** Look for the government's Energy Star labels when buying air conditioners, dishwashers and other appliances.

Example: Energy Star washing machines are at least 50% more efficient than required by federal standards.

Information about high-efficiency products: 888-782-7937 or *www.energystar.gov.*

•**Windows.** Dual panes with low-emissivity (low-e) coatings reflect heat away from the home in summer and keep it inside in winter.

If you live in a sunny climate: Consider "spectrally selective glazing" to block ultraviolet and infrared rays. This glazing will also reduce air-conditioning costs.

If you live in a cold climate: Argon or other gases sealed between the panes reduces heating bills by keeping heat in.

•**Lighting.** Compact fluorescent bulbs cost more than traditional incandescent bulbs—typically between $5 and $10—but they last up to 10 times longer and use 50% to 75% less energy.

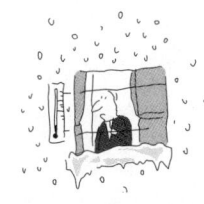

For Much Lower Heating Costs...

Spike Carlsen, executive editor, *The Family Handyman,* 2915 Commers Dr., Eagan, MN 55121, *www.family handyman.com.*

To reduce the cost of heating your home throughout the winter, follow these practical suggestions...

Consumer Confidential

- **Install and use an automatic setback thermostat** to reduce heating and cooling costs by 5% to 15%.
- **Place reflectors behind radiators** to redirect the heat that goes into the wall back into the room, and save another 5%. (Aluminum foil over cardboard will do.)
- **Insulate heating and hot-water pipes** that are exposed in areas you don't want the pipes to heat.
- **Change furnace filters every month**—or more often if needed.
- **Get a furnace tune-up** to adjust and clean burners.
- **Wrap the tank of a gas-burning water heater** in a manufacturer-approved fiberglass insulating blanket.
- **Replace worn-out thresholds** under doors and weather stripping around windows.
- **Lower the indoor temperature** to save about 2% of heating costs per degree.
- **Close the fireplace damper when not in use.** If you never use it, seal it with a plastic bag stuffed with insulation.
- **Close off rooms that are not in use,** and lower the temperature in them.

More from Spike Carlsen...

Cut Air-Conditioning Costs

The average air-conditioning duct system loses 10% to 40% of its cooling air through leaks in duct joints. If the ducts run outside the area to be cooled, this is pure waste. Sealing duct joints is not a do-it-yourself job, so call an air-conditioning professional to test the duct system in your home for leakage and, if necessary, to seal it.

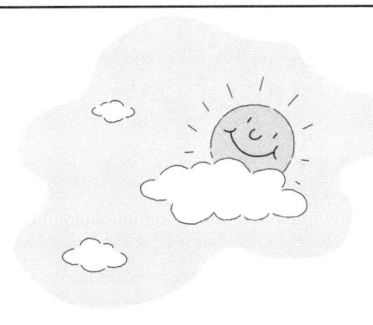

Save $100 Just by Changing Lightbulbs

Chris Calwell, vice president of policy and research, Ecos Consulting, which specializes in energy-efficiency and pollution-prevention research, Durango, CO, *www.ecosconsulting.com*.

Compact fluorescent lightbulbs are now about equal in quality and similar in color output to the incandescent bulbs. And they offer tremendous savings on home electric bills.

Compact fluorescent bulbs that screw into conventional sockets cost as little as $5 each —less if bought in bulk. But a fluorescent's greater longevity and energy efficiency can save you $30 to $60 over the life of the bulb. Fluorescents last up to 10,000 hours, versus 750 hours for incandescents, and consume up to 75% less electricity.

About 20% of the average American household's annual electric bill—about $160—goes toward lighting. Just switching a handful of a home's heavily used bulbs to fluorescents can save $100 or more a year.

Replace bulbs that get the most use...

- **Main kitchen light.**
- **Outdoor lights that are on from dusk until dawn.**
- **Living room, family room or great room lights**—wherever the family spends most of its evenings.

Halogen torchères are inefficient because they use a lot of electricity and direct light to the ceiling. Replace them with fluorescent torchères.

USING FLUORESCENT BULBS

It is a myth that fluorescent lights use so much energy starting up that it's more economical to leave them on. Turn off any bulb when leaving a room unless you will return within 15 minutes. However, it is true that frequently turning a fluorescent light on and off will reduce its life span.

BUYING EFFICIENT BULBS

Select fluorescent bulbs by looking at the number of *lumens* on the package—and not at the watts. Lumens indicate brightness level.

■ *Your Money* ■ ■

Fluorescents deliver much more light per watt of electricity.

Compact fluorescent bulbs are widely available in discount, hardware, home goods and lighting stores.

Helpful: Check the Energy Star Web site, *www.energystar.gov,* to find out if government or manufacturer rebates on fluorescent bulbs are available in your region.

Appliances That Pay for Themselves

Jennifer Thorne, research associate with the American Council for an Energy-Efficient Economy, a nonprofit organization founded in 1980 to encourage energy efficiency, *www.aceee.org*. She is coauthor of *Consumer Guide to Home Energy Savings* (ACEEE).

The newest energy-efficient appliances can cost up to $500 more than standard models. But many pay for themselves during their 12- to 20-year life spans. Virtually all major appliance manufacturers—even some of the smaller ones—offer energy-efficient models. Visit *www.energystar.gov* or *www.aceee.org* for details.

Important: Look for the blue "Energy Star" label when you shop for appliances. To earn this label, appliances must exceed government efficiency guidelines. Also keep an eye out for the Federal Trade Commission's yellow "Energy Guide" label. This provides the estimated annual energy consumption for an appliance based on typical usage.

REFRIGERATORS

The greatest progress in energy-efficient appliances has been made in refrigerators. Many models built before 1988 consume more than $100 worth of electricity a year. Those made in the 1970s can use as much as $200.

Today's standard refrigerators save an average of $50 a year in electricity. Since many new refrigerators retail in the $500 range, a new unit will pay for itself in about 10 years. The high-efficiency units can run on less than $40 a year.

Caution: The Energy Star and Energy Guide labels can be deceiving with refrigerators. The units are compared only between similar models. Thus a 22-cubic-foot side-by-side refrigerator might earn the Energy Star label, while an 18-cubic-foot freezer-on-top unit might not, even though it uses far less energy.

Refrigerators with freezers on top or bottom tend to be about 7% to 13% more efficient than side-by-side models. An automatic ice maker installed in the door can reduce efficiency by up to 20%.

Small units are more efficient than larger ones—but one large fridge is more efficient than two small ones. Don't buy something so small that you have to put the old unit in the basement for extra storage. If you do need an extra refrigerator, buy a new one.

Helpful: Consumers often feel that throwing out a working refrigerator is wasteful. But virtually every part of an old refrigerator is likely to be recycled. It is more wasteful to continue using an energy hog.

WASHING MACHINES

The typical washing machine lasts 12 years or more and consumes about $800 worth of electricity during that time.

Some new machines will consume less than half as much power, principally by using less hot water. Ninety percent of the energy used to wash clothes is to heat the water.

Buying an energy-efficient washer makes good financial sense. High-efficiency machines cost as little as $600—about $200 more than typical washers. They also deliver as much as $60 in annual energy savings, so they can pay for themselves over their lifetimes.

In addition to the energy savings, a high-efficiency machine should save 6,000 to 8,000 gallons of water per year, based on annual average family use of around 400 loads.

Front-loading machines typically are much more efficient than top loaders. They use less water, and their higher spin speeds remove more moisture, reducing the energy used by the dryer.

Energy saver: Wash clothes in cold water whenever appropriate.

CLOTHES DRYERS

Many new dryer models have temperature or moisture gauges that automatically turn off the unit when clothes are dry. Moisture sensors located inside the drum tend to be more accurate than temperature sensors. These can reduce your energy costs by up to 15%.

A typical new dryer will consume $85 worth of power a year, creating an annual savings of maybe $10. Over the expected 11-year life of a dryer, that is a total of $110.

Sensor models cost $150 to $250 more than base models. But given the energy savings, they come close to paying for the extra cost—and often do in areas where electricity is expensive.

Ask retailers which dryer models contain in-drum moisture or temperature sensors, or check for them yourself. They usually look like small, black patches located either in the back of the drum or near the lint filter.

Helpful: Replacing an electric dryer with a gas-powered model can reduce your energy bills to about 13 cents per load from about 35 cents, based on current average electricity and gas prices.

DISHWASHERS

There is now a debate regarding dishwasher energy efficiency. A number of models include a "soil sensor," which detects how dirty the dishes are and adjusts wash time and water usage. The potential energy advantage of this is obvious.

Manufacturers, however, can't agree on how much energy a soil sensor saves. The current Department of Energy tests are of little use because they test only with clean plates.

For the time being, it is difficult to say which models are best. A knowledgeable salesperson might offer some guidance. But if you need a dishwasher, check out the Energy Guide and Energy Star labels. Even without soil sensors, new models tend to be much more efficient.

Helpful: Don't prerinse dishes. Newer, more efficient dishwashers let you save time, water, electricity and elbow grease.

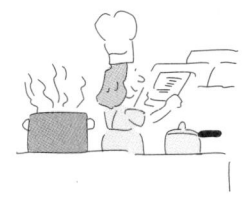

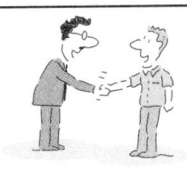

Finding a Good Contractor

Bill Keith, owner, Tri-Star Remodeling, St. John, IN, and host of the *Home Tips Show, www.billkeith.com*.

When it's time to have work done on your home, you want to locate a skilled and reliable contractor...

• **Ask your homeowner's insurance agent for contractor referrals.** It is in the insurer's best interests to have quality work done...and agents have to protect their reputations when making recommendations.

• **If you were pleased with any previous work**—a new roof, major plumbing or electrical repairs—ask the person who did it to suggest someone to do the work you now need. Contractors often are familiar with one another's work.

• **Get second or third opinions and estimates** before contracting for a major job, such as a new roof.

• **Ask your local building inspector** what he/she thinks of a specific contractor. Don't depend solely on statements that someone is licensed, bonded and/or insured. This simply means the person had money to pay the fees for such certification. Typically, no schooling or testing is required.

Important: If someone's recommendations seem odd or excessive, ask questions—a legitimate contractor will offer reasonable answers.

More from Bill Keith...

Contractor Self-Defense

To prevent problems when dealing with contractors, try following these helpful strategies...

• **Never pick a contractor from the phone book or an ad.** Referrals are best.

• **Ask references about quality and reliability.** See the contractor's work.

• **Ask for proof of licensing and insurance.** Check expiration dates.

■ *Your Money* ■ ■

• **Never pay up-front.** A common payment formula is one-third down, one-third midway and the rest of the payment on completion of the job.

Caution: Never pay in cash—you want proof of payment.

• **Ask for a *waiver of lien* in your contract.** It means you are not responsible for the contractor's debts to his/her subcontractors once you have paid him in full. The waiver must be signed and notarized once the work is done.

• **If you've given a contractor a deposit and don't hear from him,** send the contractor a registered letter—not a threatening one.

Helpful phrases: I appreciate the work you did for us…I have been unsuccessful in reaching you…To keep our relationship in good standing, I need to hear from you by (specific date) and have my work start by (specific date).

Referrals are so important to small businesses that a letter like this usually gets a response. If there's no response, you can sue in small-claims court—so long as you have a valid address for the contractor.

Also from Bill Keith…

Home Appliance Smarts

Every three months, use a rag soaked in hot, soapy water to clean the rubber door seals on your refrigerator and dishwasher. Greasy, dirty seals deteriorate, making appliances less efficient. Eventually, you would have to replace the seals, which can cost $100 or more.

No More Repair Rip-Offs

To prevent appliance-repair rip-offs, get a good idea of what is wrong before calling the repairperson—phone or E-mail the manufacturer and ask what typically causes your kind of problem. To find a good repairperson, ask neighbors for references. If the cost estimate seems high, then get a second opinion. During repairs, stick around to ask questions and take notes in case of a problem later.

David Borsykowsky, assistant attorney general, consumer and antitrust division, Office of the Attorney General, State of Vermont.

Repair Appliances Yourself

Visit *www.repairclinic.com* to help figure out what is broken on major appliances and then locate, order and install new parts. You pay only for the parts—the site is free.

Reader's Digest, Reader's Digest Rd., Pleasantville, NY 10570.

How to Hire a Moving Company

To get the best deal from moving companies, follow this practical advice…

• **Get at least three bids in writing,** preferably from firms certified by the American Moving and Storage Association.

• **Know whether you are getting a nonbinding estimate,** which is an educated guess and not guaranteed…or a binding estimate, which is a contract.

• **When you go to contract, read over the paperwork carefully**—be sure that the price includes loading and unloading.

• **Basic insurance coverage for no extra charge offers little protection.** Consider buying additional coverage.

David Sparkman, spokesman, American Moving and Storage Association, Alexandria, VA, www.moving.org.

Your Financial Future

12

Retirement Wisdom

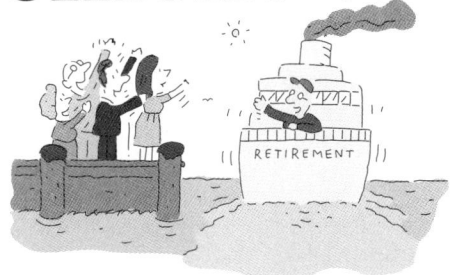

Retire on Less... And Live Well

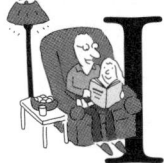

It still is possible to retire comfortably despite the last stock market tumble. Most people can reduce their living expenses by up to 30% in retirement without substantially lowering their standards of living.

Where to start...

DOWNSCALE THE HOUSE

Many people near or in retirement have one large investment that has held its value—their home. Now is the perfect time to sell your house and move somewhere less expensive.

Step down in size but not in comfort. Move to a place that is just as nice but smaller. With the kids out of the house, much of a big home goes unused.

Example: A recently retired couple sold a family home in suburban New Jersey for $450,000 and bought a small apartment just blocks from Lincoln Center in Manhattan for $300,000. They added the remaining $150,000 to their depleted retirement savings. What the apartment lacks in living space it makes up for in its interesting location.

Selling the family home also can reduce living expenses. You are likely to save on property taxes, insurance, utilities and lawn care and other maintenance. My clients who moved to Manhattan even sold their car, further trimming expenses. The savings can add up to thousands of dollars a year on top of the profit from the sale of their home.

•**Pick a cheaper region.** Most of us spend the better part of our lives living where our careers require. But in retirement, we can live wherever we like.

Bargain spots: Arizona, Florida, Nevada and Texas.

Karen C. Altfest, PhD, CFP, vice president, L.J. Altfest & Co., a fee-only financial planning and investment management company, 116 John St., New York City 10038, *www.altfest.com*. She is the northeast region chairperson for the National Association of Personal Financial Advisors. Ms. Altfest is author of *Keeping Clients for Life* (Wiley).

Everything from housing to taxes to groceries can cost substantially less. Your expenses easily can decline by 30%—or more, if you currently reside in a more expensive locale. Check *www.bestplaces.net* for a cost-of-living comparison among regions.

If you are concerned that you will feel out of touch, consider a university town. They generally have a cosmopolitan feel. Universities offer inexpensive entertainment options, including concerts, plays, lectures and sporting events.

One client of mine, a single woman in her 60s, found a wonderful way to enjoy a luxurious retirement on less than $50,000 per year. She relocated to Mexico.

Communities of US retirees are now springing up amid beautiful Mexican settings, most notably in the region of Lake Chapala. Go to *www.chapala.com*. Since the area is full of Americans, the culture shock is mitigated and dependable security and health care providers are available.

Expatriate retirees, however, still have to pay US income taxes on retirement benefits and must travel back to the US if they wish to take advantage of Medicare benefits.

You also should determine your foreign tax obligations with your tax professional. Each country is different.

STOP CARRYING THE KIDS

Many of my clients who are closing in on retirement treat their grown-up children like dependents. They help with mortgages, pay grandkids' college expenses and buy expensive gifts. That's fine if you can afford it—but most people can't.

Example: One couple nearing retirement age came to me because they were concerned about their shrunken portfolio. It turned out that they were spending more than $50,000 a year on their adult daughter—even though the daughter and her husband both had good jobs and decent incomes. My clients were not in a position to give away that kind of money without feeling a big pinch.

Explain to adult children that if you don't stop spending so much on them, they will wind up supporting you in a few years.

REEVALUATE MEMBERSHIPS

Most of my clients in their 50s and 60s have numerous memberships and attend dozens of events a year. These can add up to thousands of dollars.

Scale back on events and memberships. If you do not want to give them up entirely, inquire about senior, associate or out-of-towner membership options at lower cost.

USE SENIOR DISCOUNTS

Many restaurants, retailers, hotels and other businesses offer senior discounts, typically 5% to 15%, sometimes starting as young as age 50. You have to ask for them. If someone is willing to offer you the same product or service at a reduced rate, it is wasteful not to take advantage.

There also is no reason to give up on your retirement travel dreams. Travel very economically through senior organizations, including Elderhostel (877-426-8056 or *www.elderhostel.org*) or local seniors' groups. Groups usually get the best travel deals.

Helpful: When traveling in Europe, senior discounts are referred to as "pensioners' rates."

WORK DURING RETIREMENT

Because of the last stock market meltdown, many people who thought they were finished with work now must stay on or return to the workforce. If handled properly, this doesn't have to ruin your retirement.

Act as soon as possible if there is any chance that you will need to work. Do not procrastinate, thinking that you will go back to work in a few years if your investments don't rebound.

When you have been out of the workplace for over five years, you lose your most important asset—the people in your company and industry who know and respect your work. In many professions, skills become obsolete quickly.

Stay connected to your profession and former employer from the day you walk out the door. Then it is easier to "jump back in" and work two days a week or consult.

Example: A recently retired management consultant got rid of his office and stopped seeking new accounts when he retired. But he continues to consult on-site for existing clients. It allows him to stay active, keeps his name in circulation and supplements his savings.

Some people intend to use their retirement years to enter a "dream" profession. Even so, they should stay in touch with their old line of work in case the new profession doesn't pan out and they need to supplement their income.

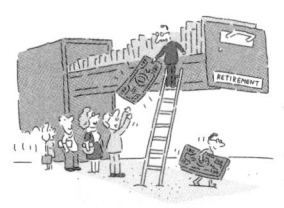

Will You Have Enough To Retire?

Jonathan D. Pond, CPA, president, Financial Planning Information, Inc. at 9 Galen St., Watertown, MA 02472, *www.jonathanpond.com.* He is author of many books on personal finance, most recently *Your Money Matters: 21 Tips for Achieving Financial Security in the 21st Century* (Perigee). He also is host of *www.yourfinancialroadmap.com,* an investment and financial planning Web site.

Despite all the warnings about the need to save, many Americans still believe that the cost of retirement will be only 35% of their current income. The majority of the 80,000 adults I just surveyed are dangerously underestimating their needs.

Reality: Middle- and upper-income Americans require at least 80% of their preretirement income during retirement. You won't be paying payroll taxes, such as Social Security, or job-related expenses. And, of course, you won't have to save for retirement. But these reductions often are offset by your medical or travel costs. Also, if you have a large mortgage your expenses could even exceed 80%.

TO PLAN SENSIBLY

•**Project your retirement *budget.*** In my survey, only 23% of people age 50 and older actually had tried to estimate their retirement spending. Yet people in this age group *should* have well-developed retirement plans.

The calculation is simple. Base your projection on the assumption that you will live to be 95. If you plan for a shorter life expectancy, you risk running out of money. *For a quick estimate, follow these steps…*

•Take your current net income, and subtract the amount you are putting into savings. If, for example, you make $60,000 a year after taxes and save $10,000, then you are spending $50,000 a year.

•Multiply that figure—$50,000—by 80%, which is the percentage of current income you'll need in retirement. In this particular example, you would need $40,000 each year.

•Multiply $40,000 by the number of years between your retirement age and 95. If you plan to retire at age 65, that would be 30 years.

Result: You would need $1.2 million to fund your retirement.

I use current spending in this calculation with no adjustment for future inflation. I assume that inflation will average 3% a year and return on your nest egg will grow at least in line with inflation.

For a more exact estimate, use one of the free Internet tools. *My favorites…*

•*www.asec.org,* from American Savings Education Council. Click on "Savings Tools," then on "The Ballpark Estimate."

•*www.smartmoney.com/retirement.* Click on "The SmartMoney Retirement Worksheets."

•**Project your retirement *income.*** Not all that $1.2 million must come from your savings. Social Security and your pension, if you will receive one, will pay some of it.

•Find out what your Social Security benefit will be. The Social Security Administration (SSA) mails you an estimate each year around your birthday. Or you can request the statement anytime by contacting the SSA at 800-772-1213 or *www.socialsecurity.gov.*

•If you will have a pension, ask your employer's benefits department to estimate your future payment. Also ask what options you have for receiving benefits.

•Ask a representative at the financial services company that manages your 401(k) plan to help you calculate how much money you eventually will accumulate and how much income it will generate.

•Assume that your other investments will appreciate until retirement—but be conservative. I now estimate a 6% return.

■ *Your Financial Future* ■ ■ ■

CLOSING THE GAP

If your calculation shows that you won't have enough money for retirement, there are steps you can take now...

• **Put your current expenses on a diet.** I frequently see even high-income people with anemic nest eggs spending about 85% to 90% of their incomes.

Debt is substantially higher for most people than it was only a few years ago, according to my survey. Money used to pay off debt is lost to your retirement nest egg.

Starting now, begin paying down your debt —and stop adding to it.

• **Delay retirement.** If you work for just one year past your hoped-for retirement age—even without adding to your savings—you increase the amount you can draw from your nest egg over the rest of your life by 10%. This is based on the compounded growth of your investment and having fewer years to spend it.

• **Break the lock on locked-in assets.** My study shows that half of most people's wealth is tied up in their homes and their possessions. In California, that figure is closer to 60%. Owning a home may make you feel wealthy, but it doesn't provide retirement income.

What to do: Pay off high-interest loans. Then devise a plan to pay off your mortgage as soon as possible in order to minimize interest payments. When the nest empties out, sell your home and buy something more modest. Add the profit to your nest egg.

Caution: Don't make extra mortgage payments until you can maximize your retirement-savings payments. Hopefully, you can do both. Even small extra payments help pay off the mortgage sooner.

Example: If you have a $100,000 mortgage balance that runs for another 25 years, you can pay it off in just 15 years if you add $100 to each mortgage payment.

Couples can take up to $500,000 in capital gains from the sale of a house without owing taxes. That's a tremendous incentive to sell your home and find someplace cheaper to live.

What I advise my clients: Buy a two-bedroom apartment. With the money you save, you will be able to put the kids up in the most expensive hotel in town whenever they visit.

KEEP YOUR NEST EGG SAFE

Many retirees take absurd risks in pursuit of high returns.

Example: A retired couple I know lost almost 70% of their nest egg because they invested heavily in technology stocks. Now they have to sell their house, eliminate vacations and curtail daily living expenses just to make ends meet.

The best allocation to earn a 6% return is the classic 60% in stocks and 40% in bonds, no matter what your age.

After several bear-market years, many retirees are horrified by the idea of having 60% of their assets in stocks. But they don't need just income —they need *growing* income. And growth in income only comes from stocks.

Here's how I would invest the 60% equity allocation...

• **20% in large-cap value.**

• **15% in large-cap growth.**

• **15% in small- and mid-cap.**

• **10% in international stock funds.**

Learning to Enjoy Your Nest Egg

Once you've achieved financial security, you need to change your mind-set from *saving* to *enjoying*. It may be difficult to shift your focus from saving and investing to doing and spending, but take pride in your accomplishment. For years, you've worked hard, planned and saved. Now you can begin living the life you've long envisioned.

David R. Reiser, CFP, and Robert L. DiColo, CLU, ChFC, senior vice presidents, investments, UBS PaineWebber and coauthors of *WealthBuilding* (Wiley).

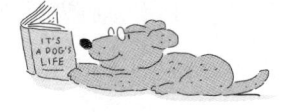

Don't Let These Financial Mistakes Destroy Your Retirement Dreams

Terence L. Reed, CFP, Livonia, MI. He is author of *The 8 Biggest Mistakes People Make with Their Finances Before and After Retirement* (Dearborn).

Retirement should mean realizing those financial dreams you've worked a lifetime to fulfill. Instead, I see many couples who will never realize their dreams because they made major errors in retirement planning.

Common planning mistakes...

Mistake: **Not putting your plans in writing.** Until you have a written plan, you haven't done all the essential investigating, fact-finding and thinking about retirement you should have. If it isn't in writing, crucial elements are certain to get overlooked.

The plan must cover every aspect of retirement—from a carefully thought out investment strategy to a realistic budget for spending. Both spouses must contribute to the plan. It can't just be the husband making decisions that the wife must live with or vice versa.

The closer you are to retirement, the more you'll want help from a financial planner in creating a written plan. Expect to spend $100 to $150 an hour. At the first session, settle how many hours it will take to produce your plan.

Mistake: **Being unrealistic about your exposure to risk.** The way Americans think about risk was distorted by the stock market bubble of the 1990s and the market crash of 2000. I see people who still have 100% of their allocation in the high-risk stocks, even though they are nearing retirement. I also see people who have moved 100% of their allocation into low-yield bank accounts. Neither group can look forward to a comfortable retirement.

Asset allocation should depend not on short-run market fluctuations, but on how many other sources of retirement income you'll have *besides* your investments.

Example: If you have a company pension plus Social Security, your allocation of money available to invest could be 80% stocks, even in retirement. If you'll have no pension to fall back on, your allocation should be limited to 50% stocks.

Even if most of your allocation is in stocks, keep your risk exposure low by keeping a good portion of the allocation in income-paying stocks.

Mistake: **Neglecting to do "dignity planning."** That means preparing a power of attorney and living will or health care proxy, which determine how much independence you can maintain in later years. Most people don't want to think about such things, so I have to work hard to get their attention.

Example: If your spouse were disabled, you would need a court order just to cash in jointly owned savings bonds—unless your spouse had signed a durable power of attorney. To make medical decisions on behalf of a disabled spouse, without court permission, you'll need a living will or health care proxy.

Once people understand that not having such documents can create big problems for their loved ones, they see a lawyer.

Mistake: **Closing the door on long-term-care (LTC) insurance.** People wrongly assume that once they're in their 60s, it's too late to buy insurance to cover nursing home stays. Actually, if your health is OK, you can buy it into your 80s. But, in your 60s, premiums are more affordable.

Caution: Don't overspend on LTC insurance, since there's a 55% chance it will never be needed. Calculate what you now spend to live at home, including food, mortgage payments and utility bills.

Say your current spending comes to $35,000 a year, while current income is $45,000. You have an annual income surplus of $10,000. If a nursing home in your area costs $50,000 a year, buy only $40,000 in LTC coverage. Let your $10,000 income surplus cover the rest. If you're under age 70, pay for a cost-of-living adjustment so the $40,000 will keep pace with inflation.

Mistake: **Failing to understand the goal of estate planning.** The biggest problem here is do-it-yourself estate planning. Without seeking professional advice, people assume the goal of an estate plan is to avoid probate.

They put everything into joint ownership so property passes to the surviving spouse.

Trap: Because all property moves outside the will, any bequests the couple had in mind can't be made. Since the couple didn't use the exemption from estate tax (now $1 million), all the property will be subject to tax when the surviving spouse dies.

The aim of estate planning is to make sure your wishes are carried out. Instead of trying to do it yourself, see an estate-planning attorney.

Important: Congress has voted to eliminate the estate tax—but not until 2010. And under present law, the tax is supposed to return in 2011. Don't let estate planning slide, assuming you no longer face any risk from the tax.

Mistake: **Stepping into tax traps that trip up retirement planning.** Fearing the money might not be there when needed, people often take money out of a 401(k) plan at retirement and put enough to live on for 10 years into CDs or Treasury bills. Since these are taxable investments, and the distribution from your 401(k) is taxable, they're diverting a huge chunk of retirement savings to Uncle Sam.

A better way: Leave your money in the 401(k) and for your fixed-income needs, buy a tax-qualified annuity. Your money builds up fully guaranteed and tax deferred until needed.

Buy a fixed annuity from a company with an A.M. Best rating of A++. Once agents know you're shopping, good deals will come out of the woodwork. One agent might guarantee your money will earn 4.5% for the next four years. Another might offer 6% for four years…and another 6% for five years.

Mistake: **Assuming you're too old for life insurance.** Seniors often assume that life insurance is only for families with young children. In fact, life insurance can be a great tool for seniors.

If you are in your 50s, you might pay $50,000 for a single-premium variable life insurance policy that carries a $100,000 death benefit. By doing so, you have *doubled* the effects of your retirement funds overnight.

Also, purchase life insurance to provide for a child with special needs…or to pay final medical expenses, which can be huge. If you don't have long-term-care insurance, use life insurance to protect your estate against Medicaid recoupment programs.

Big risk: If a nursing home stay exhausts your financial resources (other than exempt assets, such as a home), Medicaid will pick up the tab. At your death, the federal government may go after what is left of your estate to recover the bills Medicaid paid. Without money to reimburse Medicaid, your spouse could face losing the family home.

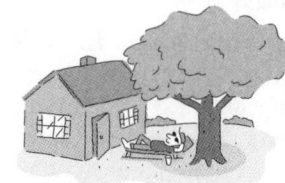

How to Guarantee Income for Life

Robert Kreitler, CFP, principal, Kreitler Associates, financial advisers and affiliate of Raymond James Financial Services, 195 Church St., New Haven, CT 06510. He is author of *Getting Started in Global Investing* (Wiley).

Many retirees rely on bond investments in their portfolios to supplement their income. Then they cross their fingers, hoping that they won't run out of money.

But immediate fixed annuities guarantee a cash flow for life—one that retirees can't outlive.

HOW ANNUITIES WORK

The immediate fixed annuities are essentially just insurance vehicles—the same as those that companies use to finance lifetime employee pensions. Most of us are familiar with deferred annuities. These annuities grow capital tax deferred for retirement.

Immediate annuities generate cash *during* retirement. The income from the immediate fixed annuity is higher than the income of government bonds because it includes repayment of principal.

Example: A 65-year-old man might make $4,400 a year in income on a $100,000 investment in a 30-year Treasury bond that yields 4.4%. With a $100,000 immediate fixed annuity, he could boost his annual cash flow for life by 68%, to $7,400 per year.

What's the catch? First, there is no principal remaining upon the annuitant's death. This is the trade-off for higher monthly payments and a lifetime guarantee. Keep the money for your heirs separate from your annuity portfolio.

Remember to obtain a *term-certain provision*. This guarantees payments for a specified number of years, usually 10, even if you die soon after buying the annuity.

An annuity is irrevocable. You can't sell it like a bond. And, like most bonds, it doesn't protect you from inflation. Therefore, keep a portion of your nonannuity portfolio in stocks.

HOW TO ANNUITIZE

Most retirees can benefit from immediate annuities. The smaller their savings, the greater the need. Generally, those who have assets in excess of $2 million probably don't need immediate annuities.

The older you are—and the shorter your life expectancy—when you buy the immediate fixed annuity, the more generous the monthly payments. Retirees can receive even more generous payments by buying a new annuity every five or 10 years, starting at age 65. Staggering terms also provides some protection against interest rates which are very low today—you hedge your bets by buying annuities in different interest rate climates.

COMPARISON SHOPPING

Research the financial health of the insurers on the Web sites of independent ratings agencies, such as A.M. Best Co. (908-439-2200 or *www.ambest.com*) and Weiss Ratings Inc. (800-289-9222 or *www.weissratings.com*). Compare the rates of top-quality insurers and take the highest rate.

Minimum investments are low, depending on the annuity. You can buy them through a broker, insurance agent or financial planner.

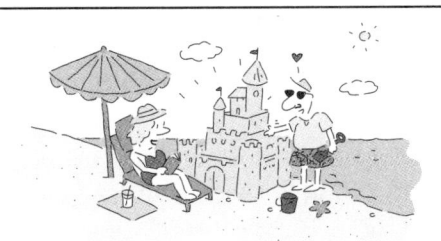

Lump Sum vs. Pension For Life

Take a lump sum at retirement if the company offers you a choice of a lump-sum payout or a pension for life. The lump sum, which you can transfer directly to an IRA, gives you control over your investments. You may be able to earn more investing on your own than from the company's choice of a fixed annuity.

Also: Most pension-for-life arrangements end at your or your spouse's death, leaving nothing for heirs.

But: Not taking a lump sum may make sense in certain circumstances, such as when you want to ensure that your spouse will have a steady income or you aren't comfortable investing on your own.

Consult a financial adviser before deciding.

Martin Nissenbaum, Esq., CPA/PFS, CFP, national director, retirement and personal income tax planning, Ernst & Young LLP, 5 Times Square, New York City 10036.

Dangerous Pension Errors to Avoid

John Hotz, attorney, Pension Rights Center, 1140 19 St. NW, Washington, DC 20036, *www.pensionrights.org*.

Carefully examine the pension you expect to receive before you make the decision to retire. If you discover a problem after you start receiving the pension, it may be too late to fix it. *Common mistakes...*

•**Taking a lump-sum payout of your benefit** because it looks like a large amount of money. Make sure the lump sum accurately reflects the value of your annuity. Forfeitures can sometimes occur when subsidized early retirement benefits are taken as a lump sum.

•**Not understanding how years of service are credited.** The specific date on which you retire can affect the calculation of your benefits.

■ *Your Financial Future* ■ ■ ■

• **Misjudging the amount of the monthly payment** you will be entitled to take.

Best: In advance of retirement, obtain the "Summary Plan Description" from your plan administrator. Review it with an adviser, then devise retirement strategies accordingly.

More from John Hotz...

Beware of the Social Security Integration Trap

When a pension plan benefit formula uses Social Security integration, it counts the Social Security benefits in your pension, so you may get less from it than you expect.

Example: Your pension plan promises $1,000 per month and your Social Security benefits will be $1,000 per month—so you expect income of $2,000 per month. But if the pension plan utilizes Social Security integration, up to half of Social Security benefits may count toward your pension. The pension itself will pay out only $500, and your income will be only $1,500.

Trap: About half of all employers use Social Security integration. Find out if yours does before you retire, so you won't be surprised.

If You Plan to Retire and Marry at the Same Time...

Getting married just before you retire can be costly. If you are married when you retire, the default payout for your pension probably will be a "joint and survivor" method. This provides less money each month in return for making payments to your spouse for life as well as to you. That may be fine—but if your spouse has his/her own pension, or if you expect to outlive your spouse, you may do better to take a pension that covers your life alone, and which may pay as much as 25% more each month as a result.

Review your pension plan *and* your future spouse's pension plan, if any, before you marry.

Find out whether your new spouse can waive survivor benefits so that you can collect larger amounts during your life. Then choose the best option available to you.

AARP The Magazine, 601 E St. NW, Washington, DC 20049.

Retirees Beware

Many companies that previously provided medical benefits to retirees are cutting back the coverage or eliminating it.

Strategy: If your company stopped providing coverage, it may be possible to fight back through a class action lawsuit, but in many cases, corporate benefit plans allow firms to make such changes.

Self-defense: Until age 65, try to remain part of your former employer's health insurance program, or call to see if you can continue your health benefits under COBRA or a similar state program.

Americans age 65 and older are eligible for Medicare, the government program that covers some but not all medical costs.

Ron Pollack, executive director, Families USA, national nonprofit organization for health care consumers, 1334 G St. NW, Washington, DC 20005.

Roth IRA Conversion Trap

Converting your regular IRA to a Roth can increase the taxes owed on your Social Security benefits.

Why: The value of the regular IRA (minus nondeductible contributions to it) is taxed as income—and the Tax Court has held that this type of income is counted when figuring taxes due on Social Security.

Planning: Make a Roth conversion before you begin taking Social Security benefits.

Robert L. Helm, TC Summary Opinion 2002-138.

Retirement Wisdom

If You Inherit an IRA...

If you inherit an IRA from anyone other than your spouse, do not remove the original owner's name. If you substitute your name on a nonspousal inherited IRA, the IRS considers the account cashed out and will assess taxes.

Self-defense: Have the IRA custodian add your name and Social Security number to the account...and make a note in account records of the date of your benefactor's death.

Lynn O'Shaughnessy, San Diego–based personal finance writer, *www.lynnosh.com,* and author of *Investing Bible* and *Retirement Bible* (both from Wiley).

Early Retirement Withdrawals Without Penalty

Retirement plan withdrawals before age 59½ are permitted without the usual 10% penalty —*under certain circumstances.* These include permanent disability, medical expenses and distributions to beneficiaries upon your death. The IRS also allows penalty-free withdrawals by calculating substantially equal periodic payments based on life expectancy. Withdrawals from accounts may also be made for education expenses, first-time home purchase and payment of health insurance premiums if you are unemployed. See your tax adviser for full details.

David Hennings, financial planner and syndicated columnist, Oak Park, IL.

Better Ways to Roll Over a 401(k) to an IRA

Avoid unnecessary commissions and fees when rolling over a 401(k) into an IRA. Find out how much it will cost you to buy, sell and hold each class of a fund's shares. Ask specifically how the adviser is being compensated so you will understand his/her bias. You also need to know about a fund's holding requirements. Typically, A shares, for which the load decreases with the amount invested, make the best sense for big sums. B shares have no front-end load, so are suitable for smaller investors. But they carry a back-end or deferred load that's payable when you sell. This fee decreases or disappears entirely the longer you hold the shares. B shares also tend to have higher 12b-1 servicing fees payable annually. Watch out for new fees being tacked on even by do-it-yourself no-load funds.

Julie Jason, JD, LLM, managing director, Jackson Grant & Co., investment advisers, 1177 High Ridge Rd., Stamford, CT 06905, *www.juliejason.com.*

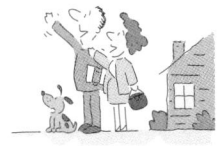

401(k) Vs. IRA Withdrawals

You are allowed to withdraw from your 401(k) *without penalty* if you leave a job to retire after reaching age 55. You will still owe tax on withdrawals, as with any tax-deferred investment. Rules for 401(k)s are different from those covering IRAs. You normally can't withdraw funds from an IRA without penalty until you turn 59½.

Ted Benna, founder and president, 401(k) Association, 2150 Dutch Hollow Rd., Jersey Shore, PA 17740.

What 401(k) Reports Don't Tell You

Long-term investment performance is missing from most 401(k) reports. Only 10% of financial services firms that offer retirement plans tell investors each quarter how much the plans have made or lost over the life of

199

■ *Your Financial Future* ■ ■ ■

their portfolios. More than half of all 401(k) providers show some form of personalized rate of return—but usually only for one quarter or year.

Self-defense: Compare your cost basis with current value to find out how much you have made or lost. A financial adviser can help you calculate the cost basis and annualized rate of return.

John Markese, PhD, president, American Association of Individual Investors, 625 N. Michigan Ave., Chicago 60611, *www.aaii.com*.

Is Your Keogh Plan Creditor-Proof?

Ed Slott, CPA, publisher, *Ed Slott's IRA Advisor*, 100 Merrick Rd., Rockville Centre, NY 11570. Mr. Slott is a nationally recognized IRA distributions expert. His Web site is *www.irahelp.com*.

Keogh retirement plans for self-employed individuals may not be protected against creditor claims by federal law when the plans do not cover employees.

Trap: Many individuals with "one person" Keogh plans (such as physicians) keep their funds in Keoghs under the mistaken belief that Keoghs are "creditor-proof" in the same way 401(k) and other qualified retirement plans are.

But such Keogh plans are protected only by state law, typically in the way that IRAs are. In many states, this leaves significant potential exposure to creditors.

Safety: If you have a Keogh plan, check its exposure to creditors under state law.

If it is as exposed as an IRA, after retiring you may do better to roll over your Keogh's funds into an IRA to take advantage of the broader range of planning options available to IRAs.

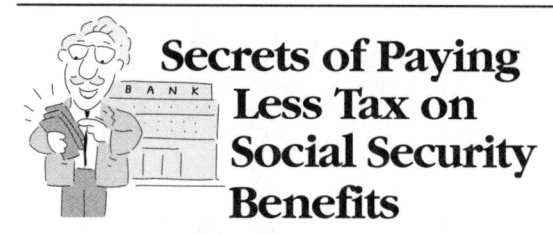

Secrets of Paying Less Tax on Social Security Benefits

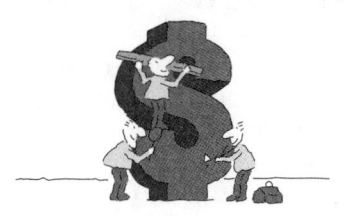

Stuart Kessler, managing director, American Express Tax and Business Services Inc., 1185 Avenue of the Americas, New York City 10036.

After many years of paying Social Security taxes on your earned income, you'll collect retirement benefits someday.

Problem: Up to 85% of those retirement benefits may be added to your other income—and taxed again.

Solution: Careful planning may reduce—or may even eliminate—the tax on your Social Security benefits.

PROVISIONAL INCOME

To determine this tax, you must first calculate your "provisional income," which is the total of...

1. Adjusted gross income (AGI) as reported on your federal income tax return.

2. Tax-exempt interest income from municipal bonds and municipal bond funds. *And...*

3. One-half of your annual Social Security benefits.

Example: With an AGI of $25,000, tax-exempt income of $4,000 and $20,000 in annual Social Security benefits, your provisional income is $39,000.

On a joint return, you can have provisional income up to $32,000 without having to pay any tax on your benefits. For single filers, the threshold is $25,000. Over those amounts, up to 50% of your benefits can be taxed.

Even worse, if your provisional income is more than $44,000 on a joint return or $34,000 filing singly, up to 85% of your benefits will be taxed.

INCOME LEVELS

As you can see, the taxability of your benefits depends on your income.

Very low income: When your provisional income is less than $25,000 ($32,000 on a joint return), you won't owe taxes on your Social Security benefits.

Very high: If that income is above $44,000 ($34,000 on a single return), there may not be much you can do to avoid paying tax on 85% of your benefits.

Middle ground: If your income is neither very low nor very high, some planning may cut the tax on your Social Security benefits.

Problem: Planning techniques may be most effective *before* age 70½. Subsequently, you probably will have to take minimum distributions from your IRA, which might push your income up to a level where taxes on your benefits are inevitable.

ANNUITIES

One solution is to use an immediate annuity for income before you reach age 70½.

Example: You retire at the age of 62 with $500,000 in a municipal bond fund that you intend to use for income. At a 4% yield, that would be $20,000 a year—all of which would be counted in your provisional income once you start to receive Social Security benefits.

Better way: Use that $500,000 to buy a 10-year term annuity. Your income from the annuity would be about $5,000 a month, or $60,000 a year.

Of the $5,000 per month you receive, only $1,000 or so might be taxable. The rest will be considered a tax-free return of capital. (The exact amounts will depend on various factors such as current interest rates and insurance company competitiveness.)

Bottom line: Instead of $20,000 worth of provisional income per year, this strategy drops the amount you will report to about $12,000. Within the income range described above, this reduction could mean 50% of your Social Security benefits will be taxed, rather than 85%. Or, your benefits might be completely untaxed.

Caution: The higher payout you get from investing $500,000 in an annuity rather than in a municipal bond fund results from your receiving a return of your own capital. Thus, you may want to spend only $20,000 a year and reinvest the rest.

OTHER OPTIONS

Additional strategies can help you reduce your provisional income and the tax you'll owe on Social Security benefits...

• **Seek shelter.** Inside deferred annuities or permanent life insurance, your earnings can build up without swelling your AGI.

Try to minimize your sales commissions and avoid surrender fees.

• **Live on loans.** Tap a home-equity line of credit or a margin account. Take out a reverse mortgage or refinance investment property. Borrow against your life insurance.

All of these techniques will provide cash flow but won't boost your provisional income.

• **Sell stocks.** Take losses on depreciated stocks and stock funds to raise cash. Not only will you avoid boosting your AGI, you'll also harvest tax losses that you can use now or in the future.

• **Stagger your income.** If you are withdrawing from your IRA or liquidating appreciated investments for retirement income, double up to skip years.

Example: You can increase your withdrawals and sales in 2004, boosting your tax bill this year. In 2005, though, you can tap this pool of cash while keeping your AGI to low levels.

A FINAL THOUGHT

Before you reach full retirement age (65 or later, depending on the year of your birth), you will face yet another problem with your Social Security benefits.

At ages 62 (the minimum starting age), 63 and 64, you lose 50 cents in Social Security benefits for every $1 you earn over $11,640 in 2004. The earned income threshold rises each year.

If you keep your earnings to that level, you'll reduce this effective taxation in addition to the actual taxation of your benefits. If your earnings will be well over $11,640, you're better off deferring your benefits. The longer you defer benefits, the larger your initial checks will be.

Once you reach your full retirement age (65 and four months for those born in 1939), you can earn any amount and still keep all your Social Security benefits. Thus, it may pay to defer compensation, including any bonuses, from ages 62 to 64 to until after age 65.

Tactic: From full retirement age to age 70, you're better off taking Social Security benefits than tapping your IRA for spending money. No more than 85% of your Social Security benefits (and perhaps less) will be taxed while 100% of any IRA withdrawals will be added to your taxable income.

Moreover, deferring your IRA withdrawals will permit you to receive more tax-deferred compounding.

Keep Your W-2s

Retain all your W-2 forms until you confirm that the Social Security Administration (SSA) has correctly recorded your earnings history. That history determines your future Social Security benefits.

How to confirm: Check the earnings history statement sent to you each year a few months before your birthday. If the SSA makes a mistake, you will need your W-2s to prove your earnings.

More information: Contact the SSA at 800-772-1213 or *www.socialsecurity.gov*.

Wayne G. Bogosian, president, PFE Group, employee communication and investment counseling firm, Natick, MA, and coauthor of *The Complete Idiot's Guide to 401(k) Plans* (Alpha).

Rehearse Your Retirement

Decide what sort of retirement life you really want to have, discuss it with your spouse and try it out about five years before you plan to stop working.

Examples: If you expect to play golf every day, take a two-week vacation and do just that—to see if you would really enjoy doing it for years. Since you and your spouse will probably be spending more time together in retirement, take a week off together and spend it at home, without any specific plans.

Also, calculate how much money you will have to live on during retirement, and try living on that amount for a time. You may find full-time retirement impractical—part-time work may be necessary.

Christina M. Povenmire, CFP, principal, CMP Financial Planning, 3960 Lytham Ct., Columbus, OH 43220.

Better Retirement Locations

When choosing a place to retire, look at the state's financial condition. Most retirement surveys rank quality-of-life factors, such as weather...sports and cultural events...medical care. But a weak economy—evidenced by low ratings for the state's bonds—can affect quality of life. It can put a crimp in services, such as senior centers and public transportation, and lead to increased crime and tax rates. In 2002, most states had budget deficits. Look to states or municipalities rated AA or AAA as possible places to retire.

Ratings can be found at *www.fitchratings.com*. Click on "Public Finance," then on "US Public Finance" and finally on "New Issue Reports."

Jim Lynch, municipal bond consultant and publisher of *Lynch Municipal Bond Advisory, www.lynchmuni.com*.

▪▪▪ Your Financial Future ▪

13

Protecting Your Estate

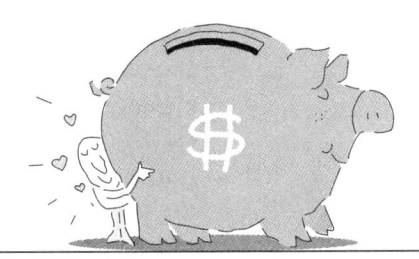

Estate Planning for Terribly Tricky Times

The recent big stock market plunge and economic recession may have reduced the resources you have to provide for your own future and that of your family.

If so, here is how to improve your estate planning in the new circumstances to protect yourself and benefit your family and heirs to the extent that you still can...

STEPS TO TAKE

First, take an inventory of your holdings now and make a realistic projection of how they may grow in the future from today's situation.

Your investments and business may both have changed in value significantly—you need to know what they are worth *now*. And if you had overly optimistic expectations of investment gains in the future, adjust them to more realistic levels.

When you know what you are worth today and have a realistic estimate of your future worth and needs, you can readjust your planning strategies. *Steps to consider...*

•**Manage children's college savings yourself.** While there are significant tax advantages to giving money to a Section 529 plan or custodial account, be sure the tax advantages outweigh your economic uncertainty. If you put college savings in a child's name—such as through a Section 529 plan, Coverdell Education Savings Account or *Uniform Transfers to Minors Act* account—you make a completed gift, although you can get the money back from a 529 plan by paying a penalty.

This can be especially risky if your job is in jeopardy or your earnings and savings declined dramatically. You can't foretell what your own

---

Martin M. Shenkman, CPA and attorney in New York City who specializes in trusts and estates. He is the author of numerous books, including *The Complete Book of Trusts* and *The Beneficiary Workbook* (both from Wiley). His Web site, *www.laweasy.com,* offers free sample forms and documents.

needs will be then, and the child may not even go to college.

You can still get tax advantages by managing these funds yourself. If you save using capital gains assets (such as mutual funds), you can cash in gains at favored long-term tax rates.

Even better, you may be able to cash in the gains at the child's lower or zero tax rate, making a gift of the investment assets to the child and letting the child cash them in to finance his/her own expenses. Children of age 14 or older aren't subject to the kiddie tax and in 2003 can take as much as $750 of investment income tax free ($800 in 2004). After that, their first $7,000 ($7,150 in 2004) of ordinary taxable income is taxed at only 10%.

You can use your annual gift tax exclusion ($11,000 per recipient, $22,000 when gifts are made jointly by a couple) to make such gifts free of gift tax.

More: If you pay tuition on the behalf of a child directly to an educational institution, gift tax does not apply at all. So, you can make an $11,000 (or $22,000) gift to the child using your annual exclusion and then pay any additional amount of tuition for the child directly to the school, free of gift tax.

Problem: Placing wealth in a child's name can also reduce the child's eligibility for tuition assistance, compared with having the same funds held by parents or grandparents. Rules vary by the kind of arrangement—and may well change in the future, so this is something else to consider with an expert before putting savings in a child's name.

•**Make loans to children and grandchildren.** Making full use of the annual gift tax exclusion to pass wealth to children and grandchildren is standard advice when one's wealth is large enough to face estate tax. Estates are taxable in 2004 when they are more than $1.5 million (lower for some state estate taxes).

But if your wealth has been reduced by the market fall, estate tax may be less of a danger and there may be more risk that you'll need the money yourself in the future.

Strategy: Help members of the younger generation by making loans to them on very advantageous terms, instead of making gifts. This way you can recover the funds if you need them—but can also make future tax-free gifts to the loan recipients that they can use to repay up to $11,000 (or $22,000) of the loans annually if it turns out you do not need the funds then.

Rules: The loans that have a below-market interest rate generally are treated by the IRS as if they carried the market rate of interest under "imputed interest" rules.

No interest is imputed if total loans to an individual do not exceed $10,000. For loans of up to $100,000, imputed interest is limited to the amount of investment income of the loan recipient. So, loans up to $100,000 can be made with no adverse tax effect if recipients with little investment income use them to buy a house, start a business or pay tuition.

•**Adjust separate bequests and spousal bypass trusts.** A married couple can use two estate tax exemptions of up to $1.5 million each (in 2004) to pass up to $3 million to heirs free of estate tax. To do this, the first spouse to die must make separate bequests of up to $1.5 million to use up his exempt amount, before leaving the rest of his estate to the surviving spouse.

Often this is done by leaving up to $1.5 million to a "bypass trust" that can pay income to the surviving spouse for life if the spouse needs it, and then distribute its proceeds to children or other heirs.

Caution: If your wealth has decreased, a will that makes a full $1.5 million of separate bequests may leave *too little* to your spouse. Even if the assets are placed in a bypass trust that can pay income to the spouse, such payouts may place the spouse in conflict with other heirs.

Safety: Increase outright (nontrust) bequests so that your spouse is well provided for first. Reduce other bequests and amounts left to any bypass trust accordingly.

•**Rebalance equal bequests.** Bequests to different heirs of different assets that once had equal value now may have very different values—such as if one was funded with shares of stock that have lost value, and another was funded with real estate that has gained value.

If you still want to make equal bequests, rebalance them now and take steps to keep them balanced in the future.

Example: After bequests of specific property are provided for, give your executor or trustee the power to distribute your remaining cash and liquid assets among heirs in a "balancing" manner.

●**Make more efficient bequests by using a "sprinkle trust."** If your wealth has been significantly reduced, bequests of equal value to several heirs may not be sufficient in size to assure the welfare of all, when heirs are in different financial circumstances.

Strategy: Leave assets in a "sprinkle trust" that gives the trustee the power to distribute its assets and income in accordance with personal needs and according to your instructions. That way, your more limited funds will be better targeted to heirs who need the money.

●**Use life insurance to fund bequests rather than pay estate tax.** People who purchased life insurance to finance expected future estate taxes should think carefully before letting the insurance lapse now if their estates have diminished so greatly that estate tax is no longer an issue.

Alternative: If you have such insurance, consider keeping it to finance bequests to heirs, now that you will be able to fund only smaller bequests from your estate. The insurance proceeds may offset the reduction of the rest of your estate.

If insurance is properly held in a life insurance trust, the proceeds can avoid estate tax.

More from Martin Shenkman...

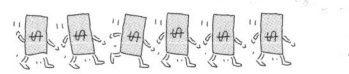

Secure Your Family's Future

The slow economy and bear market did not affect only jobs and portfolios. They also affected many estate plans. *Here are adjustments to make now to keep your family's future on track...*

UPDATE BENEFICIARY DESIGNATIONS

Outdated beneficiary designations for retirement accounts, life insurance policies, bank and investment accounts and trusts are a common and costly error.

Sometimes, accounts or policies that were set up long ago are simply forgotten, resulting in obsolete beneficiary designations.

Assets transferred to the wrong beneficiary can be expensive to redirect. When transfers are made incorrectly for IRAs and other retirement accounts, taxes may be increased needlessly.

When to update designations...

During major life changes: When you marry, have children or divorce or when a beneficiary dies.

During evolving personal circumstances: When wealth greatly increases or decreases... when children grow up and leave home.

Self-defense: Review all of your insurance policies, investment accounts and trusts to be sure that they have the intended beneficiaries. Revise beneficiary designations for IRAs and other retirement accounts with the help of an expert who is familiar with the tax rules.

KEEP THE PROPER DOCUMENTS

In addition to a will, you should draw up the following documents...

●**Durable power of attorney** that empowers a trusted individual to manage your financial affairs during any time in which you are unable to do so.

●**Living will and health care proxy** that names someone to make health care decisions on your behalf if you cannot.

●**Emergency child medical-care form.** If you have children, designate someone to make emergency medical decisions for them if you are unavailable or incapacitated.

●**Balance sheet which lists all of your assets**—insurance policies, investment and retirement accounts, etc.—so that the information (account numbers, company addresses) is in a single place.

Prepare these documents after examining *what if* scenarios.

Examples: Ask *what if* the people to whom you intended to give authority are not available... *what if* investments you plan to use to pay foreseen expenses suddenly lose value.

205

Make contingency plans, such as opening a line of credit.

Keep documents in a safe, accessible location so that they will not be destroyed in a disaster.

PROTECT YOUR BUSINESS

If your wealth is tied to a business, be sure that business is adequately protected against calamities.

Examples: The deaths of key employees …earthquake, flood or other disaster…wrongdoing by key personnel.

Also have *business interruption insurance,* which compensates for lost revenue if the business is forced to cease operations temporarily.

REVIEW BEQUESTS

Many investments lost value since the bear market began in March 2000, affecting bequest values. *Traps…*

•**Bequests meant to be of equal value may be unequal now** if they were funded with different kinds of assets—stocks versus bonds.

•**A single bequest to a person or charity may now be worth less** than you intended. The same goes for a *residuary* bequest, which is funded by what is left after all other bequests have been paid.

Review bequests periodically as your circumstances and those of your heirs change. Leave your heirs percentage shares in your estate rather than specific investments or dollar amounts.

ESTATE TAX CHANGES

Do not assume that the estate tax will be repealed in 2010 or that the personal estate tax exemption amount will increase, as the new law provides. *How to handle the uncertainty…*

•**Formula bequests.** Some wills include specific dollar amounts or formulas. Review them to avoid any unintended consequences.

Example: To use the maximum exclusion amount ($1.5 million in 2004) for a bequest, a married person might leave "the maximum exempt amount to X, with the remainder to my spouse."

Trap: The exclusion amount may change in coming years under the new law, resulting in an increased bequest to X at the spouse's expense.

Example: A formula bequest would split up a $3 million estate equally between X and the surviving spouse. But when the exclusion per person rises to $2 million in 2006, the formula clause disinherits the spouse.

•**Fiduciaries and trustees.** An executor or trustee can determine how your estate will be administered. Be sure that your estate plan provides such a fiduciary the authority he/she requires and protects him in disputes. Tell family members about the arrangements.

•**Taxes.** Assets you thought would cover estate taxes may fall short.

Big problem: The beneficiaries of assets that pass outside of the probate estate—including IRAs, life insurance and annuities—may not be required to contribute their share of taxes from their inheritances. As a result, some heirs may bear an unfair burden of the tax or face a tax assessment from the IRS.

Self-defense: Make sure your plan provides for the full payment of estate taxes.

Example: Tax-free proceeds from an insurance trust can be loaned to your estate so that it can pay the tax.

Also from Martin Shenkman…

State Death Tax Alert

State death taxes take a bigger bite out of some estates even as federal death taxes decline. More than a dozen states use a *pickup tax*—it absorbs, or picks up, the dollar-for-dollar credit allowed on the federal estate tax return for death taxes actually paid to the state. It is calculated based on death taxes as they existed in 2001 or before. Estates less than the federal exclusion (currently $1 million) will owe no federal tax—but they may owe state tax. Eleven states have *inheritance tax,* determined by who gets property and how much. Some states have tax that applies to the estate as a whole and starts at a much lower level than federal taxes.

Self-defense: Work with an estate planner to determine how to minimize death taxes.

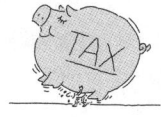

Finally from Martin Shenkman...

Estate Planning After Divorce

Most states require you to designate a minimum amount in your will to a former spouse. If you do not, he/she may have the automatic right to a portion of your estate. In many states, that means one-third of your assets. Laws differ significantly from state to state. Consult a knowledgeable attorney.

Wealth Planning for Blended Families

David S. Rhine, CPA, regional director, family wealth planning, Sagemark Consulting, a division of Lincoln Financial Advisors Corp., registered investment adviser, Rochelle Park, NJ.

Estate planning becomes especially complex—legally and personally—when one or both spouses have children from a previous marriage.

In these "blended" families, conflicts often arise among the children of different marriages, stepchildren and current and former spouses. And legal traps await, too.

Here's what to do...

HAVE A WRITTEN PLAN

You must have a written, documented plan —including a will and perhaps a living trust— to accomplish your wishes.

If you die without these legal documents in place, your assets will be divided among your spouse and children according to state law through the local probate court.

Typically, your spouse would receive half of your assets, and the other half would then be divided equally among your biological children, regardless of their personal circumstances. Your spouse's children won't be treated as your children unless you legally adopted them—so they would end up with nothing.

Division of property can be complicated by issues involving separate property you brought into the marriage and whether the community property rules apply in your state.

Since the state-law formula is unlikely to meet the specific needs of your family, it's much better to customize your property division. *You may wish to...*

- **Leave more to one child than another,** based on their personal circumstances.
- **Leave more to your children than to your spouse** if your spouse has substantial wealth of his/her own.
- **Leave more to your spouse than to your children** if they are economically successful adults.
- **Provide for your spouse's children** from a previous marriage.
- **Disinherit the economically successful children** from a previous marriage to leave everything to your spouse and minor children from your current marriage.

You aren't legally required to leave anything to children. But you cannot unilaterally disinherit your spouse. A spouse must agree to waive any estate claims by means of a prenuptial or postnuptial agreement. If you wish to minimize a bequest to your spouse, check your state's laws regarding the size of minimum spousal bequests.

QTIP SOLUTION

The estate tax exemption is $1.5 million in 2004. You will face estate tax if you own more than that—or will in the future, due to appreciation in the value of assets you own.

Basic tax planning: Assets left to a spouse pass free of estate tax. But leaving everything to a spouse may increase tax in the long run, since assets will pile up in the spouse's estate where they will get the benefit of only one $1.5 million tax-exempt amount.

Leaving everything to your spouse may also conflict with other objectives. For instance, when your spouse later dies, your children from a prior marriage may receive nothing from his estate—either because your spouse disinherited them or by action of state law if your spouse dies without a valid will in place.

Solution: Leave assets in a qualified terminable interest property (QTIP) trust to provide your spouse with lifetime income and assure the assets will pass to your children or other beneficiaries upon your spouse's death.

Property left in a QTIP qualifies for the estate tax marital deduction because only your spouse benefits from it while he lives. But on your spouse's death, the trust assets pass not according to your spouse's directions, but yours.

TRUSTS FOR CHILDREN

Assets that you leave to persons other than your spouse may require the protection of a trust as well.

•**If you leave large bequests to minor children,** you will want to create a trust to manage them for the children and control the timing of their distribution.

•**If you make bequests to minor children of a prior marriage,** your ex-spouse normally would control them as the children's guardian. So even if you make only modest bequests, but wish to control how they will be used, you may want to leave them in a trust. An account created under the *Uniform Transfers to Minors Act,* for which you name the custodian, can inexpensively serve this purpose until the child reaches the age of majority (18 or 21 in most states).

TRUSTEE SELECTION

Your choice of trustee is important because he may manage the trust's assets for a significant amount of time and have an important power over their distribution. Most often, people name a spouse or child to serve as trustee for simple estates.

If you anticipate that disputes may arise with your difficult family—a family-member trustee may be accused by others of being biased and unfair, for example—the choice can be more complicated.

Possibilities: Name cotrustees, such as a child from your current marriage and one from a former marriage, so both families feel they are fairly represented. Or name a trusted outside professional to serve as trustee and direct your estate in accordance with your wishes, immune from intrafamily pressure. Having your wishes secured may be worth the fee.

NONPROBATE ASSETS

Your most important assets may not pass through your estate at all. Such "nonprobate" assets include your IRAs, qualified retirement plan benefits, life insurance, jointly owned property and other such items that pass directly to named beneficiaries.

When dividing your estate, coordinate beneficiary designations for these items with the provisions of your will and living trust. Be sure all beneficiary designations are up to date.

If you want your retirement plan benefits to go to your children, make sure your spouse executes a "spousal waiver" with the plan's administrators. This is specifically required by federal law to waive a surviving spouse's rights to plan benefits.

If your estate is large enough to owe estate tax, be sure to provide a source of funds to pay the tax due on nonprobate assets. Otherwise, your executor would have to subtract funds from bequests he does control to pay tax due on nonprobate assets he doesn't control.

FINAL STEP

Discuss your objectives with your heirs. If they know your desires beforehand and understand why you divided your assets the way you did, this might prevent disputes among them after your death.

Review and revise your estate plan periodically in light of evolving family needs, the changing value of your probate and nonprobate assets, and changes in the federal estate tax and local estate laws.

More from David Rhine...

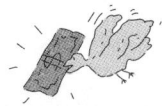

How to Help Charity And Your Family—and Disinherit the IRS

By setting up your own foundation, you can sharply cut your tax bill...and use the savings to help a charitable cause the way you want to.

Even better, you may help unite your family and garner favorable publicity for your family or business.

Plus, you may be able to leave your heirs more after-tax money than they would have received if you had made no charitable gift.

FOUNDATIONS SAVE TAXES

A private foundation is a charitable organization you fund. It is run by you and a board

Protecting Your Estate

that you put together—typically consisting of family members.

The after-tax cost of funding a foundation can be much lower than most people imagine. Moreover, tax savings can be used to buy "wealth replacement" life insurance that benefits your heirs.

Proceeds from this insurance will replace the bequests your heirs don't get when you give your assets to a foundation instead of to them. If you put the insurance policy in a trust, the proceeds will be tax free to your heirs. They can wind up receiving as much—or even more—from you after tax than they would have through a normal bequest.

Opportunity: The best asset with which to fund a foundation tax-wise is a tax-favored retirement plan account, such as an IRA or a 401(k). That's because these plans are subject to double taxation on the owner's death—the full amount in the account is first subject to estate tax, and then subject to income tax when distributed to the account beneficiary.

This double tax bill can reach 80%, including state and local taxes.

A private foundation enables you to avoid *all* these taxes—and use the huge tax savings for your own purposes.

Example: You have $1 million in an IRA, and your estate is large enough to be in the top estate tax bracket.

Without a foundation, the IRA will first be subject to 48% estate tax (if you die in 2004). That means a $480,000 tax bill.

Next, the full $1 million in the IRA will be subject to income tax in 2004 at up to a 35% federal rate when withdrawn by heirs (or by the estate to pay the estate tax on the IRA).

Partially offsetting this, the IRA beneficiaries will get an income tax deduction for the estate tax paid on the IRA—so they will owe income tax on $510,000, if the full $1 million IRA funds are withdrawn right away.

Together, the federal estate and income tax bills total more than $650,000. In high-tax states such as New York and California, local taxes may add much more.

Alternative: Create a private foundation and make it the beneficiary of your IRA. When you die, no estate tax will be owed on the IRA because of your estate's charitable contribution deduction for the gift. And no income tax will be owed on the IRA funds since the foundation is tax-exempt.

Payoff: What would otherwise be a tax bill of $650,000 is *entirely* avoided—and the full $650,000 remains available for use as you've directed.

For your heirs: When you set up the foundation, you can also create a life insurance trust and fund it with an insurance policy with a $300,000 or greater death benefit. The trust can receive the policy proceeds free of estate *and* income tax. It can use them to benefit the persons who would have been the beneficiaries of your IRA—making them "whole" with the same after-tax amount they would have received from the IRA.

The insurance policy will cost much less than the $300,000 portion of the IRA which would have remained after taxes—especially if you buy it early enough and use a second-to-die policy that pays on the death of the surviving spouse.

FUNDING WITH GIFTS

You can also make direct gifts to your foundation to get charitable contribution deductions.

Snag: Gifts to private foundations are subject to more stringent income tax deduction limits than gifts to public charities...

• **The deduction for contributions of appreciated property cannot exceed 20%** of adjusted gross income (AGI) in one year, although excess amounts can be carried to future years. The limit is 30% of AGI for gifts to public charities.

Caution: Only publicly traded stocks will net a deduction for fair market value.

• **Deductions for cash contributions to a private foundation are limited to 30%** of AGI in one year. Again, the excess amounts can be carried forward to be deducted in the future. The limit is 50% of AGI for cash gifts to public charities.

Third parties, including the general public, can make deductible contributions to your private foundation, subject to these limits. The funds don't all have to come from you.

Your Financial Future

FUNDING WITH TRUSTS

A charitable remainder trust is a popular charitable mechanism that provides multiple tax benefits and can also be used to fund a private foundation.

How it works: You transfer assets to a trust to benefit a charity. In exchange, the charity pays you income for the rest of your life or an agreed-upon term of years. At the end of that period, the principal amount of the assets passes to the charity, which could be a private foundation. *Tax benefits...*

- **If you transfer appreciated assets to the trust,** you avoid ever incurring capital gains tax on them.

Contrast: To liquidate appreciated assets on your own would probably require incurring gains tax.

- **You get a sizable charity deduction up front** for the current value of the transfer to charity that won't occur until the end of the trust term.

- **The assets left to charity are removed** from your estate, eliminating estate tax.

ADDITIONAL BENEFITS

A family foundation can promote family cohesiveness—serving to keep the family together over the long run.

Depending on how the foundation is set up, family members may serve on the board... manage investments or select an outside investment adviser...direct the foundation's charitable purpose...and select its beneficiaries.

Family members will have to work together to accomplish this. And an annual meeting that brings family members together to elect directors and perform other business can involve everyone in the family, young and old—while also serving to keep the whole family in contact for years to come.

Family members who provide services to the foundation—such as directing the foundation's investments—may be compensated by it with a reasonable amount.

A private foundation may provide favorable publicity and influence in the community—which may be useful for a family and valuable to a family business.

Expenses: The cost of establishing a family foundation is not very great. In New York, for example, the filing fee is about $150 plus an annual charge of $250. (Legal fees will also be involved.) The cost of other management tasks can be covered by having them performed by persons in the family or business that establishes the foundation, until it gets big enough to hire professional managers.

The law requires foundations to distribute at least 5% of their proceeds to charity each year. If investment returns exceed that amount, the foundation can grow in size indefinitely.

To make meaningful distributions with that level of payout, funding of $500,000 or more is probably necessary—although it need not be contributed all at one time. Funding can take place over a period of years.

Consult a professional adviser for details.

Also from David Rhine...

Self-Defense for Executor/Heirs

An executor can become personally liable for unpaid estate taxes owed to the IRS. And heirs who receive assets from an estate that was liquidated with its taxes still unpaid may be liable for them as well.

Trap: With estates of up to $1.5 million now being tax free, many people simply assume an estate won't be subject to tax, so they don't worry about it. But when insurance, retirement accounts and appreciated assets (including a home, other real estate holdings and investments in collectibles) as well as unreported or underreported gifts are tallied up, an estate may go beyond the $1.5 million mark unexpectedly.

Safety: If an estate is even close to $1.5 million, do not make any distributions (or major distributions) until the IRS has concluded its examination of the estate. The same is true for the trustee of a living trust who also may be personally liable for taxes.

Periodically value your estate and revise your estate plan accordingly—making sure adequate provision is made to pay taxes.

Finally from David Rhine...

Make Your Estate Easy on Your Heirs

Even the best estate plan is useless if key documents and information required to implement it aren't available when they are needed.

To be sure your estate plan works...

•**Draw up a contact list** that includes all the key people—professional advisers, trustees, insurance brokers, investment managers, etc.—who are involved with the plan or the management of your assets.

•**Create a list of all investments,** insurance policies, retirement plans and other assets that will be part of your estate. Include account and policy numbers.

•**Be sure all beneficiary designations for insurance policies,** retirement accounts, IRAs and investment accounts are up to date and on file.

Keep copies of all these documents, copies acknowledged as received by the institution, in your records in case the institutions that hold them lose them.

•**Collect all title documentation** for real estate and properties such as motor vehicles, so they can be properly transferred.

•**Keep all vital documents**—such as your will, power of attorney, health care proxy and the items mentioned above—in a safe location where they will not be endangered by any calamity that may strike you. If kept in a safe-deposit box, be sure your heirs and advisers know about the box and will be able to gain access to it.

Note: Safe-deposit boxes at banks are not accessible during nonbanking hours and may be sealed at your death.

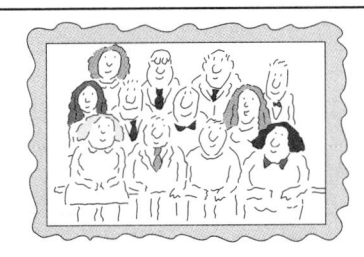

When to Revise Your Estate Plan

Revise your estate plan at least every other year—and whenever there is a marriage, divorce, birth or adoption, death of a family member, purchase or sale of a major asset or move to another state. Estate plans should also be revised in case of major changes in finances, such as a job loss, disability or serious illness and retirement.

Barbara Weltman, attorney in private practice, Millwood, NY, *www.bwideas.com.* She is author of many books, including *Bottom Line's Very Shrewd Money Book* (Bottom Line Books).

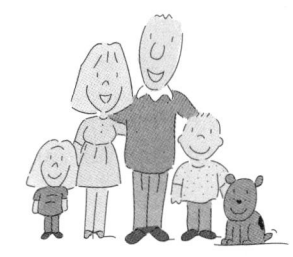

How to Pass Annuities On to Your Heirs

Lynn O'Shaughnessy, San Diego–based personal finance writer, *www.lynnosh.com,* and author of *Investing Bible* and *Retirement Bible* (both from Wiley).

An *immediate annuity,* which begins its payments as soon as it is bought, can be purchased with many payout options, some of which pass assets to heirs when the policyholder dies.

A *joint and survivor annuity* continues payments to a spouse or dependent until he/she, too, passes away.

Life annuities have five-, 10-, 15- or 20-year terms. If you die before the term ends, a designated beneficiary is paid for the remaining years.

Adding any of these options to an existing annuity will reduce the monthly payout—but not by much.

Example: A 70-year-old woman adding a 10-year term-certain period to a fixed immediate annuity might see her monthly payout decline by less than 5%.

You can compare annuity products at *www.immediateannuity.com,* or contact reputable

■ *Your Financial Future* ■ ■ ■

annuity companies, such as Fidelity (800-544-4702 or *www.fidelity.com*) and TIAA-CREF (800-842-2776 or *www.tiaa-cref.org*).

Don't Name IRA Beneficiaries Through Your Will

New rules for IRAs generally make it easier to leave an IRA to a beneficiary in a way that lets him/her keep the IRA going for many years, earning tax-favored investment returns.

But the new rules also make it clear that an IRA's beneficiary must be named by its owner in the IRA's documentation *before* the death of the owner. If a beneficiary is instead named through a will, there will be no "designated beneficiary." A great amount of tax savings may be lost to heirs.

Important: Make sure your IRA beneficiary designations are in place. Consult your tax adviser about the new rules.

Ed Slott, CPA, publisher, *Ed Slott's IRA Advisor,* 100 Merrick Rd., Rockville Centre, NY 11570. His Web site is *www.irahelp.com.*

Protect Your Legacy from A Child's Divorce

Consider establishing a living trust to administer the funds you leave to your child. He/she would have to go to a trustee to use the inheritance. In case of divorce, the money would stay in the trust for your child's benefit.

Caution: Trust assets may be counted when child support or alimony is determined. See a lawyer for details.

Jane King, financial adviser specializing in estate and retirement planning at Fairfield Financial Advisors in Wellesley, MA.

Incentive Trusts and Your Heirs

Make a bequest that directs an heir's behavior using an incentive trust to create an estate plan with teeth. Under such a trust, you can set certain goals or conditions that an heir must meet to receive a bequest. An heir who fails to do so receives a reduced bequest or nothing at all.

Example: If an heir has a problem with substance abuse, a bequest can be conditional on the heir completing a detoxification program and taking periodic drug tests, with installment payments made to the heir each year he/she remains drug free. Other conditions may be to meet educational goals or do charitable work. Consult your estate planning adviser.

Gerald Marks, Esq., partner, Gerald Marks & Associates, Red Bank, NJ.

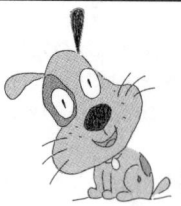

Protect Pets After You're Gone

Living trusts can protect pets after an owner dies. Legally, pets are property and cannot inherit assets. But 17 states now allow creation of trusts for pets, and some other states permit trusts to be set up in wills.

Caution: Be sure the trust is funded with enough money for your pet's entire life. Discuss the anticipated costs with your veterinarian.

If your state does not allow trusts for pets, consider a conditional gift—you leave money to a beneficiary on the condition that he/she cares for your pet.

J. Alan Jensen, Esq., attorney specializing in estate planning, Holland & Knight, Portland, OR.

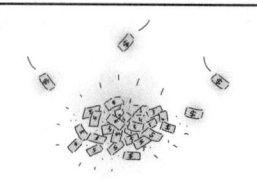

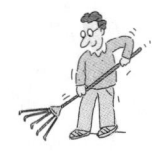

Joint Ownership Inheritance Trap

Jason S. Goldberg, Esq., partner in the law firm of Goldberg & Goldberg, PC, Melville, NY, *www.goldbergira.com*.

Be wary of placing property in joint ownership so it will pass to the other joint owner without going through probate. *Traps to watch out for...*

•**Once property is placed in joint ownership, you lose control of the interest** in that property. If you later regret the transfer, it is too late to reverse it without consent of the other joint owner.

With a will, you can change distributions up until the last minute, as long as you are competent to do so.

•**Joint property is part of your gross estate and may be subject to estate tax** unless the contribution was provided by the surviving joint owner and/or your estate is less than the tax-exempt amount.

But if most of your property passes by joint ownership, there may not be enough money in the estate for the executor to pay estate taxes. The IRS can then directly pursue any and all of the heirs who received property from your estate to collect unpaid tax up to the amount they received.

Nightmare: You place major assets in joint ownership with an heir, who later turns out to be a ne'er-do-well. You can't get the assets back without his/her consent. When you die, the heir refuses to pay his share of estate tax—perhaps he can't after squandering what he receives. The IRS goes after your other heirs to collect the estate tax due. Lawsuits abound, their cost depletes your estate and only the lawyers benefit.

Much better: Consult with an estate planning expert to set up a sound estate plan that will meet your objectives with maximum flexibility and minimum cost. Remember, your will does not govern distributions of joint accounts, and, in most cases, retirement accounts as well as any other nonprobate assets.

When There's Income Tax On an Inheritance

When a holder of EE or I savings bonds dies, income tax is due on the bonds' deferred interest—even though most inheritances are free from income tax. If a child receives bonds after a parent's death, the heir can report the interest income on the parent's final tax return or on his/her own return for the year he cashes in the bonds. Report the interest on the return with the lower tax rate.

Information: Consult your financial adviser.

Stanley Hagendorf, JD, estate and tax attorney, Hagendorf Law Firm, 2000 S. Jones Blvd., Las Vegas 89146.

Rules of Proof for Charitable Contributions

Even if you make a perfectly legitimate contribution to a charity, your deduction for it may be disallowed if you or the charity fails to follow the IRS's required documentation-and-receipt rules.

Useful: The IRS has just provided an explanation of the rules in a single publication meant for use by both donors and charities. Get IRS Publication 1771, *Charitable Contributions—Substantiation and Disclosure Requirements,* at *www.irs.gov.*

New: Charities now can provide the required written acknowledgements for contributions of more than $250 electronically—such as through an E-mail.

Doubling Up on Tax-Free Gifts

The exclusion amount for tax-free gifts is presently $11,000 per donee per year (this limit may be adjusted for inflation after 2004).

Some taxpayers incorrectly believe that they can enhance this exclusion by arranging to make a gift to a third party who then makes a gift of the same amount to the intended donee.

How this works: A father gives his son $11,000 and, at the same time, makes a gift to a neighbor of $11,000. The gift to the neighbor is made with the understanding that he will make an $11,000 gift to the son.

Caution: The IRS attacks these transactions by applying the "reciprocal trust doctrine," which treats the second gift as part of the first.

Ms. X, Esq., a former agent with the IRS who is still well connected.

Include Cost Records With Gifts

Lisa N. Collins, CPA/PFS, vice president and director of tax services, Harding, Shymanski & Co., PC, Evansville, IN. She is author of an authoritative book on tax deductions.

There is a big tax trap that the recipients of many potentially tax-free gifts may encounter.

Key: When the recipient sells the gift property, taxable gain or loss is determined using the cost records of the donor. The donor's cost basis in the gift carries over to the gift recipient. (And gift tax paid may be added in some cases.)

If the property is sold at a gain, taxable gain is determined by subtracting this carryover basis from the sale proceeds. If the property is sold at a loss, basis, for purposes of computing the amount of the loss, equals the lower of the donor's basis in it or the property's actual market value on the date of the gift.

Trap: If the donor's cost records weren't transferred with the gift and have since been lost, the IRS may treat up to the entire value of the property as gain.

Result: Taxable gain may be much larger than the real gain—and taxable gain may result even if the property is sold at a loss.

Example: You receive valuable collectibles as a gift from a grandparent and sell them for $15,000. If you can show your grandparent's basis in the collectibles was $10,000, your gain will be only $5,000. *But...*

• If you don't have records of your grandparent's basis in the collectibles, the IRS may tax up to the full $15,000 of gain.

• If your grandparent paid $20,000 for the collectibles, but you can't show this or their market value when the gift to you was made, you may owe tax on up to $15,000 of capital gains even on a sale that produced a $5,000 loss.

Safety: Whenever you make or receive a valuable gift, be sure cost records are transferred along with it. If you made or received gifts in previous years for which cost records weren't provided, try to pull together the necessary records now, before it is too late.

What It Means to Be a Health Care Proxy

Linda Farber Post, Esq., BSN, bioethics consultant for Montefiore Medical Center and assistant professor of bioethics at Albert Einstein College of Medicine, both located in the Bronx, NY.

Many people sign a document called a health care proxy, which designates a person (his/her agent) to make health care decisions for them if they are unable.

You may have been named health care agent, or proxy, for your spouse, a relative or friend. Or you may be called upon to act as an informal health care *surrogate* even though no health care proxy was signed. This role is recognized in several states.

WHEN DUTIES BEGIN AND END

Your role as a health care agent (or surrogate) starts when doctors decide that the person who appointed you—the patient—lacks the capacity to make medical decisions.

The patient may retain some capacity—for example, the ability to decide what he wants for lunch—but not the capacity to consent to surgery or to discontinue life support.

Protecting Your Estate

As an agent, you don't make the determination of capacity—medical personnel do. But if you think that the patient's capacity should be evaluated, ask the attending doctor. Often, the care team makes the determination, with input from the nursing personnel, other doctors and a psychiatrist.

Your role as health care agent ends as soon as the patient regains the capacity to make his own decisions. If incapacity is caused by a temporary condition—such as transient loss of consciousness—be prepared to step back and let the patient make his own choices as soon as capacity is restored.

If incapacity results from a permanent condition—Alzheimer's disease, for example—be prepared to act until the end of the patient's life.

WHAT YOU CAN AND CANNOT DO

As a health care agent, you essentially step into the shoes of the patient to make any decision that the patient could have made if he had the capacity. The scope of the agent's authority is determined by each state. *Typically, this encompasses...*

•**Conferring with doctors** and reviewing medical charts.

•**Asking medical questions** and discussing treatment options.

•**Requesting a second opinion** or changing physicians.

•**Consenting to—or refusing—tests and treatments,** including surgery.

•**Authorizing a transfer to another nursing home or rehabilitation center.**

•**Refusing life support.**

A health care agent is concerned solely with medical decision-making. He is not responsible for financial or other nonmedical decisions. The involvement of an agent can be limited by the patient's instructions in the health care proxy document or by state law.

You have no financial liability for acting as agent. You won't have to pay the doctor's bills for any procedures you consent to.

Your state may also give you certain post-mortem decision-making authority, such as donating organs...consenting to an autopsy... and making funeral arrangements.

MAKING GOOD DECISIONS

As a health care agent, you may have to act under trying emotional conditions. *Knowing what actions to take and where to turn for assistance will help you when the time comes...*

•**Know the patient's wishes in advance.** Since you stand in the patient's shoes, your decisions should mirror the decisions that the patient would have made.

Ideally, his preferences, values and attitudes were conveyed to you through prior discussions or in a written document, such as a living will. The person who designated you presumably believes you know him well and can be depended upon to act according to his wishes.

•**Figure out what the patient would want.** If the patient's wishes aren't plainly understood —perhaps a particular type of treatment was not ever discussed—*you'll have to determine what he would have wanted on the basis of what you know about him...*

•Solicit input from family members and others who love the patient to reach a consensus on the patient's wishes.

•Speak with the patient's physician about what treatment/care the patient may have said he would want under certain circumstances.

•Approach the patient's spiritual adviser to learn if any preferences on medical treatments or other issues were discussed.

Caution: Don't base your decisions on what you'd want for yourself. Limit your decision-making to what *the patient* would want.

•**Decide what's best for the patient.** If there are no instructions and no clues as to the patient's preferences, base your decisions on what you believe to be best for the patient. Weigh the proposed treatment against the pain and suffering it will cause. Again, talk with his loved ones to reach a consensus.

If you are stumped, ask for help from a hospital's bioethics consultant.

To avoid acting in a vacuum, prepare in advance for decision-making by discussing medical issues with the patient when a health care proxy is signed.

Helpful: *A Guide to Being a Health Care Proxy or Surrogate,* prepared by Montefiore Medical Center, Bronx, NY. Go to *http://montefiore.org/prof/* and click on "Bioethics."

■ *Your Financial Future* ■ ■ ■

AVOIDING DISPUTES

Before doing anything else, inform the medical team of your designation as the health care agent. If there's no written health care proxy appointment, you may still be able to assume health care decision-making responsibility for the patient depending on the laws in your state.

Make sure you're listed on the patient's chart as agent or surrogate. Be sure that you're consulted about all treatments. If you're kept in the loop, you should be able to avoid disputes with doctors and staff.

Be assertive in making sure that treatment coincides with the patient's wishes, what you believe are his wishes or what's best for him. Despite your best efforts, of course, disputes may arise.

To resolve disputes with doctors, talk with the hospital's bioethics committee, a patient representative or a social worker. If you can't reach an agreement and believe you're following the patient's wishes, consider changing doctors or health care facilities.

To resolve disputes with family members, remind them that, as the appointed health care agent, you're the legally designated decision-maker. This is true even if a relative is more closely related to the patient than you are.

Web Sites for Making End-of-Life Decisions

Leslie J. Bricker, MD, medical oncologist and palliative medicine specialist, Henry Ford Health System, Detroit. He worked with Michigan State University researchers to develop the *Completing a Life* CD-ROM.

Be sure to check out these helpful Web sites when looking to make end-of-life decisions...

• **Completing a Life** (*www.completingalife.msu.edu*) offers video clips of patients discussing difficult issues, such as pain control and saying good-bye.

• **National Hospice and Palliative Care Organization** (*www.nhpco.org*) helps families and patients find hospice programs and clearly communicate end-of-life wishes.

• **Partnership for Caring** (*www.partnershipforcaring.org*) offers state-specific information and downloadable documents to lay out end-of-life wishes, such as living wills and durable powers of attorney.

• **Growth House** (*www.growthhouse.org*) offers an extensive directory of end-of-life Web resources.

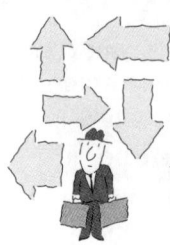

Power of Attorney Vs. Durable Power Of Attorney

Nancy Dunnan, financial adviser and author in New York City. Her latest book is *How to Invest $50–$5,000* (HarperCollins).

A power of attorney (POA) is a written document in which you grant authority to another person (your "agent" or "attorney in fact") to act on your behalf in financial matters. A POA can be very specific, such as giving the person the power to sell your car or house, or to deposit your checks and pay your bills. Or it can be broader.

A traditional POA usually terminates when you become mentally incompetent. A durable POA, however, states that you want the power to continue to operate if you become incapacitated. In some states, you can indicate that the power is to become effective *only* if you become incapacitated—that's called a "springing power of attorney."

Both types of POA must be drawn up while you are still mentally intact. More details are available from the National Network of Estate Planning Attorneys (800-638-8681 or *www.netplanning.com/consumer*).

■■■■ **Your Leisure** ■

14

Travel Tips and Traps

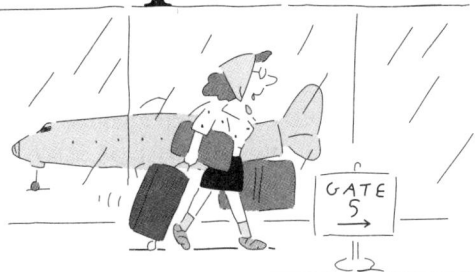

How to Get the Best Shopping Bargains On the Planet

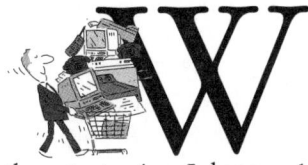

Whether you're planning to shop at the many flea markets in Paris or at the bazaars in Morocco, the strategies I learned as a buyer for the Smithsonian Institution Museum Shops will help you score real finds.

GROUND RULES

Before leaving home, take the time to prepare for shopping in a foreign country.

•**Learn from guidebooks or the Internet about the customs,** regional specialties and indigenous arts and crafts of the country.

•**Focus your shopping activities** by knowing before you travel…
 •What you'd like to buy.
 •For whom you are buying.
 •How much you can spend.

•**Take along small tokens from home,** such as pens, T-shirts and caps with logos or American symbols on them. Use them for barter or to negotiate a better price.

•**Comparison shop *before* you leave home.** If the country you're visiting has a reputation for good prices on certain items, check out prices on similar products at home. Write down those prices and take them with you.

•**Bring along a calculator or create a "cheat sheet" of the currency rates,** especially if you're bargaining in a foreign language. Also, know the value of the euro vs. the US dollar.

•**Learn about a foreign country's entry and exit requirements for goods.** In some countries, buying art and antiques may require an export license, which could result in unexpected duties or fees. *Examples…*

Kathy Borrus, Washington, DC–based author of *The Fearless Shopper: How to Get the Best Deals on the Planet* (Traveler's Tales). Ms. Borrus is the former merchandise manager for the Smithsonian Institution Museum Shops and is now a specialty retail marketing consultant.

■ *Your Leisure* ■ ■ ■

• Egyptian law prohibits exportation of any items more than 100 years old.

• In Laos, you can't take antiques or representations of Buddha out of the country.

• In Russia, you need permission from the Ministry of Culture when exporting anything made before 1945. And, exportation of antique icons is strictly forbidden.

• In South and Central America, the export of pre-Columbian artifacts is prohibited in most areas—check with the country you will be visiting to verify what their rules are.

FLEA MARKETS AND ANTIQUE FAIRS

• **Pay in cash**—it gives you better bargaining leverage.

• **Act like a seasoned buyer**—always ask the price first and negotiate from there.

• **Unless you can determine the difference between a fake and something authentic, don't buy it.** Forgeries abound—especially in bronze castings, coins and old drawings. Watch for fake jade in China and Hong Kong.

• **Be informed about prices**—carry a price guide for antiques.

• **Bargain politely**—express a willingness to buy at the right price and keep the negotiations friendly. Ask questions like, "Is this your best price?" or "Can you do better?" Or say, "I don't usually pay that much for this type of item."

• **Dress down when shopping at an open-air market.** Leave your jewelry and expensive outfits home.

BAZAARS, SOUKS AND MARKETS

You can win the bargaining game using these strategies...

• **Get a feel for the market**—look around before you buy.

• **Shop with a native if possible**—you'll get better deals. Alternatively, learn as many key phrases and numbers in the language. Learn to say "too much" and "what's the cost?"

• **Visit individual villages away from major cities.** You can often buy folk crafts directly from the artisans—prices will usually be lower and the quality better.

• **Bargain in a spirit of fun and friendliness.** *Always* reject the first offer.

• **Bring cash**—most merchants won't accept credit cards. You're in a better position if you pay with local currency (although in some places, US dollars are more desirable). Keep small bills handy.

BECOME A FEARLESS BARGAINER

Merchants know just where the profit margins are and what they can afford. *Here's how to negotiate the best deal—even when prices are already low...*

• **Before you bargain, decide what the item is worth to you.** Then ask the price—that way you'll know how much bargaining room you have.

• **See what the locals are buying** and how much they're paying.

• **If a merchant asks an absurdly high price,** offer an equally ridiculous low price—you'll probably meet somewhere in the middle. Do not be afraid to make your offer—all anyone can say is "no."

• **Be willing to walk away**—you can often get what you want if you're not attached to it. Stick to your budget and your lists.

If you're uncomfortable with the bargaining process, look for state-run cooperatives and handcraft cooperatives—they generally offer indigenous items for sale at reasonable prices.

COMING HOME

You're generally better off carrying your items home in your checked luggage than shipping them. Before buying items that will have to be shipped, factor in the shipping cost. It's no bargain to buy a $300 wooden chest in New Delhi if it costs another $300 to send it home.

The value-added tax (VAT)—the European version of a sales tax—is always included in the price of an item. Foreigners are exempt from the VAT and entitled to a refund. But getting the refund can be a hassle. You need receipts and must wait in designated customs lines at the airport.

US Customs lets you bring $800 worth of goods back to the US duty free. However, the exemption from 24 Caribbean countries is $600. Remember—you can't bring into the US any item made of ivory or turtle shell.

Travel Tips and Traps

Get your free copy of the pamphlet *Know Before You Go* from the US Customs Service at *www.customs.gov/travel/travel.htm*.

Learn How Much to Bid at Priceline

Travel bargains are available through Priceline's "name your own price" travel service. To get the best bargain, you must ask for the lowest price it will accept.

Helpful: At the new free site *www.biddingfortravel.com*, travelers who use Priceline report their successful bids.

The site also has a newsletter, offers effective strategies and reports special offers. It can help save you money on airfares, hotel rates, cruises and other travel. There's no charge to become a member. You simply register.

Malcolm Katt, antiques dealer and owner of Millwood Gallery in Millwood, NY.

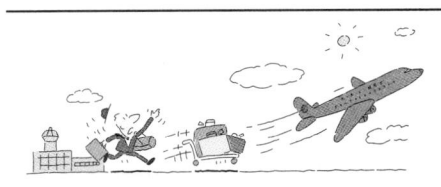

Save Big on Last-Minute Travel

The editors of Freebies *magazine, who are also authors of* The Senior's Guide to the Best Deals, Bargains, and Steals *(Lowell House).*

You can cut travel costs in half if you're flexible and willing to leave on the spur of the moment...

•**Spur of the Moment Cruises.** Sells berths for 50% or more off the published rate.

How far in advance to book: One week to three months. Free 21-page booklet of discount cruises available. 800-343-1991 or *www.spurof.com*.

•**Preferred Traveller.** Offers up to 50% off hotel rates and up to 25% off car rentals (for participating hotels and companies).

How far in advance to book: No more than 30 days and no less than 48 hours.

Cost: $96*/yr. for membership, with a free, 30-day trial. 800-444-9800 or *www.preferredtraveller.com*.

•**Moment's Notice.** Offers bargain packages to the Caribbean and Mexico, plus cruises and airfares to Europe.

How far in advance to book: Between two and 30 days.

Cost: $25/yr. for membership. 888-241-3366 or *www.moments-notice.com*.

*All prices subject to change.

When to Buy Vacation Insurance

Prepaid vacation insurance may make sense if your trip is expensive or involves multiple stops...if it is an active vacation, during which you might get hurt...if you have a preexisting medical condition...when you are traveling to an area of political unrest...or if you cannot risk problems with your trip.

When buying insurance: Read the fine print so you know the limits of your coverage. Get supplier-default protection from an independent insurance firm, not the tour company, in case the tour company fails. Check with your insurer.

Jeanne Salvatore, vice president of consumer affairs, Insurance Information Institute, 110 William St., New York City 10038, www.iii.org.

Convert Money Before You Go

You can protect the value of your dollar in the months before you take a trip by converting money to foreign currency in advance. American Express provides traveler's checks in six foreign currencies, with the exchange rate locked in the day you place your order. If your

■ *Your Leisure* ■ ■ ■ ■

trip is three months or more away, consider opening a foreign-currency savings account through Everbank (888-882-3837 or *www.ever bank.com*)—which sets up accounts in 20 currencies, often at better exchange rates than those available through American Express. If you have at least $10,000 to put aside, consider a CD denominated in foreign currency.

Business Week, 1221 Avenue of the Americas, New York City 10020.

Get Money Back When Traveling in Europe

Value added tax (VAT) is a type of sales tax charged in many countries. It is refundable to travelers from abroad when they leave the country. VAT can be expensive—up to 20% in Europe—so refunds can be significant.

Snag: The refund process is complex and varies by country, so many travelers just don't bother with it.

Help: VAT refund assistance for 32 countries—including the European nations plus Japan, Korea and Singapore—is provided by Global Refund. To learn more about how the refunds work by country, phone 800-566-9828 or visit *www.globalrefund.com* before you travel.

David Tykol, editor, *International Travel News,* 2120 28 St., Sacramento, CA 95818, *www.intltravelnews.com.*

Overseas ATMs Are No Longer Bargains

For years, ATMs offered cash at excellent exchange rates without fees. But banks are now extending currency-exchange and usage fees to foreign transactions.

Result: You may be charged an ATM fee of about $2 and a transaction fee of 2% of the amount withdrawn, depending on the bank.

Better for getting cash: Credit cards. Many charge fees of 1% to 2% for foreign currency exchanges. But some major issuers—Capital One, FleetBoston, MBNA America and Wachovia—and most community banks and cooperatives do not impose fees. Check your credit card's travel perks before leaving the country.

Also: Use credit cards for major purchases. If something goes wrong, the card issuer may help resolve the problem.

Nancy Dunnan, editor and publisher, *Travel Smart,* Box 379, Dobbs Ferry, NY 10522, *www.travelsmartnews letter.com.*

Tipping Guide

To learn how much to tip for anything, anywhere, visit *www.tipping.org,* "The Original Tipping Page." This site offers advice on how much to tip in the US and abroad for different services—bellhops, airport skycaps, concierges and so on. And if you cannot find an answer to your particular question, there is a message board available where you can post it to be answered by others.

Travel & Leisure, 1120 Avenue of the Americas, New York City 10036.

Last-Minute Airline Deals

Get the best last-minute airline deals through a travel agent. A good agent is up-to-date on airline and travel Web sites, such as *www. expedia.com...www.orbitz.com...*and *www. travelocity.com.* If you visit the sites yourself and enter your itinerary, you may get 20 pages of listings. You would need to go through every one and weigh cost against flight time and other factors. A travel agent can give you both the lowest fare and a slightly higher fare with better routing.

For last-minute leisure travel: Check out each airline's Web site. Airlines generally post superlow fares on Wednesday for travel from that Friday through the next Tuesday.

Terry Trippler, president of TerryTrippler.com, Inc., air traveler advocates, Minneapolis.

More from Terry Trippler...

Benefits of Travel Agents

Don't give up on travel agents, even though they charge fees of $20 to $45 per transaction. Most agents charge a fee because they no longer receive commissions from major airlines. An agent can work within almost any budget and provide useful information—for instance, whether you need a visa and which airlines will let you check your bags through to your final destination if you change planes. Word of mouth is still the best way to find a good travel agent.

Avoid Steep Airline Fees

Miss your flight by minutes, and many airlines now charge $75 to $100 to put you on the next flight. Don't use your advance-purchase, nonrefundable ticket on the travel day? At one time, you had a year to apply its value (minus a change fee) to future travel on the same airline. American, Delta and United still charge the change fee ($100), but you must book the new trip by midnight of your first day of scheduled travel or your ticket becomes worthless.

Consider using discount airlines, such as AirTran, JetBlue and Southwest, to avoid major airlines' steep new fees.

Rudy Maxa, publisher, *Rudy Maxa's Traveler,* 1322 18 St. NW, Washington, DC 20036, *www.rudymaxa.com.*

Getting Bumped On Purpose

If you actually *want* to get bumped from a flight so that you qualify for free tickets and other extras...

- **Find out ahead of time from reservations agents which flights are always overbooked,** and reserve seats on them.
- **Get to the airport at least *two hours* early,** so you can be one of the first to volunteer to be bumped. Be the first person on line when the gate opens.
- **Carry a flight schedule** so you can tell agents which alternative flights you want—these can be printed out beforehand from an airline's Web site.
- **If your wait between flights is more than two hours, ask for extras,** such as free airport-club admissions, meal tickets, etc.

Tom Parsons, CEO, Bestfares.com, 1301 S. Bowen Rd., Suite 430, Arlington, TX 76013.

Faster Airline Check-In

Fast airline check-in is now available at self-service kiosks in more than 100 airports throughout the US and Canada. Touch-screen machines in the kiosks let you get boarding passes, drop off luggage, get seat assignments and pay standby fees. Some airlines give extra frequent-flier miles to travelers who check in this way.

More information: Check with your travel agent or with the airline you are flying.

Condé Nast Traveler, 4 Times Sq., New York City 10036.

Travel Warnings and Help Overseas

Condé Nast Traveler, 4 Times Sq., New York City 10036.

Advance warnings of travel problems—and help if you run into trouble while overseas—is available from both government and private sources...

- **Overseas Citizens Services Hot Line** can help if you are injured or a victim of crime overseas or if you need to get in touch with a

Your Leisure

traveling relative or friend. 888-407-4747 or *http://travel.state.gov/acs.html*.

•**Ijet** tracks global events and conditions in more than 150 countries. It provides entry requirements, local emergency telephone numbers and health and security data.

Cost: $14.95* per destination. 877-606-4538 or *www.ijet.com*.

•**Overseas Security Advisory Council** posts security-related information and lists the important dates and holidays in specific countries. *www.ds-osac.org*.

*Price subject to change.

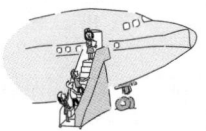

Savvier Flying

For much smoother airline travel in this changed world...

•**Don't be first in line to board the airplane**—that makes you seem too eager and just increases your chances of being stopped by security.

•**Take nonstop flights even if ones with stops are cheaper**—security delays can significantly increase stopover time.

•**Tape a business card or address label to your laptop** so you know which one is yours after it goes through security.

Upscale Traveler, 4521 Alla Rd. #3, Marina del Rey, CA 90292.

Better Airport Security

The latest airport security system has state police questioning passengers in all ticket lines. In addition to screening baggage, Boston's antiterrorism program evaluates travelers for suspicious behavior. Similar behavior-recognition programs have been extremely successful in Israeli airports since 1970 and could become more common in the US. The initial questioning takes up to two minutes per passenger. Those travelers who raise suspicion are detained for further questioning.

Major Tom Robbins, commanding officer of Massachusetts State Police Troop F, which is responsible for the behavior-recognition program at Boston's Logan International Airport.

What's Even Worse Than Airline Food?

Aircraft water tanks often contain *Salmonella* and other disease-causing organisms at levels that may be hundreds of times above government limits. If you drink water or brush your teeth during a flight, ask the flight attendant for bottled water.

The Wall Street Journal, 200 Liberty St., New York City 10281.

Recirculated Air Does Not Cause Colds

Recirculated air on modern aircraft does *not* increase the risk of contracting a cold. New commercial airplanes are designed to recirculate 50% of cabin air to increase fuel efficiency. Until now, it was not known if recirculated air enhanced the transmission of viruses.

Recent study: The incidence of colds among 1,100 passengers five to seven days after flying were similar, regardless of whether they flew on a plane that recirculated cabin air or on an older plane that used 100% fresh air.

To protect yourself from germs while flying: Wash your hands frequently and do not share drinks.

Jessica Nutik Zitter, MD, MPH, assistant clinical professor of medicine, University of California, San Francisco.

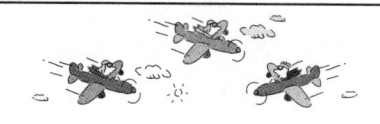

Travel Tips and Traps

When You Shouldn't Get on a Plane

Edward R. Rensimer, MD, director, International Medicine Center, travel-health specialists, Houston, *www.traveldoc.com*.

Below, a travel-health expert and physician explains the health conditions under which you should be sure not to fly...

• **If you have poorly controlled asthma,** sinusitis, pneumonia, intense allergies or an ear infection—changes in air pressure on ascent and descent can cause severe pain or breathing problems.

• **For at least 24 hours after abdominal, eye, ear or facial surgery** or extensive dental work—the swelling and bleeding can be amplified, causing sutures to rip and severe pain.

• **For one day after sustaining a concussion**—brain irritability could cause seizures when oxygen levels decline at high altitudes. Any brain swelling can cause acute neurological events in-flight.

• **For several days after undergoing a colonoscopy**—bowels may be sluggish and gas infused into body cavities may rupture or perforate intestines at high altitudes.

• **If you have a serious communicable illness,** such as measles, tuberculosis or a viral respiratory illness.

Special concerns for children: Kids with active chicken pox should not fly—the disease can be fatal to adults and is spread easily in contained-air ventilation space. Do not fly with an infant who has diarrhea—frequent diaper changes may spread germs, resulting in dysentery, especially in other children.

Refunds on Nonrefundable Tickets

Refunds on nonrefundable tickets may be available on some airlines. Travelers who buy published-fare tickets directly from the airline or through a travel agency may be able to cancel and get a refund within 24 hours of the ticket purchase. The policy does not apply to E-tickets. If you begin a trip on a nonrefundable ticket and then need to change a later segment, most airlines will allow it for a charge of $75* to $150—provided the changes meet the requirements of the original ticket.

Example: A Saturday-night stay.

Randy Petersen, publisher of *InsideFlyer*, 1930 Frequent Flyer Point, Colorado Springs 80915.

More from Randy Petersen...

How to Buy Frequent-Flier Miles

You can buy frequent-flier miles if you are just short of an award.

Price: About $27.50 per 1,000 miles—in addition to a 7.5% federal excise tax and a $25 transaction fee.

Miles are credited within five days—much faster than the six to eight weeks it can take for miles from other sources to reach your account. Check with your airline's frequent-flier program.

Also from Randy Petersen...

Don't Convert Hotel Points to Frequent-Flier Miles

Hotel points are more valuable if used for hotel stays.

Example: A three-night stay at one full-service hotel costs about 75,000 points, the equivalent of $450. Those points could be exchanged for 15,000 airline points—worth only about $300.

Finally from Randy Petersen...

New Baggage Fees

Airlines are charging bigger fees for oversized luggage. If a bag exceeds 62 inches when the height, width and depth are added together, airlines charge $80 per bag for each leg of a US itinerary—and up to $270 per bag for overseas flights.

*All prices subject to change.

■ *Your Leisure* ■ ■ ■

Self-defense: Instead of one large bag, pack smaller ones. Most airlines allow two checked bags and one carry-on. The fee for going over the two-bags-per-passenger rule often is much less than the charge for oversized baggage.

Tour Groups Beware of This Trap

Tour-group members routinely are told to leave their luggage outside of their hotel rooms so the bellman can arrange for it to be brought to the airport or the next destination. This means luggage is out of travelers' hands for several hours—and many strangers could have access to it.

Self-defense: Properly label and lock all bags. Before departing the hotel, check with the bus driver to be sure that your bags are onboard. Or just handle bags yourself.

Anat Baron, founder, Travel Fanatic LLC, travel-media company, Los Angeles, *www.travelfanatic.com*.

Send Your Baggage Separately

Bringing baggage on an airline trip is becoming much more onerous. There is less room for carry-on bags, all baggage is subject to inspection and airlines are imposing costly fees for "excess" luggage.

Alternative: New services such as Luggage Express (866-744-7224 or *www.usxpluggageexpress.com*) and VirtualBellhop (877-235-5467 or *www.virtualbellhop.com*) will pick up your luggage from your home and then deliver it to any destination.

The Mature Traveler, Box 1543, Wildomar, CA 92595.

How to Keep Airlines From Losing Your Luggage

Louise Weiss, award-winning travel writer and contributor to many travel books and publications. Based in New York City, she is author of *Access to the World: A Travel Guide for the Handicapped* (Henry Holt).

Do not let lost luggage spoil your next vacation or business trip. *Here are some things you can do to ensure that your luggage arrives when you do...*

• **Remove all old luggage tags** and stickers from previous trips.

• **On your outgoing trip,** put your destination address and phone number on your luggage tags.

• **On your return trip,** use your *business* address and phone number—if you work at an office—to avoid alerting burglars that your home is empty.

• **Tape or pin your ID**—name, home or business address, phone number—*inside* your suitcase. Include your itinerary.

• **Use colored tape to add a stripe** or simple design to the sides of your suitcase for easier identification.

• **Leave a list of the contents of your suitcase at home.** Keep a copy with you, too—but *not* in your suitcase. This will be valuable if your luggage is not recovered and you need to submit a claim.

• **Never let your bags out of your sight.**

• **Avoid obviously expensive luggage**—it's a target for thieves.

IF YOUR LUGGAGE IS LOST

OK. Now you have arrived—but your suitcase hasn't! Most "lost" luggage is found within a few days. *In the meantime...*

• **Report the loss immediately to your airline's station manager**—or ask an airport employee where to report undelivered luggage.

Do not leave the airport until you have filled out a lost luggage form and submitted it to the proper authorities. Keep a copy and get phone numbers so you can follow up.

• **Ask for an allowance to cover the cost of necessities.** The amount you can get varies by airline and situation. You may, for example, need a change of clothes—for instance, if you arrive in the Virgin Islands wearing your winter woolens, you'll need to buy something better suited to the climate.

Best: Speak to the highest ranking airline employee available. Remain calm and polite, but firm.

Better than going through all this: Take only carry-on luggage when you travel. With good planning, this is not difficult to do, even for overseas trips.

More from Louise Weiss...

The Fine Art of Travel

Some practical tips for a much smoother trip from an award-winning travel writer...

• **Carry two credit cards...separately.** If one is stolen or misplaced and the account must be frozen, you'll still have another to use.

• **Pack only as much as you can comfortably carry** up two flights of stairs.

• **Pack gloves** if you are going anywhere other than the tropics. Gloves also make carrying a suitcase more comfortable.

• **Bring film and batteries** for your camera when traveling overseas—they can be expensive and hard to find.

• **For a directory of English-speaking doctors,** contact the International Association for Medical Assistance to Travelers (716-754-4883 or *www.iamat.org*).

Pack a Whistle

Carry whistles when traveling—they can be helpful in an emergency, such as when a child is lost, someone is injured or during a robbery. Choose a model that is easy for kids or injured people to use.

Examples: Acme Thunderer 660, $1.95*...ACR WW-3 Survival, $3...All-Weather Safety Storm, $5.50...All-Weather Safety Windstorm, $4.50. Available at sporting goods or marine supply stores.

Backpacker, 33 E. Minor St., Emmaus, PA 18098.

*All prices subject to change.

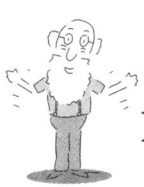

Hotel Discounts If You're Over 50

Joan Rattner Heilman, Westchester County, NY–based author of *Unbelievably Good Deals and Great Adventures That You Absolutely Can't Get Unless You Are Over 50, 2003-2004* (Contemporary).

People over age 50 can expect discounts of at least 10% at almost every US hotel. *Don't miss out...*

• **Join AARP,** other senior groups or the hotel chain's own senior club.

• **Ask about the senior discount policy** when making reservations.

• **Be prepared to make changes to your travel schedule.** Some hotels offer discounts only on a limited number of rooms and only on certain dates.

• **Confirm the discount when you check in at the hotel.**

BEST BARGAINS NOW

• **Choice Hotels** (including Clarion Hotels, Comfort Inns, Comfort Suites, EconoLodge, MainStay Suites, Quality Inns, Rodeway Inns and Sleep Inns). *60-Plus Program* offers a 10% to 30% discount with advance reservations to guests age 60 and over for bookings made via its toll-free number (800-424-6423). If you don't use this number, there is a 10% discount if you are age 50 or over.

• **Fairmont Hotels & Resorts** give 10% to 30% discounts to AARP members at most of their locations.

For reservations: 877-441-1414.

• **Hilton Hotels** has a *Senior H Honors Program* which gives discounts to those age 60 or

■ *Your Leisure* ■ ■ ■

older. First-year dues are $55* (one spouse of a couple must be 60), $40 annually thereafter.

To join: 800-548-8690.

• **Marriott Hotels** give discounts to those age 62 and older. 800-228-9290. The same applies at Renaissance Hotels, which are owned by Marriott. 800-468-3571.

• **Ramada Inns,** Ramada Limiteds and Ramada Plaza Hotels give 25% discounts to *Club Ramada's* senior program members age 60 or over. Free membership.

To join: 800-672-6232.

*All prices subject to change.

Cheaper Hotel Rates

To get the best hotel room rate—call the hotel directly, not the hotel chain's toll-free national number. Reservation agents at the hotel's front desk usually are authorized to negotiate the best prices. On-line services, such as *www.hotels.com…www.expedia.com…*and *www.travelocity.com,* can be starting points for comparison shopping—but their prices may not be the lowest. Some hotels now will undercut any price found on the Internet by 10%.

Additional cost-cutting strategies: Plan to stay when hotels have empty rooms—in cities, on most weekends…at resorts, most weekdays and out of season. Ask the front-desk attendant for their best price. When you call to reserve, make a deal for a standard double room—then ask for an upgrade for the same price. If a better room is available, you will probably get it.

Tim Zagat, publisher, *Zagat Survey,* consumer-based restaurant and hotel guides around the world, 4 Columbus Circle, New York City 10019.

More on Getting the Best Hotel Rates

Act like you don't have a reservation, even when you do, to get a better hotel room rate. Upon arriving at the hotel, ask for the best rates available. If the rates quoted are lower than your reservation rate, simply cancel your reservation and take a room at the quoted rate instead.

Arthur Frommer's Budget Travel, 350 Fifth Ave., New York City 10118.

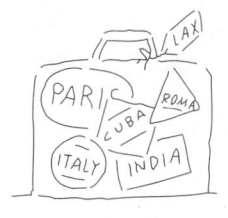

Free Hotel Rooms for Grandparents

Grandparents can stay free at Candlewood Suites hotels on 11 holidays of the year. To obtain a free hotel room on Easter, Mother's Day, Father's Day, etc.—or for a first-time stay anytime—all a grandparent has to do is pay for the night before or after. It's simple to qualify for the program—just show a photo of your grandchild when you check in.

Details: Visit *www.candlewoodsuites.com* or call 888-226-3539.

Hotel Safety

When staying in a hotel, avoid ground-floor rooms, which are easiest to break into …and rooms above the tenth floor, which fire ladders may be unable to reach. Also, choose a room closer to the elevator than the stairs—security monitoring is better. Only stay at hotels that use electronic keycards, whose codes are changed for every guest. Never prop the door open, and don't hang out the "Please Make Up This Room" sign, which signals that the room is empty. For valuables, use the in-room safe or the safe-deposit box at the front desk.

John Fannin, founder, SafePlace Corp., an independent provider of safety accreditation for buildings, 2106 Silverside Rd., Wilmington, DE 19810, *www.safeplace.com*.

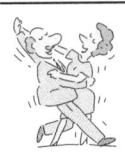

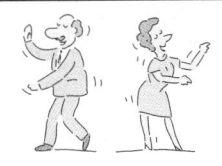

Dance Your Way to A Discount Cruise

Adele Malott, weekly columnist with *The New York Times Syndicate,* writing in *The Mature Traveler,* Box 1543, Wildomar, CA 92595.

Many cruise lines now feature volunteer "Gentleman Hosts," skilled ballroom dancers who dance with solo/independent female travelers. The hosts also greet the guests at special functions, mingle with guests during social events and perform other similar functions. Hosts generally are 45 to 72 years old, need to pass a review by a professional dance board to demonstrate their proficiency and have refined social skills. Most hosts are placed with cruise ships through The Working Vacation agency.

There is a nominal fee of $28* per day for most cruises. However, the hosts are given a cabin and meals, as well as a beverage and gratuity allowance. They also often get free shore excursions and round-trip airfare.

Details: 708-301-7535 or *www.theworkingvacation.com*.

*Price subject to change.

Cruise-Line Security

Increased cruise-line security means that passengers may be checked repeatedly. Those arriving by air must first go through all airport checks, then are carefully inspected before boarding the ship. Baggage is X-rayed and/or hand-checked...passengers pass through metal detectors and must present photo identification. Aboard the ship, sensitive locations—such as the bridge and engine room—now have restricted access for added security.

J. Michael Crye, president, International Council of Cruise Lines, Washington, DC.

Self-Defense Against Viral Illness on Cruises

Outbreaks of gastrointestinal illnesses on cruise ships have actually diminished since 1990. But exposure to illness-causing viruses and bacteria is a reality of travel. On recent cruises, the Norwalk virus infected hundreds of passengers, causing diarrhea, nausea, stomach pain and/or vomiting. The biggest risk—especially among older people—is dehydration.

Self-defense: Wash your hands frequently and thoroughly onboard *and* onshore. Information on cruise-related health issues is available from the Centers for Disease Control and Prevention, *www.cdc.gov/nceh/vsp/default.htm*.

Dave Forney, communicable disease specialist and chief of the vessel sanitation program for the Centers for Disease Control and Prevention in Atlanta.

Healthier Food on Cruises

The most healthful cruise-line food is found on Carnival, Norwegian, Royal Caribbean and Windstar ships. All offer a low-fat, high-fiber main course during breakfast...vegetarian options at lunch and dinner...and fruit for desserts and snacks.

Brie Turner-McGrievy, RD, dietitian, Physicians Committee for Responsible Medicine, Washington, DC, which rated the 10 most popular cruise lines, *www.pcrm.org*.

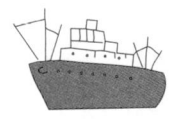

■ *Your Leisure* ■ ■ ■

Smarter Cruising for First-Timers

Before taking your first long cruise, experiment with a short two-, three- or four-night trip to make sure you enjoy the cruise experience. Bring Bonine, an over-the-counter motion-sickness medicine that appears to work better than Dramamine...or get the prescription-only *scopolamine* patch. Talk to a travel agent about the dining table choices—fixed seatings versus more flexible "freestyle" dining, first or second seating and table size preferences. Do not buy items onboard until the last day, when most things go on sale.

Jens Jurgen, editor, *TravelCompanions.com,* Box 833, Amityville, NY 11701, *www.travelcompanions.com.*

More from Jens Jurgen...

Better Cruise Ship Cabins

Avoid cruise ship cabins located below or adjacent to the disco, casino, public rest room or elevator bank—they can be noisy. Watch out for rooms near unidentified white spaces on deck plans—those spaces could be food-service areas, where food carts and early-morning activity can generate lots of noise. Cabins near the gangway or the anchor chain can also be noisy at times. On older ships, the views from some outside cabins may be hidden by lifeboats.

Self-defense: Examine the ship's deck plan carefully. Discuss cabin location choices with a travel agent. Midship cabins will have the least motion during storms, so they are best for minimizing seasickness—but they usually cost more.

Also from Jens Jurgen...

For the Lowest Hotel Rates...

If you do not have a hotel reservation when you arrive in a city, go to the convention and visitors' bureau or tourist office. These offices often keep lists of last-minute room availabilities. AAA Auto Club offices book hotel rooms, and state welcome centers along major US highways also have hotel information.

For the lowest rates: Visit *http://travel.price line.com,* even for some same-day reservations before 6 pm. If you don't have a computer on hand, use one at a local library. Also carry a list of the major hotel chains' toll-free numbers to make a last-minute reservation.

When traveling in larger European cities: Use the hotel booking offices at major railway stations and airports.

Jens Jurgen on bump vouchers...

Save an Expiring Bump Voucher

If you agree to be bumped from an overbooked airline flight, in addition to a seat on another flight, you may receive a valuable voucher that you can apply to the cost of a subsequent flight.

Snag: Vouchers have expiration dates—usually one year—and can't be sold or transferred.

Money saver: You can use the voucher to pay for an airfare for another person.

Self-defense from Jens Jurgen...

Protection Against Travel-Company Bankruptcies

To protect yourself from travel-company financial problems or tour disruptions...

●**Try to book tours with reasonable and flexible cancellation terms**—be sure to read the fine print.

●**Ask your travel and insurance agents about a policy** to cover the chance the tour operator will go bankrupt.

●**Buy trip-cancellation insurance** from an independent company—most policies bought from tour operators may not provide coverage against their default.

●**Before booking, research the company on the Internet** to see if it has had any recent financial problems. Check the Better Business Bureau's Web site at *www.bbb.org* to get a complaint history for a tour operator.

Reminder: Always pay for travel costs with a major credit card so you can dispute charges more easily.

Finally from Jens Jurgen...

Avoid Rental-Car Rip-Offs—Here and Abroad

The most common car-rental rip-off is pressuring you to purchase unnecessary Collision Damage Waiver (CDW) insurance. If you have a personal gold or platinum credit card and your own auto insurance policy, you are most likely covered for the full cost of any rental-car damage.

Caution: Make sure your card includes this feature and its coverage extends to the model you are renting in the country you are visiting for the duration of your rental.

Note: Most corporate cards do not include car-rental insurance.

Smarter Car Renting

Visit car-rental company Web sites for bargains—they often offer the best deals. As a trip date approaches, call the company again—rates may decline after you make your initial reservation. If traveling to Europe, check *www.easycar.com.* Based in England, it undercuts regular car-rental companies in 16 European cities. Outside of the UK, it only accepts reservations via the Internet.

Arthur Frommer's Budget Travel, 350 Fifth Ave., New York City 10118.

Road Trip Know-How

More people are vacationing by car. To prepare for your next road trip...

- **Check brakes,** tires, lights, battery and windshield wipers.
- **Check levels of engine coolant,** motor oil and brake fluid.
- **Bring a cell phone.**
- **Pack a first-aid kit,** jumper cables, toolbox and flares.
- **Be sure the car's registration,** inspection and insurance are up to date.
- **Make lodging reservations in advance.**
- **Pack clothing for the right climate** to avoid having to shop when you arrive.
- **Borrow audio and travel-game books for kids** from your local library.

John Nielsen, director, AAA-Approved Auto Repair Network, Heathrow, FL, *www.aaa.com.*

Protect Your Health While Traveling

Mark Wise, MD, Toronto–based family practitioner who specializes in travel and tropical medicine. Mr. Wise is author of *The Travel Doctor: Your Guide to Staying Healthy While You Travel* (Firefly). His Web site is *www.drwisetravel.com.*

Few things are more frightening than suffering a medical problem while you are away from home. Fortunately, good planning can prevent most health mishaps.

When overseas travelers become ill, it's usually because of an infection or disease that is contracted in a foreign country. But both international and domestic travelers are vulnerable to unexpected complications arising from preexisting medical conditions.

ARE YOU AT RISK?

Not everyone planning to board an airplane needs to visit his/her doctor. However, it may be important if you have a current medical problem. *Check with your doctor before flying if you have...*

- **Anemia.** If your hemoglobin level (measurement of a protein in red blood cells) is less than 8.5 grams per 100 milliliters, you may need supplemental oxygen during the flight because of the cabin's reduced oxygen level. You must arrange this with the airline at least 48 hours in advance.
- **Heart disease.** If you suffer from unstable angina, serious arrhythmias or congestive heart

failure, you may not be fit to fly. If you've had a heart attack, wait at least two weeks before flying. All heart disease patients should consult their doctors before flying.

If you have recently had abdominal surgery, such as laparoscopic gall bladder removal, you should avoid flying for a few weeks. Any air that might have been introduced into your abdominal cavity during surgery will expand at higher altitudes, where cabin pressure is lower.

By the same token, a recently applied cast, which contains air bubbles, may become dangerously tight during flight as those bubbles expand and impede blood circulation to that area. Wait at least 48 hours after being fitted with a cast before flying.

DANGER ZONES

Certain travel destinations can also cause medical problems. A high-altitude location—whether it is a Colorado ski resort, Nepal or Peru—may be dangerous for those patients with heart or lung disease. The air is thinner at high altitudes, which means there is less oxygen available to breathe.

Asthmatics should check with their doctors before visiting heavily polluted cities, such as Bangkok, Beijing and Mumbai.

Even healthy people are at increased risk for illness while traveling. Nearly 30% of those visiting Mexico, the Caribbean and other popular tropical destinations experience "traveler's diarrhea"—even when staying at top resorts.

Self-defense: Avoid local water (including ice cubes) as well as uncooked or undercooked food. Bring *loperamide* (Imodium), which will help decrease your symptoms if you do become ill.

If you're traveling outside of North America, find out if there are any required or recommended inoculations. For more information, contact the Centers for Disease Control and Prevention (877-394-8747 or *www.cdc.gov/travel*).

For more information on inoculations and medications for traveling, contact The International Society of Travel Medicine (770-736-7060 or *www.istm.org*) to locate a travel clinic in your area. Or see your doctor at least two months before your departure if possible.

Important: Pack all of your medical supplies in *carry-on* baggage, rather than in checked luggage. Many medications and batteries can freeze in the baggage compartments.

If you are carrying syringes, make sure you have a signed, stamped note from your doctor explaining why you need the syringes.

If you have a chronic disease, such as diabetes, emphysema or cancer, consider bringing a copy of your pertinent medical records.

If you have heart disease, bring a copy of your latest electrocardiogram.

Don't Get Sick On Your Vacation

People often get sick while on a vacation. That's because when stress levels rapidly subside, resulting biochemical changes lower the body's immunity.

To prevent this effect: Relax slowly by exercising lightly, even while on vacation.

Helpful: Short bursts of exercise—a quick jog or brisk walk, for 10 minutes two to three times each day during the first and second days of vacation—can activate the body and boost immune response.

Marc Schoen, PhD, teaching faculty, department of psychiatry, Cedars-Sinai Medical Center, Los Angeles.

Stock Up Before You Go

Buy extra medicine before you go on a trip, and ask your doctor for duplicate prescriptions in case your medication is lost or stolen. Also, carry prescription medicines with you—not in your suitcase. And bring medicines in their original bottles. If you use sedatives, tranquilizers or other narcotics, take along a letter from your doctor that explains why you need them—this will help prevent problems at border crossings.

Donald Sullivan, RPh, PhD, travel-medicine specialist, Columbus, OH, and author of *A Senior's Guide to Healthy Travel* (Career Press).

Natural Treatment for Traveler's Diarrhea

In a recent study, volunteers who drank three cups of milk a day for 10 days and were then infected with the bacterium *E. coli* had diarrhea for just one day. Those who drank low-calcium milk had diarrhea for three days.

Theory: Calcium increases growth of the diarrhea-fighting bacterium *lactobacillius* in the gut.

Good news: Calcium supplements (1,000 milligrams daily in divided doses) may also do the trick for people who don't drink milk.

Ingeborg M.J. Bovee-Oudenhoven, MD, scientist at the Wageningen Center for Food Sciences/Nizo Food Research, Ede, the Netherlands.

How to Handle Illness After a Trip

When illness strikes after an overseas trip, get immediate medical attention. *Be sure to see a doctor...*

If you have been to a region in which malaria is present and you develop a fever above 100°F, even if you took antimalaria pills—they do not always work...if you experience intestinal problems that last longer than one week or are accompanied by severe pain, fever or dizziness ...or if you develop skin lesions.

Brian Terry, MD, travel-medicine specialist, The Travel Medicine Clinic, Pasadena, CA, *www.healthytraveler.com*.

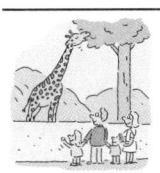

Safer Adventure Vacations

Peter Guttman, New York City–based travel journalist and photographer.

Before embarking on an adventure vacation, make sure your guide knows how to keep you safe.

Adventure vacations—which include risky activities such as whitewater rafting, mountain climbing and canyoneering—can result in disaster if safety is not uppermost in the minds of those running them.

Self-defense: Look for a company that has at least 10 years of experience in the activity. Inquire about its insurance coverage—an indication that the company has a solid record. Ask for references from previous customers—and check them.

Also ask the operations director about the requirements for trip leaders and guides. In addition to being familiar with the geographic area, they should have medical training.

Most important: They should be certified as Emergency Medical Technicians (EMTs).

Best company now: Mountain Travel Sobek (888-687-6235 or *www.mtsobek.com*) a pioneer river-rafting and adventure travel company with 30 years' experience.

Have Fun Traveling Solo

Eleanor Berman, New York City–based travel writer with 20 years' experience traveling on her own. She is author of *Traveling Solo* (Globe Pequot).

Many people fear the loneliness and awkwardness of traveling alone. But those on their own can have fun, dine at great restaurants and even find a group with which to travel. *A few tricks to make it work...*

EATING ALONE

Perhaps the most uncomfortable situation for solo travelers is eating alone in restaurants.

Your Leisure

Also, busy restaurants often are reluctant to give tables to lone diners since seating two generates twice as much revenue. *Smart strategies...*

•**Find restaurants with *dining bars*,** where customers eat at counters rather than tables. These are increasingly common, even at high-end restaurants. To find one, ask your hotel concierge...consult a *Zagat* guide...or go to the sushi bar at a Japanese restaurant.

•**Dine at small neighborhood restaurants.** These usually have more people eating alone, so you're less likely to stand out.

•**Make lunch your big meal.** Restaurants have more solo diners at lunch than at dinner. Prices usually are cheaper as well.

•**Eat at a nice hotel restaurant**—even if you are not staying at the hotel. These, too, attract many solo diners.

•**Ask your concierge to book the table.** If you would like to eat at a high-end restaurant but fear that it won't take a reservation for one, enlist the concierge's help. Restaurants rarely turn down reservations placed by the concierges who send them business.

BED & BREAKFASTS (B&Bs)

Hotels typically charge solo guests the same prices they would charge pairs. Many B&Bs cost significantly less for one person than for two. Plus, they are generally friendly places where you can easily find someone to talk to.

ATTENDING EVENTS

Since most people are interested in purchasing two or more tickets, single travelers often are in a position to benefit. Call ticket offices to see if there are any single seats remaining for otherwise sold-out events.

GROUP TRAVEL

Single travelers often join groups or tours so that they won't be alone. Before you do, contact the tour organizer to make sure you're not the only solo traveler amidst couples or families. *Best bets for single travelers...*

•**Adult-education programs.** Many colleges offer summer programs for adults. Attendees often come on their own. You stay in dormitories, eat in cafeterias and have fun while learning. *Examples...*

•Cornell University (Ithaca, NY) offers weeklong courses in topics ranging from the history of photography to US–Cuba relations. 607-255-6260 or *www.sce.cornell.edu/cau*.

•St. John's College (Santa Fe, NM) provides weeklong seminars on many subjects, including classic literature and opera. 505-984-6117 or *www.sjcsf.edu*.

Call other colleges or check their Web sites to see what programs they offer.

•**Skill-development workshops.** Interested in photography? Cooking? Solo travelers make up a large portion of attendees. *Examples...*

•Maine Photographic Workshops, in Rockport on the Atlantic coast, conducts more than 200 photography seminars each summer. 877-577-7700 or *www.theworkshops.com*.

•Going Solo in the Kitchen, a cooking class, is held throughout the year at the Pelican Inn on Dog Island, off the coast of Florida's panhandle. 800-451-5294 or *www.thepelicaninn.com*.

•**Club Med** has many resorts that cater to single adults. Those over age 50 will be in the minority but not alone. 800-258-2633 or *www.clubmed.com*.

•**Elderhostel** has educational travel opportunities for the 55-and-over crowd. Programs range from spelunking in the Southwest to learning about the culture of Chicago. 877-426-8056 or *www.elderhostel.org*.

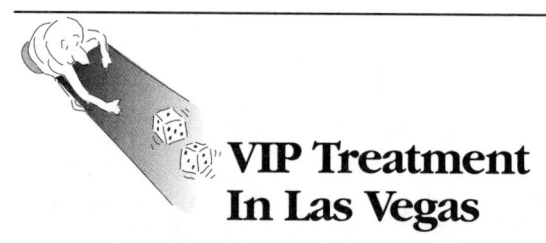

VIP Treatment In Las Vegas

You can avoid buffet and coffee shop lines in Las Vegas. While gambling, ask floor personnel for *line passes*—one for that day and one for the next. Make each for four people, even if you are alone. Line-pass holders enter at the VIP entrance. If you decide not to use the pass, consider giving it to an elderly person or a family with small children.

Thomas B. Gallagher, CEO, Thomas Casino Systems, 5380 Overpass Rd., Santa Barbara, CA 93111.

Your Leisure

15

Just for Fun

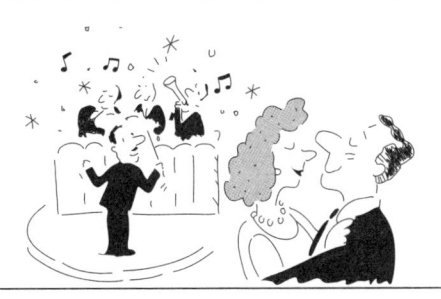

How I Won More Than 500 Sweepstakes And Contests

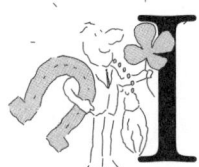

I have won thousands of dollars in cash and prizes from promotional contests. My latest prize was an all-expense paid trip for two to Jamaica.

Here are my top secrets for bettering your chances of winning a national sweepstakes or a local store giveaway. I spend only 20 minutes a day at it.

MAIL-IN SWEEPSTAKES

Big sweepstakes usually blindfold the selectors. Smaller contests, such as those at stores, are less formal. *Learn to exploit the differences...*

- **Use large or oddly shaped envelopes.** Some sweepstakes require a specific envelope or postcard size. If not, the more surface area that can be grabbed by a selector, the better. I use large padded envelopes on occasion, though the cost can be prohibitive.

- **Send colored envelopes.** A brightly colored envelope is several times more likely to win a local sweepstakes, for which the selector might not be blindfolded. I haven't found any one color to be most successful.

- **Decorate your envelopes.** I add stickers, glue-on glitter, even fingerpaint to the outside of my sweepstakes-entry envelopes, especially those for local sweepstakes. This helps my envelopes stand out from the rest.

I usually limit my number of entries to just a few per sweepstakes. It is better to enter several sweepstakes than to put all your eggs in one basket.

IN-STORE DRAWINGS

You usually drop entries into a box for store contests. *To better your odds...*

- **Fold entry cards.** An entry card folded into an interesting shape is more likely to be

---

Steve Ledoux, author of *How to Win Lotteries, Sweepstakes, and Contests in the 21st Century* (Santa Monica Press). He has won hundreds of sweepstakes prizes and is a freelance television graphic artist and writer living in Studio City, CA.

■ *Your Leisure* ■ ■ ■

grabbed than one lying flat, hidden in a stack of entries. Accordion-style folding has proven particularly effective for me.

●**Take entry forms home.** Fill them out, and return with them later. Few people have the patience to fill out more than one or two entries while standing in the store. Boost your odds by entering many times—assuming the rules permit it.

I like to drop off my entries on several occasions, so they don't wind up together. It's also best to spread entries among more than one store location.

Example: When one local supermarket chain ran a sweepstakes for a vacation to Puerto Rico, I filled out 200 entries and dropped them off at a dozen stores. While there was only one grand prize, each store was giving away a television. I won the vacation *and* three TVs.

CONTESTS

Contests differ from sweepstakes because skill is required. But you can win even with little skill.

For essay-writing contests, saying positive things about the company sponsoring the contest is more important than writing well. I won a contest sponsored by the LA Dodgers by describing my fantasy of pitching for the team —and striking out its opponents. The prize? The honor of throwing out the first ceremonial pitch before 38,000 fans, as well as tickets to the game for friends.

SWEEPSTAKES TO AVOID

Don't bother with…

●**Most Internet sweepstakes.** Enter only those sponsored by familiar companies. Otherwise, the only guaranteed return has been to fill my E-mail account with junk E-mail.

●**Sweepstakes that require entrants to make purchases.**

●**Sweepstakes with long entry periods.** Anything longer than a few months will have large numbers of entries and much smaller odds of winning.

●**Contests or sweepstakes with "strings" attached.**

Example: Car giveaways in the shopping malls generally insist that you listen to a sales pitch before your entry becomes valid.

TAX DEDUCTION

Track postage and envelope expenses for each sweepstakes or contest. When you win, consult your accountant. The amount you spent on postage and envelopes is deductible up to the amount you won during the year.

FINDING SWEEPSTAKES

Many advertisers promote sweepstakes in the coupon section of newspapers. *Other good sources are magazines, TV and radio ads and newsletters…*

●**Rags to Riches Sweepstakes Newsletter,** Box 891, Derry, NH 03038, *www.ragstoriches.com.*

●**SweepSheet,** 105 Town Line Rd., #329 wb, Vernon Hills, IL 60061, *www.sweepsheet.com.* Two free on-line newsletters…

●**www.sweepstakesonline.com**

●**www.sweepthenet.com**

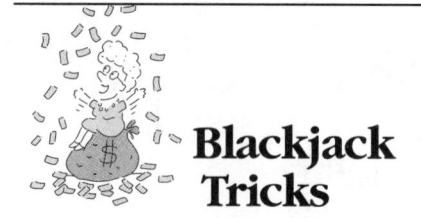

Blackjack Tricks

Thomas B. Gallagher, CEO, Thomas Casino Systems, 5380 Overpass Rd., Santa Barbara, CA 93111. The company conducts blackjack and craps seminars nationwide and publishes instruction guides, including the *Blackjack Survival Kit*. Call 800-333-5608.

Blackjack seems like a very easy game—if you can count to 21, you should be able to play. But there's a big difference between playing and playing *well.*

A savvy blackjack player can cut the house's edge from 5% to less than 1%. Unfortunately, only one player in 1,000 bothers to learn basic strategy before playing. The other 999 will lose money needlessly.

The following are my top 10 winning blackjack strategies…

BEFORE THE DEAL

●**Buy a blackjack strategy card,** and use it at the table. In a perfect world, players would learn all the intricacies of the game before walking into the casino. Since few are willing to invest the time, spending $1.50 on a strategy card at the casino gift shop is the next best option. These cards offer the proper strategy for every blackjack situation. Most casinos allow the use of the cards, particularly at low-stakes tables.

Students in my blackjack seminar often complain that referring to a card during a game makes them feel stupid. I reply that anyone who makes the casino richer by playing poorly should feel stupid. And do not worry about slowing down the game. It's in your best interest. The more bets per hour, the more the casino's mathematical edge works against you.

•**Play at a full table.** A full table slows down play, reducing the number of hands—and thus the house's edge—and again giving you more time to consider strategy.

•**Sit on the dealer's right.** The player on the dealer's left is the first to receive cards. Sitting near the dealer's right gives you additional time to weigh each decision.

•**Look for a casino that offers a "surrender" option.** A few casinos allow players to surrender their hand after the initial deal in exchange for half of their wager. Casinos allow this because they know many gamblers surrender the wrong hands and lose money.

Surrender should be used when the dealer is showing an ace, nine, 10 or face card, and you are dealt a *hard* 16. A hard 16 means another card could break the total (go over 21). A *soft* 16 means another card could not break it—for example, if you have an ace (which counts as a one or 11) and a five. Surrender should also be used when the dealer is showing a 10 and you are dealt a hard 15.

Two Las Vegas casinos that usually allow the surrender option are the Flamingo Las Vegas Hotel and the Stratosphere Casino Hotel and Tower. Other casinos offer and repeal this option often. Call the casino's blackjack pit, and ask a pit boss if surrender is offered.

•**Get "rated."** Ask a casino host for a rating card, which tracks how often you play and how much you spend. Give this card to the dealer when you sit down to play any game at the casino. The more time you spend at the tables—and the more you bet per hand—the more comps the casino offers you. Even if you're only betting $5 a game, you might get a free ticket for the buffet. A $25 player might get a room discount, free meals, tickets to shows or other perks.

DURING PLAY

•**Never split pairs of fives or 10s.** If the first two cards you're dealt are a pair, you have the option of splitting the cards into two separate hands, then playing and betting on each hand independently. Do not exercise this option if the pair in question is made of fives or 10s.

Reason: A pair of 10s adds up to 20, a likely winner. A pair of fives also offers better odds of success together—since 30% of the cards in a deck have a value of 10.

•**Always split pairs of aces and eights.** A pair of eights adds up to 16—too high to take another card, too low to be a likely winner. It is better to break them up. An ace can be one or 11. Either one is a better starting hand than two or 12 (two aces).

•**Never take *insurance* or *even* money—**even if you have blackjack. When the dealer's up card is an ace, players are then offered the opportunity to lay a side bet that the dealer has blackjack. Called *insurance* or *even money,* the bet is equal to half the amount the gambler has risked on the game and pays off at two to one. Unless you're able to count cards and determine how many 10s are remaining in the deck, it is a sucker's bet.

•**Stand on hands as low as 13 or 14—**if the dealer shows a small card (two, three, four, five or six). Few novice blackjack players stand on a total as low as 13 or 14, but it's the smart play.

Reason: If you have a 13, any card of nine or above pushes you over 21, breaking your hand. That makes hitting a risk. When the dealer has a six or lower, it's virtually certain the dealer will take a card as well (the dealer must hit on a hard 16 or less and stand on 17). That means the odds are reasonable that the dealer's hand could be broken as well.

235

▪ *Your Leisure* ▪ ▪ ▪ ▪

When both you and the dealer are in a situation in which being broken is a significant possibility, the smart play is to stand. If you both are broken, you lose because the player acts first...dealer, last.

•**Double down on 10 and 11.** When you double down, you double your bet and receive one card face down. Doubling down can be a moneymaker. Always double down with a total of 10 except when the dealer shows a 10 or an ace. Double down on a total of 11 except when the dealer shows an ace.

Slot Machine Myths

Steve Bourie, president, Casino Vacations, Box 703, Dania, FL 33004, and author of *American Casino Guide* (Casino Vacation).

There are many myths associated with slot machines. *Check out some of the most common below...*

Myth: **Machines are reset to favor the house on weekends** or when big conventions are in town.

Reality: This would require changing an internal computer chip and complying with numerous regulations—a full-day process. It isn't done.

Myth: **The best-paying machines are on the aisles.**

Reality: Same-denomination machines—nickel, quarter, etc.—have the same payouts, no matter where they are located.

Myth: **You can predict hot and cold payout cycles.**

Reality: All payouts are random. A machine that just paid a jackpot could pay another on the next play—or not for a long time.

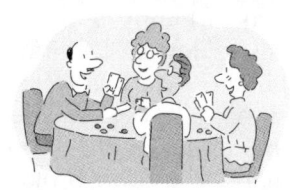

Win at Baccarat

Frank Scoblete, Malverne, NY–based author of numerous gambling books, including *The Baccarat Battle Book* (Bonus). He spends more than 100 days a year playing in casinos. His Web site is *www.scoblete.com*.

Baccarat is so simple to play and offers some of the best odds of any casino game. But it is ignored by most American gamblers, who may view it as a sophisticated, high-stakes European game.

HOW TO PLAY

Two cards each are dealt to the player and the bank. A face card or 10 is worth zero points ...an ace is worth one point...and other numbered cards are worth face value. The winning hand at game's end is the one that adds up closest to nine—counting only the final digit.

Example: A hand with a seven and a nine has a score of six—not 16—since only the last digit of the total counts.

If the player or bank—or both—has a score of eight or nine (nine beats eight) after the deal, the game ends right there with a winner or tie declared.

If neither the player nor the bank has a score of eight or nine, more cards may be dealt. *Unlike blackjack, in which the gambler decides if he/she wants another card, specific rules dictate the action...*

•**The player automatically gets a third card** if his hand has a score of less than six. If he has six or seven, the hand stands.

•**The bank automatically gets a third card** if its score is two or less.

•**The bank may or may not receive a third card** if its score is between three and six. This depends on a complex set of rules that incorporates the bank's score, the player's score and whether the player was dealt a third card. The details are unimportant. It does not affect your chances of winning.

HOW TO BET

The only real strategy involved in baccarat occurs before the deal, when each gambler decides whether to bet on the bank, the player or a tie...

- **Bank.** This is your best bet. A winning bet on the bank pays out at 1:1, while a winning bet of $25 pays back your bet plus $25. Successful bets are charged a commission, usually 5%—so the profit on a winning bank bet of $25 is $23.75.

The house has a 1.06% advantage on bets placed on the bank. That means for every $100 a gambler bets on the bank, the house makes an average profit of only $1.06, a low take by casino standards.

- **Player.** A winning bet on the player also pays out at 1:1. Betting on the player is reasonable because the house advantage is a still-slim 1.24%.

- **Tie.** This is a sucker's bet. Winning bets on a tie pay out at 8:1—bet $25 to win $200. But the house has a whopping 14.36% advantage.

Plan on needing $1,000 to play at a $25 table...$4,000 for a $100 table.

BEWARE OF MINIBACCARAT

Casinos offer two versions of baccarat. Rules and odds are the same, however, the stakes and speed of play are different.

In minibaccarat, you bet less per hand—the minimum bet might be $10, versus the $25 or $100 minimum common at traditional baccarat tables. But in minibaccarat, casino employees deal the cards and keep the action moving—120 to 200 hands per hour.

In traditional baccarat, the gambler deals the cards, so the game moves more slowly—50 to 60 hands per hour. The tremendous speed of minibaccarat makes it riskier on a potential-dollars-lost-per-hour basis.

Helpful: Don't be intimidated by having to deal the cards when you play traditional baccarat. Casino employees are usually quite willing to help.

PLAY ON WEEKDAYS

On weekends, you probably won't find a traditional baccarat table with a minimum of less than $100. But during the week, when crowds are smaller, many casinos have $25 tables. This makes playing more affordable.

Strategy: When at a $25 table, bet the minimum on the bank. The casino will take the 5% commission on a successful bank bet—$1.25 on a $25 win.

Many casinos round down to the nearest dollar when taking commissions. Then the real commission is only $1. Ask to pay your commission after every successful hand rather than after the *shoe*—a set of six or eight decks of cards. Some casinos won't let you do this—but at those that do, the quarters you save will add up.

Not every casino has $25 baccarat tables even on weekdays. Fancy casinos, such as Bellagio or Venetian in Las Vegas, rarely offer anything less than $100. And some casinos don't have baccarat at all.

In Las Vegas, try Bally's, Sahara, Stardust or Treasure Island. In Atlantic City, try Bally's, Caesars Palace, Hilton, Showboat or Trump Taj Mahal.

Casino Safety

To protect your belongings in a casino, follow this practical advice...

- **Do not carry a purse or bag.**

If you must: Keep it securely between your legs or on your lap when playing.

- **Do not be distracted.** Thieves use loud noises or other distractions as an opportunity to grab chips, coins, bags, etc.

- **Hold your belongings tightly** if anyone bumps or spills a drink on you...or says, "You dropped some money." Check your belongings before looking around.

- **Cash out your chips before leaving the casino.** If you win a large amount, ask for a check or deposit the funds at the cage rather than carry cash.

- **Ask the casino for a security escort** if you are carrying a lot of cash.

Basil Nestor, columnist, *Casino Player,* 8025 Black Horse Pike, Pleasantville, NJ 08232. He is author of *The Unofficial Guide to Casino Gambling* (Wiley).

■ *Your Leisure* ■ ■ ■

How to Hook a Big One

Tom Mann, three-time professional bass-fishing world champion, member of the National Fishing Hall of Fame and owner of Tom Mann's Fish World in Eufaula, AL. He is a cohost of the weekly syndicated TV show *Tom & Tina Outdoors, www.tomandtinaoutdoors.com*. Mr. Mann is also author of *Think Like a Fish: The Lure & Lore of America's Legendary Bass Fisherman* (Broadway).

Fishing is very relaxing, whether or not you catch anything. But nothing beats coming home with a big one to impress friends and family—and to cook for dinner.

Here are the most common mistakes fishermen make, plus tricks to catch four favorite sport fish...

COMMON MISTAKES

•**Holding the rod too low.** Former President Jimmy Carter was a pretty good fisherman when I met him—but even he made this mistake. Hold your rod nearly straight up, perpendicular to the ground. The rod's flexibility will make it harder for a fish to snap the line.

•**Setting the hook too forcefully.** When they feel a fish tug, many fishermen use their whole forearm to set the hook, which could pull the hook free. A simple flick of the wrist and one-half revolution of the reel is enough. The sharpness of the hook—not the strength of the set—does the work.

•**Ignoring the current.** If the water is flowing swiftly—after a hard rain, for example—try fishing in the shelter of obstructions, such as pilings and rocks, that protect fish.

•**Looking for big fish in deep water.** Big fish eat small fish. They often head for shallow water, where small fish hide.

•**Assuming powerboats scare the fish.** Plenty of fishermen disagree with me on this, but powerboats do *not* scare off fish.

In fact, I have found that motors can work to a fisherman's advantage. Drive the boat through the reeds and lily pads that provide cover for small bait fish. Flushing out the bait fish will bring bigger fish out of hiding.

HOW TO HOOK THESE POPULAR FISH

•**Largemouth bass.** You can find largemouth bass just about everywhere people fish in freshwater in the US, except Alaska. More than 75% of largemouth bass are caught in less than seven feet of water.

As with any of the shallow-water fish, you are most likely to catch bass during the early morning, late afternoon and on cloudy days. Heat and bright light drive them to deep water. If you must fish at midday, you may find them in shady areas under overhanging trees.

The best bait for bass are plastic lures, including soft plastic worms and plastic minnows. Stick with topwater lures so you can keep the lure at or near the surface. Do not add weights.

•**Walleye.** This popular sport fish is found in the freshwater rivers and lakes of the upper Midwest, from Minnesota and Wisconsin up into Canada. Walleye are bottom fish, so you will have to fish within a foot or so of the bottom. A boat equipped with an electronic fish finder is very helpful.

You can fish for walleye all day. You can even fish for them at night, when they are likely to feed near the surface, especially around rocks and pilings.

Walleye like moving lures. Use a trolling motor, if you have one, to keep moving very slowly. Otherwise, use your reel to keep the lure moving. Best artificial lures include shad wraps, eerie deeries and crank baits.

•**Speckled trout.** These are found in coastal waters from Corpus Christi, Texas, all the way up to New Jersey. They live in freshwater near the mouths of rivers, in saltwater or in brackish water. Similar to bass, speckled trout like the shallow water. Unlike bass, speckled trout migrate, so finding them depends on the season.

When the weather warms up, speckled trout then head to the brackish waters around the grass flats to spawn. They stay there through the summer.

At this time of the year, use the same soft plastic lures you would use for bass. Or use grubs, MirrOlures or Chub Bugs. Keep the lure near the surface.

After the first cold snap of the season, generally around October, speckled trout head upriver and go deeper. In these conditions, try a type of weighted artificial lure known as a lead-head jig with a grub.

•**Crappie.** You can find crappie in freshwater throughout the South. They bite on minnows and small jigs, particularly feather jigs.

Fish around pilings and under old bridges. A great time to catch them is after dark with a handheld glow light, available at most fishing-supply stores. The light attracts insects, and insects attract crappie. On some lakes, there are so many people fishing with glow lights that the whole area is lit up like a city.

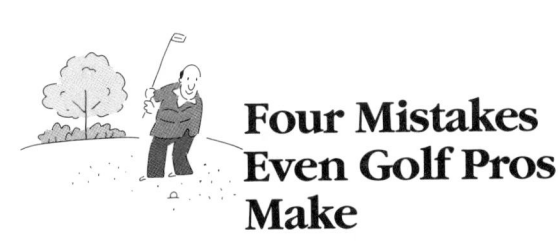

Four Mistakes Even Golf Pros Make

Billy Casper, professional golf legend, PGA Hall-of-Famer and PGA Tour Player of the Year in 1966 and 1970. He is considered one of the greatest putters of all time and is senior adviser to Billy Casper Golf, a golf course management and consulting firm in Vienna, VA, *www.billycaspergolf.com*.

Some putting mistakes are so difficult to shake that even professional golfers can fall victim to them…

•**Raising your head.** This is the most common putting mistake. I still catch myself doing it occasionally. It is a natural tendency to lift up your head to see where the golf ball is going. Unfortunately, it can throw off your stroke and send your putt off-line.

Better: Focus your attention on the ball. If you don't see your putter strike the ball, you are moving your head too soon.

•**Lifting the putter on the backswing.** Aim for a level backswing. If the head of your putter comes up, you will hit down on the ball, giving it spin. This reduces the chances that it will roll where you want it to.

•**Too much right hand**—or left hand, if you are left-handed. To strike a putt properly, a right-handed golfer's left hand should do most of the work.

Focus on using the left hand (right hand for lefties) to perform the backswing and most of the forward motion.

Allow only the right hand to take charge just before you hit the ball, when you need to add power for a long putt. It sometimes helps to pretend that the back of the left hand is the clubface. When you direct the hand, the putter face should follow.

•**Stay in rhythm.** It is easier to putt properly if you putt from habit and don't need to think about the mechanics every time. Practice keeping your putting stroke slow and low—and the same every time.

Anxiety can knock even a pro out of sync. If you are nervous before a big putt, step back, take three deep breaths and start over.

Kite-Flying Secrets From a National Champ

Phil Broder, Burlington, IA–based coordinator, National Kite Month, *www.nationalkitemonth.org*, and director at large, American Kitefliers Association. Mr. Broder is a former national-champion stunt-kite flier.

Whether you are just starting out or seeking to perfect your skills, you will have more fun flying a kite if you follow this advice from a master…

•**Wait for the right wind.** Novices do best with wind speeds of five to 15 miles per hour (mph). More advanced kite fliers use different kites for different winds—ultralight models for light wind…vented kites for high wind.

To find wind speed: Wind speed is listed in your local newspaper and on The Weather Channel and its Web site, *www.weather.com*.

Helpful: Wind-speed estimates often come from airport wind socks in exposed areas off the ground. Reported wind speeds of 10 to 20 mph equate to actual wind speeds of five to 15 mph.

•**Avoid turbulence.** You are most likely to find turbulence around buildings, trees and other obstructions.

Follow the *rule of sevens*—if a tree or building is upwind, position yourself away from the obstruction by at least seven times its height.

■ *Your Leisure* ■ ■ ■

Example: A 20-foot tree requires 140 feet of distance.

• **Don't run.** Novices often think the best way to launch a kite is to run with it. Not true.

Better: One person holds the line. Another takes the kite 50 feet downwind and tosses it in the air. The wind does the work. If you are alone and there is enough wind, you should be able to launch the kite right from your hand.

PICK THE RIGHT KITE

• **Beginner.** *These kites fly in almost any wind and usually come packaged with a reel and string...*

• Delta kites. Until about 15 years ago, the most common beginner kite was the diamond. But the ease and stability of the triangular delta have pushed it to the front of the pack.

• Pocket parafoils. Parafoils look like small parachutes. They have no wood or plastic spars. That means no assembly required and nothing to break.

• Box kites. These are trickier to assemble and fly, and they are more prone to damage than deltas and parafoils. Still, they are within the capabilities of most novices.

• **Advanced.** *Expert kite fliers have many options available...*

• Stunt kites can perform precise and intricate maneuvers.

• Design kites resemble anything from a biplane to a giant squid.

• Japanese fighting kites, called *rokkaku*, combine kiting with professional wrestling. Fliers try to knock down other kites or cut their strings. The last kite flying wins.

WHAT TO PAY

With kites, you get what you pay for. A $5 discount-store model falls apart fast. Go Fly a Kite (800-243-3370 or *www.goflyakite.com*) is a reliable brand for entry-level kites. Expect to pay about $20 to $50 or more.

For more advanced kites, buy quality brands, such as Gomberg, Premier, Prism Designs or Sky Burner. Stunt kites sell in the range of $60 to $400. Handcrafted models can cost as much as $4,000.

Buy quality kites at kite and hobby shops or at better toy stores. Also, try Into the Wind (800-541-0314 or *www.intothewind.com*) or The Kite Loft (800-682-5483 or *www.kiteloft.com*).

Better Scrabble Strategy

Try these winning tips the next time you play Scrabble...

• **If you have three tiles of the same letter on your rack,** use or exchange at least one.

• **Try to think of three possible moves** before making one.

• **If you are behind when the game is half finished,** take more risks to get points and open the board for high-scoring plays.

• **If you are leading at the halfway mark,** try to close the board so your opponents can't play all their tiles.

Sheree Bykofsky, literary agent, New York City, and co-editor of *The Big Book of Life's Instructions* (Galahad).

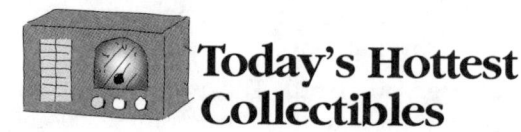

Today's Hottest Collectibles

Harry L. Rinker, president, Rinker Enterprises, 5093 Vera Cruz Rd., Emmaus, PA 18049. He is the host of *Collector Inspector* on Home and Garden Television (HGTV) and author of *The Official Harry L. Rinker Price Guide to Collectibles* (House of Collectibles).

Looking to start a collection or add to one that's already established? *Here's what serious collectors are on the lookout for...*

• **Vintage radios.** *Especially popular are...*

• Console radios from the 1920s (by manufacturers such as Zenith). Prices range from $50 to $1,000.

• Table radios from the 1930s and 1940s (manufactured by Bendix, Emerson, Fada and Garod, among others). Prices can range from $50 to $1,000.

• Transistor radios from the 1950s and 1960s, which were often tossed out when they stopped working. *Example:* A Sony Model TR-63 sells for about $150.

High-end: Colorful Bakelite radios—particularly those with an Art Deco design—can bring $2,500 and up.

Also keep an eye out for instruction manuals, vacuum tubes and other radio-related items that might interest radio collectors.

- **Golden oak furniture.** The oak furniture industry peaked in the 1890s, so pieces have now achieved antique status—more than 100 years old.

An armchair with spindles shaped to look like rope can be had for about $200...a bookcase with a carved or scrolled backsplash for around $1,500...and a sideboard with mirrored sections and carved doors for about $1,000.

In demand: Oak dental cabinets with drawers, sliding shelves and a folding top sell for around $2,000.

- **Gas station collectibles.**

  - Solid glass gas-pump globes with etched graphics. These could be found atop gas station pumps from about 1910 to 1970. As they become harder to find, prices are rising. Globe collectors will pay thousands of dollars for the right one.

  Brightly colored globes in good condition with unusual graphics or shape, such as the one-piece, raised-letter Texaco Star globe, can bring as much as $5,000. A Texaco Sky Chief globe with a glass body and glass-insert globe goes for about $400.

  Pump globes have been extensively reproduced, so watch out for fakes.

  - Gas station signs, motor oil cans, advertising displays, clocks, thermometers and even wall calendars are also very collectible. *Example:* A pre-1945 one-quart motor oil can displaying a brand name, such as Mobil or Shell, can bring as much as $600.

- **Flow blue china.** Made in England and America from 1830 to 1900, this china—distinguished by blurred blue designs on white earthenware and ironstone china—has long been a favorite of collectors. *There were three periods of production and style...*

  - Early patterns (1835–1860) would feature Chinese-inspired landscape designs.

  - Middle patterns (1860s–1870s) generally had Japanese motifs and floral designs.

  - Late patterns (1870s–1900) used Art Nouveau designs.

  Prices range from $60 for a relish dish to $200 to $1,000 for a platter, depending upon period and design.

- **Silverplated figural napkin rings.** This American invention was patented in 1869 and made up until the 1920s. The most popular of them depict girls originally created by artist Kate Greenaway, as well as birds, cherubs and domestic and wild animals.

  Major manufacturers included Barbour Silver, Meriden Britannia and Derby Silver. Most are marked with the manufacturer's name and mold number.

  Caution: Beware of reproductions. Look for manufacturer marks that are die-stamped—fakes are marked in the cast.

  Prices for originals range from $200 to $2,000. Reproductions cost as little as $20 to $45.

- **Fishing collectibles.** Fishermen are always looking for old rods, reels, flies, nets, decoys, creels and tackle boxes.

  Old creels can be priced from $80 to $400, depending on size and condition. Rods made by H.L. Leonard, C.F. Orvis and Thomas & Thomas can bring as much as $10,000. Look for lures made by Pflueger, Heddon, Hastings, Shakespeare and Southbend—some sell for several hundred dollars. Reels by Hardy Bougle and vom Hofe bring top dollar.

- **Old slot machines.** Introduced during the 1880s, the original models have three or more reels, a handle that makes the reels spin and a mechanism that dispenses the payout when the right combination appears in the windows.

  Manufacturers include Mills Novelty Co., Jennings, Caille Brothers and Watling Manufacturing Co.

  Prices go as high as $30,000 for a Caille Centaur, 5¢, 25¢, double-upright slot machine in an oak case. A Mills Bursting Cherry, 5¢ slot machine with a cast aluminum front and wood sides sells for $900.

- **Jukeboxes.** Manufactured by Seeburg, Capehart, A.M.I., Wurlitzer and Rock-Ola, units from the "golden age"—1940s and 1950s when the most colorful and innovative designs were produced—can be pricey. You can pay $7,000

■ *Your Leisure* ■ ■ ■ ■

for a Wurlitzer model 1015 and $15,000 for a model 850.

Most valuable: Jukeboxes produced from 1938 to 1948 that play 78-rpm records.

Most affordable: Jukeboxes that play 45-rpm records. You can get a common Seeburg for less than $1,200.

●**Beer and soda trays.** A form of advertising, colorful, lithographed metal serving trays were made in the 1890s for American breweries and soft drink companies. Look for older trays in good condition, with interesting graphics.

Top-of-the-line: The "Drink Coca-Cola, Relieves Fatigue" tray from 1907 sells for around $5,000.

Beer trays from the 1930s to 1950s sell for $25 to $50. Watch out for reproductions.

"SHABBY CHIC" RETURNS

Even if you aren't a serious collector, you may find items at flea markets that you can turn into art or functional pieces to fit your personal taste. Called "shabby chic," it is one of the most popular decorating trends today. *What to look for…*

●**Old furniture that can be fixed up.** Slap on some white paint for the cottage look so popular these days.

●**Chandeliers and lamps.** Just rewire and repaint them.

●**Vintage fabrics.** Use as curtains, furniture covers and wall decor.

●**Bread boxes,** tin pie cupboards, firewood and coal carriers, and crocks. Use as functional accent pieces (spice shelves, magazine racks, etc.).

●**Old doorknobs,** locks and hinges. Recycle as coat hooks or furniture accents.

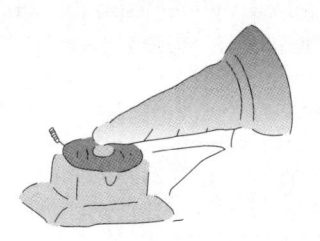

Baseball Cards Are Hot Again

Leila Dunbar, senior vice president and director of the collectibles department at Sotheby's in New York City. Ms. Dunbar is also an appraiser on the PBS TV series *Antiques Roadshow.*

The baseball card market has been surprisingly strong recently. People have latched onto collecting baseball cards as a nostalgic escape from all the troubles of today. You can find cards everywhere, from yard sales to eBay.

Here's what you should know to maximize your return on the fun…

●**Players from the 1930s through the 1950s are hot.** The children who grew up rooting for these baseball players are now retiring. They have time, cash and nostalgia for their childhood.

Particularly popular: Goudy Gum cards of the 1930s…Play Ball cards of the late 1930s and early 1940s…postwar Bowman cards…and Topps cards of the early 1950s.

Mickey Mantle cards have traditionally overshadowed all others from the 1950s. A 1951 Bowman Mickey Mantle rookie card can run as high as $275,000. But recently, the cards of other 1950s Hall-of-Famers—Hank Aaron, Yogi Berra, Eddie Mathews and Satchel Paige—have begun commanding higher prices.

Example: Ten years ago, Satchel Paige cards were worth $50 to $500 each, depending on their condition. Today, these cards run $100 to $8,000.

●**Exceptional cards don't have to be of exceptional players.** But cards must be in mint condition, with crisp corners and edges, bright colors and no nicks, stains or scratches.

One 1980 Rickey Henderson rookie card in mint condition recently sold for $10,000, an astonishing price for a relatively recent card—and more than 100 times what it would sell for in only near-mint condition.

A mint 1952 Topps Andy Pafko card recently sold for more than $80,000. Pafko was never a great player. But his card was the first in the set that year and thus was particularly vulnerable to damage from packaging and shipping—and children who put rubber bands around their collections.

Store cards in plastic or Mylar sheets in notebooks, away from heat and light.

•**Avoid modern *Collector's Edition* cards.** Since the 1980s, cards have been produced in increasing quantities, often in "collector" sets. There are too many around to be valuable. But rookie cards may be worth saving in case a player becomes a star.

•**Buy still-affordable cards of the early 1960s.** Cards featuring such Hall-of-Famers as Hank Aaron, Harmon Killebrew and Willie McCovey currently sell for a few dollars to a few hundred dollars. In 10 years, the people who grew up with these cards will begin to retire—and prices will go up.

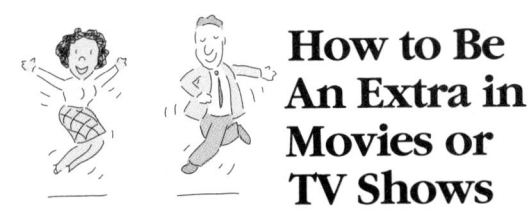

How to Be An Extra in Movies or TV Shows

Robert Demkowicz, author of the E-book *Anyone Can Be a Movie Extra* (*www.firstprint.com*). He lives in East Winthrop, ME.

You don't need to live in Hollywood to be in a movie. You do not even need any acting experience. I have a full-time job in Maine, and I've appeared in more than two dozen movies and commercials that were filmed during weekends, evenings and vacation days—and I did not ever have to leave New England.

Studios film on location around the world. They often need local "extras" for nonspeaking background roles. Usually, extras stand in the back of a shot doing an everyday thing, such as walking a dog or eating lunch.

What you get paid varies. Reimbursement ranges from free meals for independent films to a few hundred dollars for the big-budget productions.

Beware of all "opportunities" to become an extra that require you to pay the film company. These are most likely scams.

FINDING ROLES

Look for newspaper reports of open casting calls in your region. Unless you live in a big city, a film company coming to town is sure to make the papers.

Check out the national extra Web site *www.beinamovie.com*. Or contact your state's film commission. In a search engine such as *www.google.com*, plug in your state's name and "film commission" or "film office."

Some recent TV and movie filmings that needed extras…

•***CSI* and *Six Feet Under*,** Las Vegas. These TV series need extras on a regular basis. 702-252-8382.

•***Everwood*,** Ogden, UT. This Warner Brothers' TV series requires extras on a regular basis. 801-256-1637.

•***50 First Kisses*,** Honolulu. Film that features Adam Sandler and Drew Barrymore.

•***Stuck on You*,** North Miami Beach. A film from the Farrelly brothers, with Matt Damon, Meryl Streep and Cher.

•***The Alamo*,** Austin, TX. A Ron Howard film. Hispanic men were in great demand.

FINDING AN AGENT

Once you have been an extra a few times, you might look for a local agent who can keep you apprised of roles. Avoid signing with any agent who asks for payment in advance. Most agents take a 10% to 20% commission only after they find paying jobs for clients. Get agent referrals from local theater actors, or look in the *Yellow Pages*.

GETTING SELECTED

At an open casting call, you will be asked to fill out a form with information about yourself, including clothing sizes. A Polaroid or digital photo will be taken. If many would-be extras show up, the odds of being selected can be low. You might boost your chances by learning more about the film. If the movie is based on a book—many are—read the book. Then see how your skills match up.

Examples: If the setting is a casino and you can deal cards like a pro, bring a deck to

■ *Your Leisure* ■ ■ ■ ■

the casting call and show off your skills. If there is a big scene in a bowling alley and you are a longtime bowler, include this on your form.

ON THE SET

Read filming schedules very carefully. Three o'clock might mean 3 am. Movies often shoot at odd hours, when office buildings or other settings are available.

Expect to spend hours on the set—even if your screen time amounts to a few seconds. Bring a book or a CD player with plenty of batteries. On the bright side, the food tends to be excellent.

Avoid speaking to any professional actors unless the actor initiates the conversation. You might be accused of bothering the stars and get thrown off the set. On a multimillion-dollar production, time is money. Asking for autographs and taking photos are frowned upon.

This isn't to say that extras never get to rub shoulders with stars. On the set of *Message in a Bottle,* I had lunch with Paul Newman—but only after he joined my table. It would have been inappropriate for me to scramble for a seat next to him.

Helpful: Don't look directly at the camera during your scene unless told to do so by the director. When an extra looks into the camera, whole scenes must be reshot. That won't make you any friends.

Write Your Memoirs

Writing regularly can be fun and fascinating. Share your memoirs with your children and grandchildren—they will marvel at what the world was like when you were their age. Writing letters to friends and relatives is also a stimulating learning experience. These letters will be especially cherished at a time when letter-writing is a lost art.

Jack and Phoebe Ballard, founders, Third Half of Life Institute, Highstown, NJ. They are also coauthors of *Turning Points: Create Your Path Through Uncertainty and Change* (1stBooks).

Better Autograph Collecting

Serious autograph collectors concentrate on signed documents, letters or manuscripts—not on signatures alone. The more significant a document, the higher its value. If you collect only autographs, focus on those of famous people who did not often sign their name, such as Abraham Lincoln and Franklin Roosevelt. Avoid signatures of recent presidents signed by autopen. Authenticate any autograph with a handwriting expert before you buy it.

Jordan E. Goodman, president, Amherst Enterprises, former financial analyst and Wall Street correspondent, Scarsdale, NY. He is author of *Everyone's Money Book* (Dearborn Trade).

Save a Pet via the Internet

If you're in the market for a pet, find what you are looking for and save a homeless one at the same time through the Petfinder Web site (*www.petfinder.com*).

This nationwide clearinghouse for animal rescue organizations can provide you with any kind of pet—dog, cat, bird, reptile, etc. You can find specific breeds, such as Siamese cats, through its links to organizations that specialize in them, such as *www.siameserescue.org*.

Also: Post want ads…research the kind of pet you are interested in.

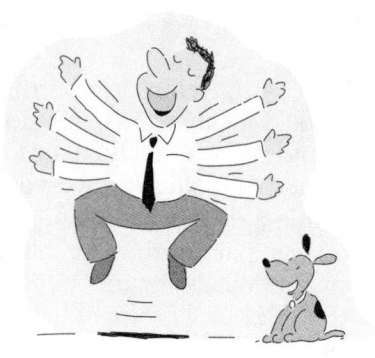

..... **Your Leisure** .

16

Car Care

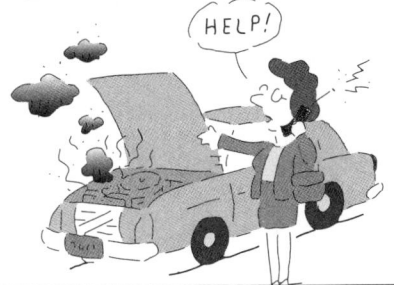

The Biggest Mistakes Car Owners Make

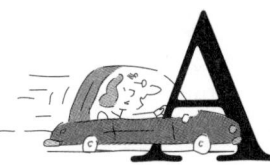

A car is often our most expensive possession, second to our home. But we rarely treat cars the way we should, dramatically hurting their performance, longevity and value.

Mistake: **Not warming up the car.** The most wear and tear on an engine occurs during the first few minutes of operation. Even in warm weather, let your car warm up for at least one minute before driving or turning on the air conditioner. On frosty mornings, let your car warm up for two minutes.

I also recommend synthetic oil, which flows more easily and provides faster lubrication during start-up than nonsynthetic oil.

My favorite: Redline 100% synthetic oil.

Mistake: **Changing the oil every 3,000 miles.** If you usually drive less than 10 miles each time you use the car, step up your oil changes. Short-trip driving puts severe stress on the car. Instead of changing the oil every 3,000 miles, do it every three months—regardless of mileage.

Mistake: **Using poor-quality oil filters.** There is a wide variation in the quality of oil filters, which can affect engine longevity. If you frequent fast-lube oil-change shops, you may not be getting the best quality. Purchase an oil filter ahead of time, and ask that your filter be installed.

My favorites: Purolator PureOne, WIX, NAPA Gold or factory filters. Change the oil filter every time you change the oil.

Mistake: **Not changing air and fuel filters.** These are often neglected, yet changing them is a cheap way to prevent problems. Change the air filter every 30,000 miles and the fuel filter every three years or 50,000 miles, whichever comes first.

David Solomon, certified master auto technician and director, Nutz & Boltz, a consumer automotive membership organization, Box 123, Butler, MD 21023, *www.nutzandboltz.com*.

My favorite: Bosch filters.

Mistake: **Failing to lubricate grease fittings.** Many vehicles—especially light trucks and sport-utility vehicles—have grease fittings on the steering linkage, such as tie rod ends. Ask your mechanic to lubricate these. Failure to do so can cause the part to break. Door hinges need lubricating to prevent springs from snapping and creaking.

Mistake: **Just assuming that the fluid-change intervals in the owner's manual are accurate.** Often, the listed change intervals are unrealistic for the way people drive. *My suggestions…*

• **Coolant/antifreeze.** Two years or 24,000 miles, whichever comes first, for older vehicles with green-colored coolant. And three years or 36,000 miles, whichever comes first, for vehicles with new, long-life coolant.

Best: Bring several gallons of distilled water to your mechanic to mix with the coolant. Otherwise, tap water, which might cause radiator-clogging deposits, will be used.

• **Brake fluid.** Two years or 24,000 miles, whichever comes first, for newer vehicles with antilock brake systems (ABS). Three years or 36,000 miles, whichever comes first, for older vehicles without ABS.

• **Power-steering fluid.** Every three years or 50,000 miles, whichever comes first.

• **Transmission fluid.** For vehicles with automatic transmissions, it should be changed every three years or 36,000 miles, whichever comes first. For those with manual transmissions, every 100,000 miles.

Mistake: **Replacing your spark plugs at 100,000 miles.** The factory often recommends replacing spark plugs every 100,000 miles. This is unrealistic for 90% of today's drivers who drive in stop-and-go traffic or short distances. It leads to premature breakdown of expensive ignition components. A more realistic change interval is 60,000 miles. If your vehicle also has spark plug wires, have them replaced at the same time.

Mistake: **Excessive idling.** When you're at a long stoplight, shift into neutral to reduce engine wear. If you are stopped for more than two minutes, shut off the engine.

Mistake: **Ignoring the timing belt.** Failure to change the timing belt can result in an unexpected breakdown and even catastrophic engine damage. Instead of you paying $300 or more to have the timing belt replaced, the repair bill may be as much as $10,000. When you need to change the timing belt varies. Check your owner's manual.

Mistake: **Not using gasoline additives.** Gasoline does not contain enough deposit-controlling additives. Using high-test gasoline does not help. Put a few ounces of deposit-controlling additive in your gas tank every time you fill up.

My favorite: Redline SI-1 injector and valve detergent.

Mistake: **Driving on underinflated tires.** This drastically shortens a tire's life. Also, for safety, replace tires when the tread is worn halfway down—when about $5/32"$ of it is left. Measuring tools are available in auto-parts stores. Have tires inspected and rotated every year or 10,000 miles, whichever comes first.

Mistake: **Not replacing the battery.** Modern engine compartments are crowded and hot, which takes a toll on the battery. If battery acid boils over, it can result in expensive damage to important electrical components. Replace the battery six months before its warranty is up. Be sure to install a sealed gel-cell battery.

My favorite: Optima.

Mistake: **Failing to protect paint.** Even the paint on new cars needs protection from environmental fallout, such as acid rain, and the sun's harmful UV rays. You should apply a paint-protection product every time you wash your vehicle. Test on a small area first.

Easy to use: Eagle One Wax As-U-Dry.

More from David Solomon…

Tire Blowout Smarts

If a tire blows at high speed, hold the steering wheel firmly and slowly remove your foot from the accelerator. If possible, allow the vehicle to decelerate on its own to less than 30 miles per hour before braking. Look for somewhere to pull off the road safely.

Also from David Solomon...

Even Four-Wheelers Need Winter Tires

Winter tires are still necessary—even for four-wheel-drive vehicles that have all-season tires—in areas that get snow, sleet and freezing rain. All-season tires are a compromise of tire factors, such as dry and wet traction, durability and fuel economy. Winter tires are made with softer rubber that grips well in cold weather and have deep treads to improve traction. Consider buying a set of winter tires and a set of rims for them. Tire prices vary widely. Rims cost anywhere from $40 each for used ones to $280 each for new ones.

Finally from David Solomon...

Tinted Glass Saves on Gas

Coated or tinted glass boosts gas mileage by reducing heat buildup inside the car. Air conditioning does not have to work as hard, so mileage may increase by up to two miles per gallon. Windshield solar glass coatings are available as an option when you buy a new car or can be installed by auto specialty shops. Coated glass has a tinted film applied that is removable. Tinted glass is permanent.

Beware: Windows that are treated to more than 35% opacity are illegal.

Gas-Pump Alert

Static electricity can cause a fire when fueling your car in cold weather. Almost all gas-pump fires caused by static electricity start when someone gets back into the vehicle while pumping gas, then gets out and touches the nozzle. The fire starts when gasoline vapors connect with static charges.

Self-defense: Never get back into the vehicle while gas is pumping. If you do, close the door when you get out and touch the metal at a spot far from the fueling port before going anywhere near the pump.

Also: Don't use your cell phone while pumping gas—the battery also may spark a fire.

Robert N. Renkes, executive vice president at the Petroleum Equipment Institute, which represents manufacturers, installers and sellers of equipment used in service stations, terminals, fuel oil and gasoline delivery, Tulsa, *www.pei.org*.

Don't Delay Fixing Your Windshield

Many people put off repairing small cracks until they spread and the entire windshield has to be replaced. This is dangerous. A minor impact, even a stone hitting your windshield, could cause the crack to spread suddenly while the vehicle is in motion. Most chips or cracks smaller than a dollar bill can be repaired for less than $75—and many insurance companies will waive the deductible, making the repair free.

John Zinno, assistant vice president, glass department, Geico Inc., one of the largest property/casualty insurers in the US, Fredericksburg, VA.

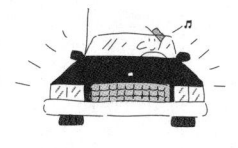

Mold Danger In Your Car

Mold, mildew and fungi in cars can make you sick. Allergens stick to engine grime and are pulled into passenger areas through air intakes. Food particles and pet dander on seats and carpets attract and grow bacteria. Moisture that gets in through weather stripping or window seals can lead to mold growth. And, fungi can grow in the air-conditioning system, producing airborne spores.

Self-defense: Maintain your car well, and keep the inside clean. Keep car windows open

■ *Your Leisure* ■ ■ ■

slightly for 10 minutes after starting the air conditioner, and direct vents away from your face.

Linda B. Ford, MD, certified asthma educator and allergist, The Asthma and Allergy Center, 401 E. Gold Coast Rd., Papillion, NE 68046.

Better Car Repairs

Being charged for unauthorized work is the most common car-repair problem.

Best defense: A written estimate signed by you and the mechanic is a legally enforceable contract. Insist on approving any additional work before it is done. If unauthorized work is done and you must pay to get your car, do so. Then ask your state consumer protection agency to help you get your money back.

Donald Johnson, supervisor of the California Bureau of Automotive Repair's San Jose field office, which monitors repair garages for compliance with state consumer-protection laws.

Avoid Hassles by Going On-Line to Buy a Car

Stephan Wilkinson, automotive editor in Cornwall-on-Hudson, NY, who has test-driven and reviewed cars independently for more than 20 years.

These days, savvy car buyers are using the Internet. They're researching models and prices on-line and actually buying—and selling—cars on-line. The on-line auction house eBay sold more than $3 billion worth of cars in 2002 from its new automotive sales division, eBay Motors.

Car shopping on-line eliminates the need to go from dealer to dealer hunting for the right car at the right price. And shopping on-line can spare you the hassle of haggling over prices.

You can save, on average, between $300 and $400 by researching and/or buying a new car on-line, according to auto industry research firm J.D. Power and Associates.

BEGIN YOUR RESEARCH

One of the most comprehensive directories of automotive resources on the Internet now is Where-Can-I-Buy-A-Car-Online.com (*www.where-can-i-buy-a-car-online.com*). *This Web site lets you conduct the following searches...*

• **I know I need a car,** but I have no idea beyond that.

• **I know what kind of car I want,** but not which cars meet my criteria.

• **I have narrowed my search** down to three or four cars, and I would like to compare them.

• **I know exactly what I want,** but I need to research it fully.

OTHER ON-LINE RESEARCH RESOURCES

• **AutoTrader.com** (*www.autoconnect.com*) helps you to narrow down your choices from hundreds of car models. You'll get a list of vehicles ranked by how closely they fit your criteria and a review of each model.

• **AutoSite** (*http://autosite.com*) lets you research and compare new and used cars—then links to three car-buying sites.

• **CarSmart.com** (*www.carsmart.com*) enables you to select criteria, such as price, safety features and resale value, then presents a list of cars that meet your selections.

Additional helpful sites: AutobyTel.com (*www.autobytel.com*), Car and Driver (*www.caranddriver.com*), CarsDirect.com (*www.carsdirect.com*), Edmunds (*www.edmunds.com*), Kelley Blue Book (*www.kbb.com*), Microsoft's MSN Autos (*http://autos.msn.com*) and Road & Track (*www.roadandtrack.com*).

Important: Read a range of reviews of cars you're focusing on because they vary from site to site. Also look at manufacturers' sites—type in the name of the manufacturer (for example, *www.subaru.com*) or use a search engine to locate the manufacturer's Web site.

If you are considering a used auto, Carfax at *www.carfax.com* can provide you with a complete history of a particular vehicle—ownership transfers, serious accidents in every state and minor accidents in most states. The charge is $19.99* for a single history report and $24.99 for unlimited history reports.

*All prices subject to change.

Car Care

BUYING ON-LINE

There are two kinds of Internet service for car purchasers—dealer referral and direct Internet service.

- **Dealer referral.** Autobytel.com is the major player here. Instead of an immediate price quote, you submit a free, no-obligation purchase request, which is sent to the company's 5,000-plus dealer network.

The Internet manager at a local dealership will usually contact you within one business day, giving up-front pricing and delivery information. If you like what you hear, you visit the dealership to buy the car at the agreed-upon price.

Caution: Each dealership has an exclusive territory so you will get a price for only that dealership. That dealer may not have exactly what you want or be able to provide it within a reasonable time. You may have to try another dealership.

- **Direct Internet service.** With CarsDirect.com, for example, you supply information on the car you want and get an immediate, nonnegotiable price quote—backed up by a guarantee. If, within three days after buying the car, you find a lower price for an identically equipped car, the company will refund the difference between the price you paid and the lower price.

You may be matched with an authorized dealer, depending on where you live. In that case, the price isn't guaranteed and you must negotiate it with the dealer.

If you're buying a used car, CarsDirect.com can put you in touch directly with the seller (a dealership or individual) in your area. Autoby-Tel can also put you in touch with a seller.

Most buyers using a direct Internet service get delivery within a few days. Nearly one-third get their cars within 24 hours.

Strategies for better Internet car buying...

- Shop for more than one price quote.
- Get competing bids from more than one car-buying service.
- Check used-car prices from more than one price service.
- Shop for more than one vehicle—there are usually several comparable competitors.
- Keep your options open. If you don't find the vehicle with the exact features you want, stay flexible.

OTHER ASPECTS OF CAR BUYING

- **Trade-ins.** To trade in your old car, you must go to a dealership, whether you use a dealer referral service or a direct Internet service.

Suggestion: Sell the car yourself—you may be able to get more money than you would on a trade-in.

- **Financing.** Most Internet research and car-buying services have partnered with—or are linked to—on-line finance and insurance companies. *Examples...*

  - E-LOAN (*www.eloan.com*) has annual percentage rates lower than most dealers—as low as 3.79% on a new car for 36 months. You receive loan documents on-line or in the mail that you can use to obtain financing to purchase almost any vehicle from the franchised dealer of your choice.

  - PeopleFirst.com (*www.peoplefirst.com*) is America's largest on-line vehicle lender. It will make an approval decision within 15 minutes (during Pacific Standard Time business hours), overnighting to you a check that's payable to the seller.

- **Insurance.** You can buy insurance on-line at competitive rates. *Examples...*

  - Esurance Inc. (*www.esurance.com*).
  - Progressive Casualty Insurance Co. (*www.progressive.com*).

Shop around by visiting several car insurance company sites that provide rates for a number of companies (both Esurance and Progressive give rates for up to three competitors).

More from Stephan Wilkinson...

Safer Cars

If you are concerned about car rollovers, consider models by Audi, BMW, Mercedes-Benz, Saab, Volvo and Volkswagen. The best European cars have stronger roofs than American and Japanese autos. Don't expect US manufacturers to follow suit—it would cost them hundreds of millions of dollars to make their car roofs stronger.

■ *Your Leisure* ■ ■ ■ ■

New-Car Checklist

Ashly Knapp, CEO, AutoAdvisor.com, a nationwide vehicle-buying and consulting service, Seattle.

Be sure to go through this helpful new-car checklist before you drive away from the dealer…

•**Examine your car carefully** before signing the papers. Inspect it inside and out in daylight. Look for scratches, dents and broken glass.

•**Check the price sticker** on the window to make sure the car has all the features you ordered. Be sure the vehicle identification number matches that listed on the paperwork.

•**Check the equipment list** against your purchase order to be sure the car has everything you want.

•**Read the odometer.** More than 200 miles suggests the car was used as a demonstration model. If it was and has significant mileage, ask for a discount of 1.5%.

•**Ask the salesperson to demonstrate everything.** Climate controls, navigation systems and electronic displays can be complex.

Notice something wrong? Dealers usually can correct most problems right away. Get it right *before* you leave the dealership.

Whiplash Protection

New auto designs protect against whiplash. *Active restraints* move into position when your car is hit from the rear. As your back pushes in toward the seat back, the restraint moves forward and up so it is closer to your head and makes contact at a higher point.

Cars offering this: Buick LeSabre…Nissan Maxima…Saab 9-3 and 9-5.

The *whiplash injury protection system* has a hinge built into the seat. During a rear-end impact, the seat back will make a controlled tilt toward the rear. This, combined with a good head restraint, helps prevent whiplash.

Cars offering this: All new Volvo models.

Stephen Oesch, senior vice president at the Insurance Institute for Highway Safety, 1005 N. Glebe Rd., Arlington, VA 22201, *www.highwaysafety.org*.

Dangerous Backseats

Children riding in the rear seating compartments of compact extended-cab pickups, such as the Toyota Tacoma, are nearly five times more likely to be hurt in a crash than kids riding in other vehicles. Car manufacturers also warn that children under the age of 15 should not ride in side-facing jump seats found in some sport-utility vehicles—they are exempt from certain federal safety standards.

Flaura Koplin Winston, MD, PhD, director, Trauma Link, Children's Hospital of Philadelphia, and leader of a study by Partners for Child Passenger Safety of 71,229 crashes involving 110,423 child occupants, published in *The Journal of the American Medical Association*.

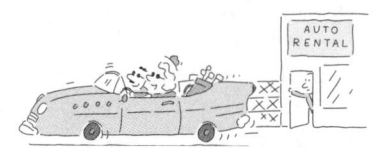

Better Driving with Your Spouse

How to avoid tension when driving with your spouse…

•**Let the more cautious person drive.**

•**If you disagree about something unrelated to safety,** such as parking technique, let it go.

•**Don't let an argument escalate** in the car and distract the driver.

•**If you can't get along when driving together,** drive separately or work out a different transportation arrangement.

Mark Goulston, MD, psychiatrist and senior vice president at Sherwood Partners, a business consulting firm in Los Angeles, *www.shrwood.com*. He is author of *The 6 Secrets of a Lasting Relationship* (Perigee).

Your Leisure

17

Home and Family Life

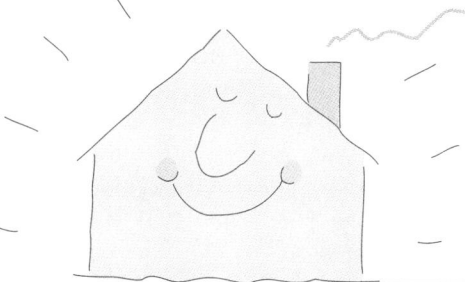

How to Avoid the Biggest Dangers at Home

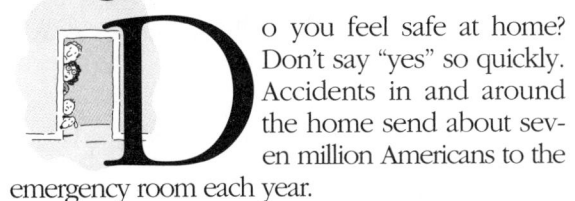

Do you feel safe at home? Don't say "yes" so quickly. Accidents in and around the home send about seven million Americans to the emergency room each year.

Most home injuries can be prevented. *Here, an emergency physician reveals some of the biggest dangers...*

FROZEN FOODS

Cutting any frozen food is risky, but frozen bagels are especially dangerous because they are round and hard to grip. It is easy for the knife to skate off the slick surface into your finger or hand.

A few years ago, a man who had been trying to separate a roll of frozen hamburger patties with a utility knife ended up in the emergency room. He cut his left thumb so seriously that it had to be repaired in the operating room.

To stay safe: Soften frozen foods—breads, meats, etc.—in the microwave before cutting. Knives will be less likely to slip. Never hold something in one hand that you are cutting with the other. Always use a cutting board. If you eat a lot of bagels, buy a holder that keeps them upright while you cut.

PLASTIC PACKAGING

The tough plastic packaging around toys, auto parts and other items often has to be cut open. People tend to grab the first sharp thing handy, such as a kitchen knife or utility blade, and end up cutting themselves.

To stay safe: Examine the package—cut lines are usually clearly marked. Use shears or round-nosed scissors.

ELECTRIC HEDGE CLIPPERS

People sometimes use their free hand to steady the blade and end up getting a finger caught. Or they lose their balance and the

---

Richard O'Brien, MD, spokesman for the American College of Emergency Physicians and an emergency physician at Moses Taylor Hospital, Scranton, PA.

■ *Your Leisure* ■ ■ ■

clippers mangle an arm or leg. These clippers can easily snap a bone.

To stay safe: Put on heavy work gloves... long trousers, in case the blade grazes your leg ...and sturdy shoes, so you don't slip while working. Keep your hands behind the safety guard. Do not overreach—you can lose your balance. Stop working when you are tired—most injuries occur when people are fatigued.

The safest clippers automatically shut off when you release the trigger. Avoid models without this feature.

FLYING DEBRIS

When you're working on your home, it's easy for specks of fiberglass or paint to get in your eyes. Rust, with its razor-sharp edges, is especially dangerous.

In the emergency room, I have had to remove specks of rust from people's corneas with a tiny medical drill. We use topical drops for anesthesia. Eyesight usually is restored if we get out all of the debris and no infection takes over.

Even mowing the lawn and weed whacking fling dangerous debris.

To stay safe: Wear protective goggles. Regular eyeglasses don't provide side protection.

SPLINTERS

They can be painful and easily infected. Splinters in the feet are especially dangerous because there are lots of sweat glands there, which create a warm, moist environment for germs to grow.

To stay safe: Always wear shoes when you are walking in the yard or on wooden decks. Wear gloves when working with wood or in the garden.

Use tweezers to remove splinters that stick out. Don't soak a wood splinter. Wood absorbs water and then swells, making the splinter even harder to remove.

You can soak a metal or glass splinter to clean it, but that generally doesn't aid removal.

Do not try to dig out a deeply embedded splinter with a needle or tweezers. See your doctor instead. It's almost impossible to sterilize the metal properly, making it more likely that the wound will become infected. Applying alcohol afterward doesn't kill germs below the skin.

Also, using an instrument sterilized by a flame can push carbon under the skin, creating a permanent tattoo.

UNDERCOOKED MEAT

Undercooked meats are vulnerable to *E. coli, salmonella* and other pathogens that can cause intense nausea, diarrhea and dehydration. Just a few drops of undercooked meat juice can harbor millions of harmful organisms.

One year, at a local food festival, a chicken dish served by a vendor had salmonella. Dozens of attendees ended up in the hospital.

To stay safe: Marinate meats in the refrigerator. Don't let juices from raw or undercooked meats drip onto plates or salads. Thoroughly wash cutting boards.

Use a thermometer to make sure meats are sufficiently cooked. Hamburger should reach at least 160°F...chicken, 170°F...and steak, 145°F. Don't let meats sit out.

POISON IVY

Exposure to poison ivy, oak and/or sumac can cause a painful, itchy rash. Severe cases may require treatment with oral steroids.

To stay safe: Wash with soap and water right after exposure. Soap breaks down *urushiol,* the oil that causes the allergic reaction. Wash tools, clothes, jewelry, etc. in warm, soapy water. Urushiol retains potency for years. I once saw a fireman with a severe rash on the back of his neck. Over a three-month period, three more firemen came in with the same problem. A rubber coat shared by the men had urushiol on the collar—it had probably gotten there when they were fighting a fire in the woods.

HOUSEHOLD CHEMICALS

The most dangerous are products to clean toilets and unclog drains. Chemicals can splatter or boil if they are used improperly. Even brief exposure can cause serious, disfiguring burns, even blindness.

To stay safe: Read the instructions carefully. Wear goggles, long pants, a long-sleeved shirt and gloves. Never mix chemicals. For example, automatic toilet-bowl cleaners kept in the tank make the water acidic. Adding an alkaline drain opener can trigger a chemical boil and release toxic fumes. Also, never mix bleach and ammonia. It forms a toxic gas that is deadly if inhaled.

If you get splashed with a chemical, rinse the area with running water for 10 to 15 minutes. If there is still stinging or you have a wound or a cough, go to the emergency room. Don't try to neutralize chemical splashes with baking soda —it can worsen chemical burns.

CATS AND DOGS

Even friendly pets can bite when they are startled or encounter strangers. About half the animal-bite cases I see are caused by the victim's own pet. Dog bites are serious—but cat bites are worse because they involve deeper, narrower puncture wounds that seal quickly.

To stay safe: Keep your distance from dogs and cats until you are sure that they are not aggressive. Petting cats can work them up, and make them more likely to bite. A dog wagging its tail is probably friendly—but wagging can also mean a dog is excited or high-strung and more likely to bite.

If you are bitten, wash the area thoroughly. See your physician—he/she may prescribe a course of oral antibiotics.

Allergic to Your Pet?

If you have cat allergies, a diluted version of the animal sedative *acepromazine,* added daily to the cat's fresh water, changes the chemical composition of the cat's saliva. This makes its dander less likely to cause allergic reactions in humans. The highly diluted tranquilizer does not affect the cat's mood or activity level. It usually takes one to three weeks for the drug to take effect, depending on how much the cat drinks. It works for all types of cats.

Cost: About $12/month. Available only from veterinarians.

For dog allergies, some people get relief by washing their pets weekly with Allerpet D, a dry shampoo available at most pet stores. It's good for all breeds.

Cost: From $8.99 to $11.95.

William Lutz, DVM, veterinarian, Whitehouse Animal Hospital, Whitehouse, OH.

Little-Known Pet Danger

A roundworm infection called *toxocariasis,* untreated, can cause blindness. But there could be no early symptoms—or only vague ones, such as eye redness or swelling and fever or cough. The infection appears most often in crawling babies and toddlers, who tend to put fingers and toys in their mouths. The period between infection and vision problems may be months or even years.

Self-defense: Have your pet checked and treated for roundworms regularly...do not let children play in any uncovered sandboxes to which pets and other animals have access... have kids wash hands after playing with pets, on the floor or outdoors.

Robert Baltimore, MD, professor of pediatrics at Yale University School of Medicine, New Haven, CT.

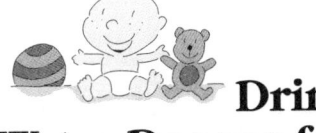

Drinking-Water Danger for Kids

Young children who reside in communities that treat their water with *fluosilicic acid* or *sodium silicofluoride* are significantly more likely to have damaging lead levels than children in communities using sodium fluoride or not fluoridating at all. Increased levels of blood lead can harm intelligence and self-control.

Self-defense: Check with your water authority to see if either of these chemicals is added to the water supply. If so, you can protest this use with the water authority. You may also want to drink bottled water.

■ *Your Leisure* ■ ■ ■ ■

To test for lead: Have your physician perform a head-hair analysis on your child.

Cost: About $49. Check with your health insurer about coverage.

Roger Masters, PhD, research professor, Dartmouth College, Hanover, NH, and president, Foundation for Neuroscience and Society, and Myron Coplan, registered chemical engineer, Natick, MA. Their study of lead concentrations in children was published in *Neurotoxicity*.

Examine the Trees Around Your House

Check the trees around your house annually to determine whether they could fall onto your house. Cut off dead wood, and check for cracks extending through the bark into the tree. Watch for weak branch unions, where similar-sized branches grow so closely together that bark grows between them. The bark may wedge the branches apart.

Also, watch for any signs of decay, such as fungus, crumbly wood and deep cavities...and cankers—parts of stems or branches where the bark is missing. Finally, check a leaning tree for newly exposed roots—it could fall over.

If you find several problems on a single tree, have it professionally inspected and pruned or, if necessary, removed.

Patricia Barnes-Svarney and Thomas Eugene Svarney, science writers, Endwell, NY, and authors of *A Paranoid's Ultimate Survival Guide* (Prometheus).

Mold Warning

Indoor mold can ruin furnishings, damage a building's structure and cause health problems. The problem cost US insurers $1.3 billion in 2001 alone.

Signs: Musty odor...discolored or cottony patches on walls, ceilings or furniture...indoor allergy symptoms.

Treatment: Repair leaks, damp basement, etc.—and clean the mold with diluted bleach (one part bleach to 10 parts water). Extensive or persistent mold problems may require professional removal.

Information: www.cdc.gov/nceh/airpollution/mold/links.htm.

Stephen Redd, MD, chief of air pollution and respiratory health branch, Centers for Disease Control and Prevention, Atlanta.

Mr. Fix-It's Nine Things Every Home Owner Should Know

Lou Manfredini, who has spent over 18 years in the construction business. Mr. Manfredini is a contributor to NBC's *Today* show and "House Smarts" columnist for *USA Weekend* magazine. He is also author of *Mr. Fix-It Introduces You to Your Home* (Ballantine).

Buy a $25 toaster, and you get an owner's manual. But a $300,000 house doesn't come with instructions. It's easy for home owners to let small problems turn into big ones.

Nine "vital signs" every home owner needs to monitor...

FURNACE, CENTRAL AIR-CONDITIONING AND WATER HEATER

Most home owners don't worry until these items stop working. After 15 years, furnaces and central air-conditioning systems are so energy-inefficient they should be replaced. If you spend $1,500 a year on fuel for an old furnace operating at 60% efficiency, a new, 90%-efficient model that costs $3,500 will pay for itself in seven years, based on a $500-a-year savings on fuel. Water heaters should be replaced after seven years.

Cost: Approximately $500 or more, including installation.

ATTIC INSULATION

If you do not have enough, you are wasting money on heating and air-conditioning. Every home's insulation should be rated at least R-30. (R values measure thermal resistance.) That's a minimum of eight inches of standard fiberglass insulation. Homes in the colder regions should have insulation that is rated R-40 or even R-50, a minimum of 12 inches. Take a ruler up to your attic and measure.

Upgrading a typical home from R-15 to R-30 can save hundreds of dollars a year, depending on the cost of heating fuel and the local climate.

Cost: About 80 cents to $2 per square foot, depending on the R value and the construction of your attic space.

ATTIC VENTILATION

On a hot day, hold an outdoor thermometer in the middle of your attic. If it registers more than 20 degrees above the outside temperature, you have a venting problem. Install attic fans or ridge or mushroom vents.

SEPTIC SYSTEM

If your drains have been backing up, the septic tank needs to be pumped. Have this done every three to five years.

Cost: About $200 each time.

Don't put it off, particularly if you are planning a large gathering. Left unattended, the solids in the tank could spill over into your draining system and clog up the leaching field. You might have to spend thousands to replace the system.

Smart: Don't use liquid drain openers to unclog pipes or chlorine bleach in laundry. These can kill bacteria in the tank that break down solid wastes. Use a snake or plunger instead…or call a plumber.

SEWER

If every drain backs up, the main sewer line is probably clogged. A plumber can feed a camera through the line to spot breaks or blockages. Insist on a live view, not a videotape. An unscrupulous plumber might play tapes of other people's broken sewer lines to home owners who have less serious problems.

Cost to repair a sewer line: $500 to $5,000, depending on the problem.

PLUMBING

Some home owners pay dearly for plumbers to solve problems that they very easily could solve themselves…

• **Low flow from a faucet.** This is usually caused by a buildup of sediment inside the faucet's aerator. Just unscrew and wash it off.

• **Loud, banging water pipes.** This indicates that all the air has worked its way out of the system. Most home owners don't realize that water pipes work better when they contain air pockets.

To drain the system: Shut off your main water valve. Open up every faucet, and flush every toilet. Reclose all the faucets. Finally, reopen the main valve. With air back in the system, the banging should stop. If it doesn't, call a plumber.

• **Lead pipes.** Homes built before the 1940s may have lead—not copper—pipes. The word lead scares most people, but *lead* pipes probably don't need to be replaced. Very little lead leaches into running water. Still, you might want to run the tap for three minutes before taking a drink or cooking, to let water that has been in the pipe for several hours flow through.

Also: Store clean water in a bottle in your refrigerator.

If you are still concerned, take a water sample to an independent testing lab.

FOUNDATION

It is natural for concrete to develop hairline cracks as it dries and settles. A problem occurs when these cracks allow water to enter. Moisture could produce mildew in the basement or rot the wooden structure of the home. If unchecked, a crack could expand, endangering the structural integrity of the house.

Examine the foundation walls in your basement. Cracks smaller than one-half inch that are not letting in water probably don't require action. But check them yearly to make sure they aren't growing. For larger cracks, call a foundation specialist. For as little as $500, an epoxy injection can bond to the concrete and prevent a crack from spreading.

If your home has a brick or stone foundation, monitor moisture entering through the mortar, especially after heavy rains. Eventually, perhaps even after several decades, it will be necessary to replace the deteriorating mortar, a procedure known as tuck-pointing. Expect to pay thousands for a large job.

To locate a foundation specialist, ask your real estate agent or home inspector…or try the *Yellow Pages*.

Your Leisure

ROOF

Asphalt shingles, architectural shingles, concrete tile and cedar shingles all can be fine. The real cost of the roof is in the installation.

•**Slate roofs** can last more than 100 years, but they cost 10 times as much as traditional asphalt. Top-quality installation is even more important with slate because slate is so expensive. Don't jump at the lowest bid.

•**Asphalt-shingle roofs** last about 15 years. Many home owners put a layer of shingles on top of an old one instead of replacing the roof. Roofs with multiple layers might have hidden problems, such as leaks and rotted sheathing, in the wood below the shingles. Costs vary depending on size and location, but the difference is small—for example, $2,500 to $3,000 for a new layer, versus $3,000 to $4,500 to strip off the old and start fresh.

Signs a roof should be replaced: Cracked or buckled shingles, shingles blowing off during storms, granule loss from the surface of asphalt shingles, leaks.

To preserve the life of your roof...

•Cut away tree branches that rub against or hang over it.

•Remove moss. It can trap moisture and rot shingles in just a few years. Mix equal parts chlorine bleach and water...spray it on the affected area...and scrub gently with a brush. Do this yourself only if you feel comfortable climbing ladders and working on a roof. Check and repeat every four to five years if necessary.

•Clean gutters once or twice a year, depending on how often they get clogged with leaves. Or install leafless gutters.

Cost: $10 to $20 a foot, versus $4 to $7 a foot for traditional gutters.

ELECTRICAL SYSTEM

Most homes built before the 1950s have inadequate 60-amp service, versus 100 to 200 amps for modern homes. The service rating for your electrical system should be written on a sticker attached to your circuit-breaker box. Expect to pay about $10,000 to update the electrical system in the entire home.

Check the box every few years for rusted circuit breakers. Rust can prevent a circuit from shutting off when overloaded, creating the risk of fire. Call an electrician if you find rust or a breaker that won't budge.

What You Must Know About Chimney Care

Ashley Eldridge, director of education at the Chimney Safety Institute of America, Plainfield, IN. He is a former technical director of the National Chimney Sweep Guild and has 20 years of experience as a chimney sweep.

Neglect your chimney, and a small problem can become a big repair or even a safety hazard. The chimney can become clogged with creosote or develop cracks, both of which may allow carbon monoxide into the house. Creosote can cause chimney fires, which can spread through the house. *To stay safe...*

•**Call in a professional chimney sweep annually.** A chimney should be inspected even if the fireplace is rarely used. In most homes, the furnace or water heater vents into the chimney.

Expect to pay $50 to $150 for a cleaning and inspection, depending on your region and the size and complexity of the chimney. If you have a woodstove in your fireplace, expect to pay about $50 more because the woodstove attachment must be removed and reattached.

The nonprofit group with which I am associated, Chimney Safety Institute of America (800-536-0118 or *www.csia.org*), certifies chimney sweeps.

•**Install a stainless-steel chimney cap.** A cap prevents birds and animals from nesting or becoming trapped in your chimney and creating a dangerous blockage. It also helps keep out water, which can shorten the life of masonry. Stainless steel can last as long as the house, so it is better than galvanized steel, which can rust in just a few years.

Cost: $100 and up.

•**Think about installing a new chimney liner if you replace your furnace.** Home owners will often replace oil-burning furnaces with gas-burning models. If the furnace vents into the chimney, the combination of chemical residues from burning both oil and gas can degrade the masonry significantly in a short time—in some cases, just a few months.

A new liner made of stainless steel or cast-in-place masonry prevents this buildup. An average liner costs around $2,000, depending on the chimney.

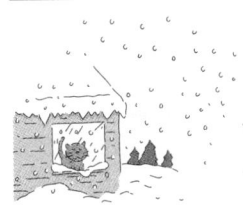

Weatherproof Your Home

Bill Keith, owner of Tri-Star Remodeling in St. John, IN, and host of the *Home Tips Show*. His Web site is *www.billkeith.com*.

Spend just a few dollars and hours now on home maintenance to prevent expensive repairs and save on heating bills.

INDOORS

•**Check window and door seals.** Air leaks mean higher heating bills. Refasten any loose weatherstripping. To replace stripping, purchase a weather-stripping kit.

Cost: Less than $10 per opening.

•**Deep-clean carpets.** When the windows are closed, kicked-up dust will recirculate in the air. Renting a carpet cleaner costs $20 to $30 per day, plus about $10 for cleaning solution.

•**Clean the furnace.** This is important for furnace efficiency—whether it burns oil or gas.

Have your furnace professionally inspected and cleaned every autumn.

Cost: $50 to $100.

Also change the furnace filter two or three times per year (actual frequency depends on the climate in your area). Filters are located before the cold-air return, usually on the side of the furnace. If you're not sure how to do it, ask a technician to show you. Standard filters cost about $1 each.

If you have a humidifier next to your furnace: Make sure the technician changes the pads at the annual inspection. Clean pads improve efficiency and prevent dirty air from circulating.

OUTSIDE

•**Clean gutters.** I get two or three calls a month to replace rotted wood. This problem can be prevented by keeping gutters clean.

If you are uncomfortable standing on a ladder, hire someone.

Cost: $35 to $100 per cleaning.

•**Check your roof every two to three years.** You can pay a roofer to inspect and repair the metal flashings, problem shingles and cracked seals around vents. Or do it yourself with a caulking gun and silicone sealant for less than $10.

If necessary, a professional should replace flashing or shingles.

Remove leaves and sticks from the roof to prevent rot and eventual water leakage.

•**Cover your air conditioner.** Protecting it from the elements in the cold months will extend its life. Covers, sold at hardware stores, are available for window and central-air units.

Cost: About $15 for window units...more for central air-conditioning units.

•**Reseal your asphalt driveway.** Sealant keeps water from seeping into the asphalt, causing it to crack and crumble when water freezes and expands.

Reseal your driveway every two years—more often if it becomes dull gray instead of shiny black. This takes three to four hours.

Cost to hire a professional: $100 to $200 for a standard driveway.

In warmer climates, the sun deteriorates the surface. So even if you reside in a climate that stays above freezing, reseal your driveway every four to five years.

•**Aerate your lawn.** An aerator looks like a push lawn mower with spikes instead of blades. It removes plugs of grass and soil and distributes them on the surface of the lawn, allowing rain to penetrate the ground.

Result: A healthier lawn in the spring.

It only takes about a half-hour to aerate an average lawn. Go in with some neighbors, and rent an aerator for $50 to $80 for eight hours. Or pay a professional to do it.

Cost: $80 to $100.

■ *Your Leisure* ■ ■ ■

•**Trim tree branches and bushes so they don't touch your house or roof.** Wind can cause branches to scratch away paint and/or roofing material, inviting mold and wood rot.

•**At least a dozen other colors now are available,** in addition to the traditional white and brown.

Stephen Elder, home inspector/home repair specialist, Pittsboro, NC.

Arsenic-Free Decks

Prompted by the Environmental Protection Agency, deck makers have discontinued consumer sales of pressure-treated lumber preserved with arsenic. Lumber treated with other preservatives and nonwood alternatives is now on the market.

Examples: Wolmanized Natural Select, treated with copper azole...Preserve and Preserve Plus, treated with alkaline copper quaternary. Ask your deck builder which preservatives are available in your area.

Caution: Even decks built with wood substitutes require pressure-treated lumber for load-bearing areas.

David Deegan, spokesman for the Environmental Protection Agency, Washington, DC.

Buying the Right Roof Gutters

If you're in the market for new roof gutters, keep these tips in mind...

•**Thicker gutters cost more** but are less likely to bend or dent when clogged.

•**Downspouts, or leaders, don't have to be as thick as the gutters** themselves since they don't bear the weight of water.

•**Standard gutters have five-inch channels for water,** but homes with large or steep roof areas would do better with six-inch gutters —though they can cost three times as much.

•**Hidden hangers attached to the building with screws are better** for gutter attachment than nails, which can pull out.

Better Lawn Mowing

For more effective mowing, mow only dry grass and leave grass two-and-a-half inches high so that it shades out weeds and resists drought. Mow in a different direction every other time, and mow diagonally once in a while. Also, keep the mower blade sharp. You can leave clippings on the ground, so the lawn recycles them. Finally, always wear protective footwear and sunglasses or safety goggles.

Zac Reicher, PhD, associate professor and turf grass extension specialist, department of agronomy, Purdue University, West Lafayette, IN.

Keeping Deer Out Of Your Garden

To deter deer, consider using plants that they are not likely to nibble on...

Trees and shrubs: Daphne...dogwood... forsythia...lilac...pine...shadblow.

Perennials: Astilbe...bleeding heart...butterfly weed...fern...foxglove...liatris.

Flowering bulbs: Allium and daffodils.

Deer love most other plants...and if food is scarce, they will eat almost anything, even the plants listed here.

Michael Harvey, director of horticulture at Bartlett Arboretum, Stamford, CT.

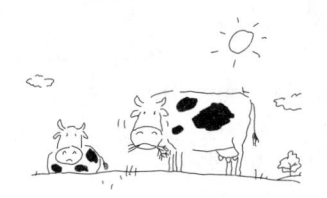

258

Disinfect with Your Microwave

To disinfect sponges, soak in a mixture of water and white vinegar or lemon juice. Then, heat in the microwave on high for one minute. Use an oven mitt to remove the hot sponge from the microwave. To disinfect plastic cutting boards, wash well, rub with the cut side of a lemon, then heat for one minute.

Real Simple, 1721 Avenue of the Americas, New York City 10020.

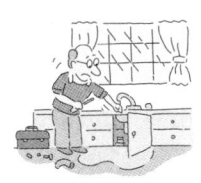

Home Tricks For Do-It-Yourselfers

Some quick tips for do-it-yourselfers from Mrs. Fixit…

• **Wrap a rubber band around a ruler** to mark a measurement you will use several times.

• **Use a quarter to open a can of paint**—just put it in the lip of the can and turn it.

• **Sharpen a dull utility knife** by sliding the blade back and forth against a matchbox strike panel.

• **No rubber mallet?** Cut a slit in an old tennis ball and put it over the head of any hammer you have.

• **Pull a saw through a bar of soap before using it,** to reduce sawdust on the blade.

Terri McGraw, host of the syndicated TV show *Mrs. Fixit Easy Home Repair.* Based in Syracuse, NY, she is author of *Mrs. Fixit Easy Home Repair* (Pocket). Her Web site is www.mrsfixit.com.

Decorating for Next to Nothing

You want your home to look better than it does, but spending thousands of dollars to hire a decorator and buy new furniture is out of the question. What do you do?

Professional room arrangers create a new look using the furniture and accessories you already own. They typically charge $100 per hour…$300 to $500 per room.

We asked 10 interior arrangers to share their favorite decorating tricks…

ARRANGING FURNITURE

• **Find the room's natural focal point.** Most rooms have an architectural feature that draws the eye—often a window or fireplace. Arrange furniture around that feature. If you add an additional focal point, such as a TV, position it near the architectural focal point.

• **Separate "heavy" furniture.** If a room contains a dark armoire and a dark-colored couch, place them on opposite sides of the room. Left together, they can make a space feel unbalanced.

Joanne Hans, A Perfect Placement, an interior-arrangement firm located in Mechanicville, NY, www.aperfectplacement.com.

• **Turn an oversized room into two or more activity areas.** If a room is so large that you can't have a comfortable conversation sitting at opposite ends, turn a corner into its own cozy space with two chairs and a table arranged for private conversation.

Sarah Susanka, Raleigh, NC–based author of *Not So Big Solutions for Your Home* (Taunton). www.notsobighouse.com.

• **Pull the sofa away from the wall.** Then place a table behind it to create depth and interest. The table should be a little shorter than the sofa and 12 inches deep. Because the table will be hidden behind the sofa—and perhaps covered in cloth—even a cheap table will do. Sears and JC Penney have them for about $100. Top them with plants, books and framed photos. If the table isn't hidden, put a basket with a fern underneath.

Gina March, of the St. Louis–based interior rearrangement firm It's Your Stuff! Professional Home Styling, www.itsyourstuff.net.

• **Borrow from the dining room if you don't have enough seating in the living room.** Many dining-room sets come with two armchairs that sit unused. It's perfectly acceptable to put these chairs elsewhere in the house. Borrow from other rooms, too. A

■ *Your Leisure* ■ ■ ■

nightstand can become an end or hall table. A bathroom mirror can be used in the hall.

Wendy Dilda, Real Enhancements in Westlake Village, CA, *www.interiorarrangement.com*.

●**Never position furniture so you have to walk around it to enter a room.** It makes the room uninviting.

Chayse Dacoda, featured designer on TLC's room-makeover series *While You Were Out*. She runs Dacoda Design in Beverly Hills, CA, *www.dacodadesign.com*.

RUGS

●**Put an angled area rug in a small room.** Small rooms can be a decorating challenge because they often leave few options—you might have no choice but to push all of the furniture up against the walls. To add interest, place an area rug at an angle to the dimensions of the room. Area rugs can be placed on wall-to-wall carpeting as well as on wood or tile floors.

Judy Alto, Interior Expressions, LLC, in Annapolis, MD, *www.judyalto.com*.

WINDOWS

●**Buy curtain rods that are up to three feet wider than the windows.** Hang curtains that cover the extra inches on each side. This makes a room look grander. Hang the curtain rod higher than the top of the window—this makes the ceiling appear higher, too.

Chayse Dacoda.

ART AND MIRRORS

Most home owners hang art and mirrors too high. *Better...*

●**Consider the room's function.** In a hallway, hang wall decorations at standing eye height—five to six feet high. In a dining or living room, art should be closer to seated eye level. Art hung over furniture should be only five to 12 inches above the top of the furniture.

●**Place mirrors so they reflect a view or piece of art.** Mirrors often are hung so high that, for people seated, they reflect nothing but the ceiling. (This does not apply to hall and bathroom mirrors, which serve a more utilitarian purpose.)

●**When hanging groups of pictures,** leave the width of four fingers between them. It doesn't matter how many pictures are being hung or their sizes—leave about two-and-a-half inches between them.

Tara Smith, Design Alternatives in Yorktown, VA, *www.designalternatives.net*.

●**Move beyond traditional artwork.** Hang old architectural elements, such as windows or ironwork, or housewares, such as old plates and platters.

Terry Hicks, co-owner of Rearranges and Changes Interiors in Cincinnati, *www.rearrangesandchanges.com*.

●**Don't put small art on large walls.** The art disappears. Groups of small pictures are only slightly better. Put your biggest piece of art on your biggest wall, even if it isn't your favorite.

Lisa Billings, president and cofounder of the Interior Arrangement and Design Association at *www.interiorarrangement.org*, and owner of Lisa Billings's Artful Arrangement in Dallas, *www.lisabillings.com*.

LIGHTING

●**Use three lamps per room (in addition to ceiling lighting).** Three lamps will light most rooms well, yet still be subdued enough for cozy warmth. Arrange lamps in a triangle, not a line.

●**Choose lamps of different sizes.** If you have matching lamps, swap one with a lamp from another room. This will make the room visually more interesting.

Grace Kelly, founder of Grace Kelly Designs in Medford, NJ, *gkellydesigns@fcc.net*.

●**Put can lights in corners.** These cylindrical lights—six to nine inches tall and four to six inches wide—sit on the floor and shine up. Placed in dark corners, they give a room a cozy glow. They're available for as little as $10 at such stores as The Home Depot or Lowe's.

Gina March.

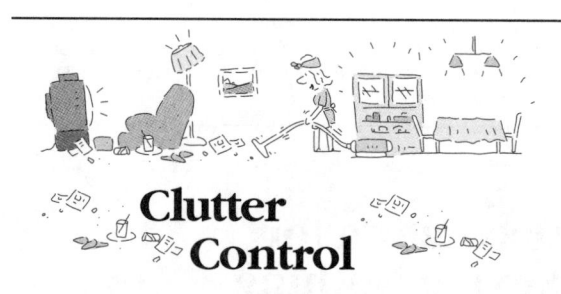

Clutter Control

To minimize clutter that tends to build up around the house...

●**If you collect keepsakes,** keep just *one* that best represents a particular occasion.

Home and Family Life

- **Set a specific goal to encourage you to arrange things.**

  Example: An organized kitchen makes preparing meals easier.

- **Start with a single room.** Finish that area before moving on.

- **Create specific places for things** so they do not wind up all over the place.

  Example: A place where the mail always goes until you sort it.

Lorraine Chalicki, owner, Personal Systems, which helps clients to eliminate clutter and organize work and living spaces, Seattle, *www.youneedme.com*.

How to Make Much More at Your Yard Sale

Cindy Skrzynecki, author of *50 Ways to Make the Most Money Having a Garage Sale* (CMS).

You will make the most money from a yard sale by running it efficiently. *Take a look at the following tips…*

- **Check with your local permit office** about rules for sales and sign placement.

- **Make up signs from brightly colored poster board,** using a thick black marker. Give them the drive-by test for readability.

- **Put signs up the night before** and take them down after the sale ends.

- **To help sell clothing,** have a full-length mirror available.

- **Attract buyers by prominently displaying furniture,** sporting goods, tools and your most colorful items.

- **Keep money in a fanny pack** or carpenter's apron, not a cash box.

- **Price used items at 10% to 25% of retail value** and unused items at no more than 50% of retail.

- **Price in multiples of 25 cents** so change is easy to make.

Strategies for a Smooth Move

Home, 1633 Broadway, New York City 10019.

If you're relocating to a new home, be sure to check out these helpful suggestions for a trouble-free move…

- **Ask the moving company for a *not to exceed estimate,*** which guarantees that the final price won't be greater than the estimate.

- **For easier lifting,** pack heavy items in small boxes, light things in large boxes.

- **Set up all services and utilities in your new home**—including phone, electricity, cable and security systems—before you arrive.

- **File change-of-address forms** with the post office on-line at *www.usps.gov.*

- **Back up all important computer files.**

- **Move irreplaceable items,** such as photos and financial papers, yourself.

- **Take a current phone book** and *Yellow Pages* to your new home in case you need a number in your former town.

- **Unpack everything as soon as possible after arrival,** so you will know if there has been any breakage.

- **Keep the written contract,** called the *bill of lading,* until the move is completed and any claims are settled.

Dramatically Increase The Value of Your Home Without Spending a Lot

Robert Irwin, author of more than 50 books on real estate, including *Improve the Value of Your Home Up to $100,000—50 Surefire Techniques and Strategies* (Wiley). He lives in Westlake Village, CA.

Some of the best value-boosting strategies for your home don't cost a cent—just time and effort. And, if you plan very carefully, you can keep the cost of major improvements to a minimum.

NO-COST IMPROVEMENTS

•**Join a homeowners' association.** The key to real estate value is, of course, location. Buyers target neighborhoods before they zero in on individual homes. You can't change your home's location, but you can try to enhance a buyer's perception of the neighborhood.

If your neighborhood has a homeowners' association, join it. Attend meetings. Speak out in favor of action that will improve the neighborhood—better street lights, more trees, etc. If the association is inactive, help reactivate it.

Emergency fix: If you're selling soon and your neighbor's yard is a mess, ask if you can help to clean it up—mow the lawn, remove debris, plant shrubs, etc. A little friendly help can translate into a higher home price for you.

•**Form a neighborhood action committee.** If there is no homeowners' association where you live, form your own informal group to work for neighborhood improvement.

While a homeowners' association can take legal action to force members to comply with its rules, neighborhood action committees use persuasion to encourage improvements. *Productive strategies...*

•Get a local real estate agent to show the association how similar homes in better-looking neighborhoods sell for more.

•Form a board to decide on a course of action. This may include getting help from charities or government agencies for beautification or similar projects.

•**Work to improve the neighborhood schools.** The quality of the schools is the single most important influence on a neighborhood's home values. Great-looking homes in an area with poor schools won't sell for what they would fetch in an area with better schools.

But good schools cost money and take time to improve. *Action...*

•Vote for bond issues that will upgrade area schools, even if it means tax increases.

•When selling, use good test scores to promote the sale. If scores are low, present them to your homeowners' association as a wake-up call that something needs to be done.

•Attend school board meetings. Consider running for a position on the board.

•**Go after eyesores.** Find out who owns the industrial and commercial properties that have become eyesores. Speak to them about these problems. If necessary, complain to the town planning board, health department, etc.

•**Get city hall on your side.** Go to the planning commission or city council to state your opposition to proposed negative changes in the neighborhood, such as construction of a strip mall.

•**Contact your public works department.** Make sure your city or town knows that roads need to be improved, sidewalks need fixing, streetlights upgraded or streets cleaned.

LOW-COST MAKEOVERS

•**Make over the front of your home.** Curb appeal is critical, so update your front lawn, driveway and entrance. New door accents, such as a new brass knocker, door knob, etc., can cost as little as a few hundred dollars.

•**Improve floors.** Buyers spend a lot of time looking down, so clean wall-to-wall carpeting or replace it.

Cost for new carpeting: $7,500 or more for 2,000 square feet. Inexpensive carpeting, if you're selling right away, can be bought for about $3,000. If you have wood floors refinished, it will cost you $2,000 to $3,000.

•**Repaint the entire interior.** Do this before listing your home for sale.

Cost: About $3,000 for 2,000 square feet. Use light, neutral colors that buyers won't find objectionable.

•**Remove acoustical ceilings made of cellulose fiber.** They depress the home's value. Expose the underlying wallboard and retape and paint it.

Cost: About $2,500 for 2,000 square feet.

Caution: If the ceiling contains asbestos, get asbestos removal experts to handle the job.

Cost: $5,000 and up for 2,000 square feet.

MORE EXPENSIVE PROJECTS

•**Make over your kitchen from top to bottom.** The one room of your home that experts agree will improve your home's value is the kitchen—what you put into it will be returned to you when you sell.

Home and Family Life

A typical makeover includes replacing appliances, cabinets and countertops, putting in new lighting and flooring, and repainting the entire kitchen.

The minimum figure for a complete kitchen makeover is $25,000, but this can vary considerably (depending on your choice of cabinets, fixtures and appliances and whether you make structural changes to the room).

Rule of thumb: Spend no more than 10% of your home's value on a kitchen makeover.

How can you tell if your kitchen needs a makeover? If the kitchen is more than seven years old, it will need—at the very least—a partial makeover because of changing technology and fashion.

Consider adding a trash compactor. Buyers associate them with upscale homes.

- **Do just a partial kitchen makeover.** You can increase your home's value at a fraction of the cost of a complete kitchen makeover by limiting the work to putting in a new kitchen floor and countertops, and refinishing cabinets.

Mixed media is a popular style today, with countertops that combine ceramic tile, Corian and granite.

For floors, consider wood laminates. They cost a fraction of what real wood costs. For existing tile floors, regrouting may be all that is needed—but sometimes you are better off replacing old tile.

Caution: Linoleum is not the way to go for increasing home value.

If wooden cabinets are structurally sound, just refinish the surface. Or simply replace the doors and handles. This can be done for a fraction of the cost of entirely new cabinets. Consider glass doors with fancy handles or doors made of specialty woods.

Cost for refinishing floor, countertops and cabinets: $10,000 to $20,000.

- **Do a bathroom restoration.** Second to a new kitchen, a bathroom makeover improves a home's value the most. But don't sink a lot of money into the project. A basic bathroom restoration may do the trick. Unlike a kitchen, where modernization is key, success in the bathroom is a question of style.

Example: In an older home, consider redoing the bathroom in the style of the time in which the home was built.

Cost: An entirely new bathroom can cost $25,000, depending on the selection of fixtures and the extent of renovation required.

Rule of thumb: Spend no more than 5% of your home's value on a bathroom restoration.

For simple makeovers…

- Replace countertops and flooring with inexpensive tile. *Cost:* $1,000 to $2,000.
- Replace the sink and faucet. *Cost:* $300 to $700 for both.
- Reglaze the tub. *Cost:* $200.
- Retile the shower. *Cost:* $1,500.
- Add new towel racks, repaint and put in new light fixtures. *Cost:* $200.

- **Convert an attic or basement.** Enlarge your home by converting an unused attic or basement into a living space. But be sure the area looks like part of the home.

Cost: $10,000 to $25,000.

Caution: Hire a contractor and an engineer to determine if the project is feasible.

More from Robert Irwin…

Better Condominium Buying

If you're looking to buy a new condominium, keep in mind that the upper floors tend to be quieter and less accessible to intruders. Also, purchase a unit with the best possible view—it will be more pleasant to live there, and reselling will be easier.

If you are concerned about noise: Visit the condo at various times, such as 7 am, dinnertime, on a weekday and during the weekend. Avoid units near the street, a parking lot, laundry rooms or open-air recreation areas.

Open House Trap

Holding an open house to sell your home may help your broker more than you. Only a very small percentage of open houses are successful at attracting a buyer.

■ *Your Leisure* ■ ■ ■

Problem: Many people who attend open houses aren't really interested in buying a home. They show up to learn more about the market, such as if they have a home that *they* want to sell. But every open house attendee is a potential customer for your broker, who will be sure to give his/her business card to all. So be wary of promoting your broker's business at your expense.

Sean McNeill, independent broker at McNeill Real Estate, New York City.

How to Price Your Home for Sale

When pricing your home for sale, price it at just 3% above its fair market value. For example, if you think your home is worth $350,000, put it on the market for $360,500. In today's market, would-be buyers will not look at homes with inflated prices. But a modest price may start a bidding war.

Lisa Linzer, proprietor of L&S Realty, which is located in Stamford, CT.

Compare Available Homes On-Line

DataQuick.com charges $9.95* for a report that includes recent sale prices and offers additional details on a geographic area at extra cost. A total analysis is available only through real estate brokers—on-line versions do not disclose the seller's identity, reason for selling or other information.

Blanche Evans, associate editor of *Realty Times,* a free on-line real estate news service, *http://realtytimes.com,* and author of *Homesurfing.net: The Insider's Guide to Buying and Selling Your Home Using the Internet* (Dearborn).

*Price subject to change.

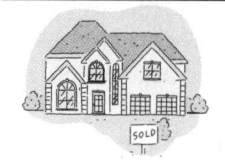

Check Zoning Rules Before Buying

Before purchasing a house, personally check out the zoning rules. A broker or seller may not mention local zoning rules, or say that you can do things with the property that you can't. If you don't find out about the rules until after you make a prohibited improvement, you may be forced to remove it—and incur the out-of-pocket costs involved.

SmartMoney, 250 W. 55 St., New York City 10019.

Midlife Is the Right Time To Improve Your Marriage

Steve Brody, PhD, and Cathy Brody, MS, both psychotherapists in private practice in Cambria, CA. They are authors of *Renew Your Marriage at Midlife: A Guide to Growing Together in Love* (Perigee).

The rocky shoals of midlife can generate stress in your marriage, leading to disharmony, conflict—even divorce.

But the later years can also be a time of renewed bonds and greater understanding—a time when your marriage grows stronger and more intimate, as well as more rewarding than ever before.

STAYING IN BALANCE

Marriage is like a mobile. Each aspect of the relationship is arranged in such a manner that the whole thing hangs together in equilibrium. *Any change in you or your life, including those that come with age, disrupts the balance...*

●**One spouse gets sick,** and the other—the formerly "dependent" one—must assume a stronger role.

●**Your spouse retires,** and you suddenly spend much more time together.

●**Your youngest child goes off to college.** Struggling to keep things the way they were is a losing battle. Instead, you must continually redefine your relationship in order to reach a new equilibrium.

It's a challenge, but also a matchless opportunity to step back and take a closer look at yourselves and what you mean to each other.

Marriages that negotiate such challenges inevitably come out stronger.

ADJUST YOUR EXPECTATIONS

Unrealistic expectations undermine even strong marriages. Movies and songs promote a "happily ever after" fantasy in which love brings perfect harmony…partners understand each other all the time…and every difference is easily overcome.

In the past, you may have been too busy with the demands of an active work and family life to think much about the ideal partner. But now that the kids are gone and you're face to face every evening, you may wonder, *Is this all there is? All there's ever going to be?*

Accept that your partner has limitations—just as you do. But also acknowledge that this is *not* the end of the world. You can be very happy anyway. Cherish what is wonderful in your relationship, and develop other aspects of your life.

HOW TO AVOID CONFLICT

In most marriages, the same circumstances create conflict, over and over again. The key to harmony is spotting these "circuit breakers" and taking care to avoid tripping them. *Use this four-step approach…*

1. Know the trigger. What is it that "pushes your button," and starts a chain of negative thoughts and reactions that inevitably bring on strife?

Common triggers: Your spouse isn't ready on time…complains…is indecisive.

2. Identify your faulty assumption. Are you misinterpreting the triggering event in a way that leads to bad feelings?

Common faulty assumptions: Your partner is doing it out of disregard for your needs …or he/she does not really care about your feelings…or is just being selfish.

3. Analyze the consequences to your relationship. How do your reactions start a cycle that ends in conflict?

Example: You become testy or withdrawn or do something to get even.

4. Substitute a realistic interpretation that will enable you to act differently and preserve harmony. Accept responsibility for your own feelings, rather than attempting to alter your partner's feelings.

Example: One woman loved having a house full of grandchildren at holiday time. Her husband insisted on keeping their visits short. She took this personally, thinking he was trying to impose his will on her. She became irritable and resentful, and arguments ensued.

Then she recognized that her husband was just uncomfortable with the chaos at home. She became more sympathetic, and found ways to see the grandkids more on her own.

HONE COMMUNICATION SKILLS

Understanding one another often means the difference between love and discord. *Make the most of all the time that you have together by working on static-free communication…*

●**Listen well.** When we think we're *listening*—especially to someone we know well—we're often *thinking* instead. We're responding inwardly to the first thing we hear, planning a reply. The other person feels unheard and not understood.

Instead: Focus completely on what the other person is saying. If your mind wanders, bring it back to your partner.

Silence is the key. Agreeing, sympathizing, suggesting how a problem can be solved are all positive responses—but *not* if they come before the other person has said what's on his mind. Wait until there's a natural pause before taking your turn. Otherwise, he'll feel cut off.

Encourage your partner nonverbally—nod…make eye contact. Also, repeat back what you understand him to have said. *Then* respond.

●**Assert yourself smartly.** Each partner needs to know what the other is thinking and feeling. One common mistake is to talk about your partner instead of yourself.

Example: "Why didn't you ask me before making plans? You acted selfishly."

Assertiveness means providing information about yourself in a firm but calm way—"I felt

■ *Your Leisure* ■ ■ ■ ■

hurt when you left me out. I thought you didn't care." This makes it possible for your spouse to give his own information, rather than simply fighting back—"I thought I had told you I was planning to come home late. I'll make sure next time."

It takes courage to admit vulnerability, but it's the basis of real intimacy.

Hope for Unhappy Marriages

Two-thirds of unhappy marriages become at least moderately happy within five years. Of this group, 19% divorce.

Also: Common feelings during unhappy marriages, such as depression and low self-esteem, rarely change after divorce.

Surprising: The unhappiest marriages had the greatest turnarounds, with 78% of people who stayed in marriages they had called "very unhappy" calling themselves "happy" just five years later.

Reasons for the turnaround: Couples talked problems through, often with professional help…"hung on" and outlasted their problems…or gave the marriage less importance in their lives.

Linda Waite, PhD, sociologist, University of Chicago, and leader of a study of 5,232 married adults, prepared for the Institute of American Values, New York City.

"What Did I Just Say?" And Other Things *Not* to Say to Kids

Denis Donovan, MD, medical director, Children's Center for Developmental Psychiatry, St. Petersburg, FL. He is coauthor of *What Did I Just Say!?!* (Owl).

Tired of trying to get your children to behave? *The problem might be simply a matter of miscommunication…*

•**Don't use a question instead of a command.** Parents often question their kids instead of telling them what to do.

•Don't ask "empty" questions—that don't even hint at what you want the child to do. *Example:* A woman who wants her son to stop pushing boxes around in a toy store asks, "Do you want a spanking?" The child keeps pushing. Louder, she asks, "What did I just say?" Still no response. The child does not connect her questions with his actions. She should directly state what she wants her son to do—"Stop pushing those boxes."

•Do not pose negative questions—which invite negative responses. *Example:* When you ask your child, "Can't you clean your room?" he/she is likely to respond with a simple "no." Or he will think, "Sure. But I don't want to." Again, just tell him, "Clean your room."

•Don't end statements with "okay?" or "all right?" Parents who do this may be looking for acknowledgment that the child has heard them—"Put on your boots, okay?"…"We're going to be leaving soon, all right?" But the child thinks he is being asked for his permission. Simply state what you want your child to do—"Put on your boots."

•**Don't speak as "we."** When you use "we," you take part of the responsibility for the very behavior you are trying to influence. Your child hears "we" and will decide that no action is required of him.

Example: "We're going to do better on our homework next time."

Say "you" when you want your child to take responsibility.

•**Don't refer to yourself as "Mommy" or "Daddy."** Parents tend to do this as a way of maintaining a connection with their children. It is easier to say, "Don't talk that way to Daddy" or "Don't pull on Mommy's hair" than it is to admit that your child is not being nice to you.

Children over age two-and-a-half use and understand personal pronouns, such as "I" and "me," and possessives, such as "my" or "mine." You can say, "Do not talk that way to me" or "Do not pull on my hair."

•**Don't depersonalize objectionable behavior by saying "it."** When you use the word "it," you are not specific about what

266

your child did. Describe exactly what bothered you so your child can take responsibility.

Examples: Instead of saying, "It was a terrible day," say, "You misbehaved all day." Instead of "It was one of the most embarrassing experiences I ever had," say, "When you told your teacher to bug off during the parent-teacher conference, I was really embarrassed."

•***Don't explain.*** Some parents will always explain why they are asking children to do something—"Don't run into the street or you'll get hit by a car"…"Stop interrupting. It's rude."

Always giving kids reasons trains them to automatically ignore any command that is not accompanied by an explanation. They will always ask, "Why?" before they listen. Issue the command with no explanation. If your child asks why, reply, "Because I say so." Many parents are surprised to find that children accept this—and listen.

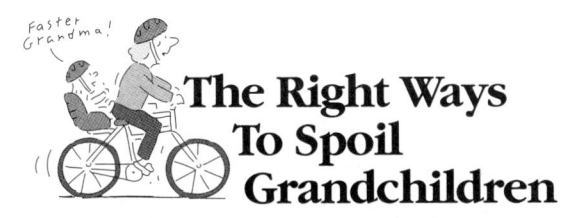

The Right Ways To Spoil Grandchildren

Nancy Samalin, founder and director of Parent Guidance Workshops in New York City, *www.samalin.com*. She is author of several parenting books, including *Loving Without Spoiling: And 100 Other Timeless Tips for Raising Terrific Kids* (McGraw-Hill/Contemporary).

A strong grandchild/grandparent bond can enrich the lives of both generations. It provides a powerful source of unconditional love, but it requires a partnership between grandparents and parents. Their common goal should be to foster a closeness between child and grandparent without putting the parents in an awkward position.

Here are common trouble spots and advice for grandparents and parents…

OVERINDULGENCE

It's natural for grandparents to shower gifts on grandchildren. But this can put parents in a difficult spot if they are trying to cut down on the "gimmes."

Grandparents: **It's fine to spoil grandkids a little bit.** Overdoing it, however, can make parents look like the bad guys. Before bringing expensive gifts, ask the parents.

Parents: **If grandparents overindulge your child, let them know how important they are in his/her life,** but emphasize that affection and attention are more important than gifts. You might say, "You don't have to bring Roger a new toy whenever you visit. What he really loves is going to the playground with you."

RULES

Grandparents and parents should try to follow similar rules. It can be difficult for Mom if she says, "It's time for bed," and Grandpa says, "Oh, just let her stay up for another hour." Similarly, it's hard on Dad if child and grandparent align themselves against him, as happens when Grandma slips the child candy and says, "Don't tell your dad."

Grandparents: **Learn what the parents' rules are, and don't undermine them.** If you would like the parents to make an exception, ask them about it ahead of time.

Example: If bedtime is 9 pm at home, parents could approve a 10 pm bedtime when the child stays overnight at the grandparents' on the weekend.

Parents: **You may want to relax some rules when grandparents are around—**but make it clear to your kids beforehand that these are special occasions.

Example: "When Grandpa visits us this weekend, you won't have to go to bed quite so early." Or, "You may have some special treats you don't usually have."

CRITICISM BETWEEN PARENTS/GRANDPARENTS

In some families, grandparents carry around old criticisms of their child ("You're still so disorganized"), while parents hang on to lifelong views of their parents ("You're too rigid").

Voicing critical remarks in front of children can be harmful, particularly when the discord focuses on how parents raise their children.

Grandparents: **Keep your counsel to a minimum.** Express it in nonblaming terms in private. Don't start out with the phrase, "How can you let her...?" That puts parents on the defensive. Instead, try saying, "What do you think about...?"

***Parents:* Accept that your parents are unlikely to change.** Listen to their advice—it may be helpful. If the criticism seems unwarranted, reply noncommittally, "Thank you for your input. I'll think about it."

CRITICISM OF THE CHILD

It is common for grandparents to voice disapproval of grandchildren's behavior, yet this can damage the bond between them.

***Grandparents:* Times have changed.** Your grandchild undoubtedly talks, dresses and behaves differently than kids did a generation ago. You don't have to lie and say that you like body piercing, but keep your disapproval to yourself. Criticism usually leads to defensiveness and hurt feelings. Focus on your grandchild's positive attributes. Comment on how well Suzie performed in the school play. She will be thrilled.

***Parents:* Remind grandparents in a nonconfrontational way that criticism is detrimental.** "I know you dislike the way Suzie dresses, but it hurts her feelings when you make comments about it. She cares so much what you think of her."

PLAYING FAVORITES

It is impossible to like all grandchildren equally. Some grandparents are more comfortable with girls than boys or enjoy older rather than younger kids. Many grandparents may not realize that they are hurting the less-favored child. The solution can be as simple as becoming aware of the situation.

***Grandparents:* If you notice that you spend more time with one grandchild than another,** find ways to be more attentive to the less favored child. Start out by playing games, going out to dinner or going to a movie alone with that child.

***Parents:* If you notice that grandparents are more attentive to one child,** suggest some simple activities that they might do with the other child. Over time, this relationship may grow or another grandparent may step in to show more attention to that child.

DIFFERENT EXPECTATIONS

Many parents have an image of the ideal grandparent who adores the grandchildren, bakes cookies and always wants to baby-sit. Today's grandparents, however, often have full, active lives of their own.

Both parents and grandparents should try to strengthen the bond between child and grandparent in ways that are comfortable for both.

***Grandparents:* Find some things your grandchildren enjoy that you enjoy too,** and try to interact through those activities. If you live far away, E-mail short notes, stories, jokes or photos. Send audio- or videotapes. Tape yourself reading one of their favorite stories.

Don't assume that your grandchildren don't need you. They want you to be involved.

***Parents:* Find activities that match the grandparents' interests.** If Grandpa favors golf, he might enjoy taking the kids to a miniature golf course. If Grandma loves to read, she could take the kids to the library.

Don't give up if your efforts to strengthen the grandparent/grandchild bond stall. As children grow up, both generations may find more common interests.

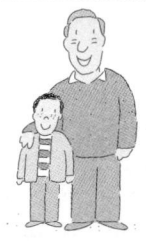

Predict How Tall Your Child Will Grow

To predict how tall your child will grow, find a projected height calculator for children in the health calculators section at WebHealthCentre.com (*www.webhealthcentre.com*). For a calculator designed specifically for children age four or older, check the calculator provided by ParentCenter.com (*www.parentcenter.com*).

Your Leisure

18

Winning Ways

How to Say "NO!" When Others Ask Too Much

Many of us suffer needlessly because our sense of duty toward others leads us to ignore our equally great responsibility to acknowledge our own needs and desires. Sometimes it becomes necessary to say "no" to requests. When we respond "yes" to too many commitments, we become stressed and can harm our own well-being.

If you feel that you may be losing control over the tasks you do out of a sense of duty, ask yourself the following questions about each task…

•**Do you carry out the task cheerfully—**but later feel exploited or angry?

•**Do you do it because you really want to—**or because you feel obligated?

•**Do you spend a lot of time thinking about the task** before and after doing it?

•**Do you dread having to do the task?**

•**Even when you try your best,** do you still get criticized about how you carried out the task?

•**Are you resentful that others do not help with the task?**

If you answered affirmatively to even one of these questions, it's time to sit down with the people you're performing the task for and have a constructive discussion. If this is not possible, decide whether you simply need to make some changes in the way you approach the task or whether you should abandon it.

SET BOUNDARIES

If you are lucky, the people around you appreciate you and are able to communicate

---

Vera Peiffer, analytical hypnotherapist (therapy that identifies emotional problems by hypnotic regression), and principal of The Peiffer Foundation in London, *www.verapeiffer.com*. She gives courses and workshops in England, Germany and Italy, and is author of *How to Say NO When You Feel You Ought to Say YES* (Sterling).

■ *Your Leisure* ■ ■ ■

with you constructively whenever a problem arises. But if they treat you like a child or try to force their opinions on you, be prepared to stand your ground.

When you are at odds with family members, it is important to negotiate a set of rules that satisfy the needs of each person. Have your needs been overlooked? Point that out. You may have to be persistent in the negotiating process, because it is often difficult to change old ways of doing things in a family.

Be on guard to ensure that people do not relapse into their old, familiar behavior patterns.

The amount of control you have over your life is a crucial element in how you look at yourself and others. Acknowledge other people's boundaries by treating them politely and with respect—and expect the same in return.

If you recognize your own wishes, needs and threshold for emotional pain, you will have greater control over your life and will be able to ask for what you want without feelings of guilt.

NEGOTIATING WITH INTEGRITY

Problems seldom go away by themselves. But people often choose passivity and suffering over negotiating a solution—because they believe that asking for what they want will bring conflict. However, once you establish the habit of tackling problems head-on, in a constructive way, it is amazing how much you can achieve.

Negotiating a better deal for yourself can dramatically improve the relationship between you and your negotiating partner—provided that you air your grievance in an appropriate manner and prepare yourself well. *Basics of effective negotiation...*

•**Know what you want.** *Before you begin negotiating, answer three questions...*

•What is the ideal outcome?

•What is a realistic outcome?

•What are the minimum concessions that the other person must give you to make the discussion worthwhile?

•**Don't blame or manipulate.** *No matter how the other person has treated you in the past, or how close you are to him/her...*

•Be composed before you start negotiating. Don't enter negotiations when angry or upset.

•Agree on a convenient time when you can speak in private. Set aside enough time to discuss the matter in full.

•Switch off the radio, TV and any other sources of distraction.

•Express yourself in a firm and clear way.

•Speak only about facts, not opinions.

•Don't blame the other person in an attempt to get him to change his ways. That may cause him to withdraw instead.

•Recognize the other person's feelings to encourage him to show consideration for yours.

•Don't lecture or try to psychoanalyze the other person. Listen to what he says.

THE LAST RESORT

Negotiation is usually the most effective tool to help you escape from the duty trap, but there are some situations when it is unlikely to succeed. These include cases where your negotiating partner has a violent temper...has been known to physically attack others...has threatened you...has a substance-abuse problem...has mental illness...has used past negotiations to belittle or ridicule you...has disregarded past agreements.

In these cases, consider seeking professional counseling and/or ending the relationship.

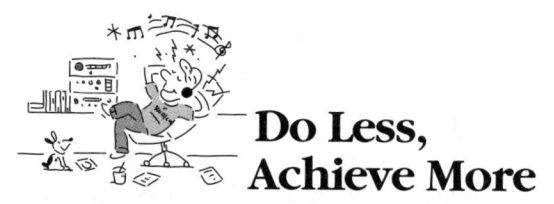

Do Less, Achieve More

Chin-Ning Chu, expert on Asian business psychology and chairperson, Strategic Learning Institute, which provides education on integrating Asian philosophies into Western personal and business practices, Box 2986, Antioch, CA 94531, *www.strategic.org*. Her books include *Do Less, Achieve More* (HarperCollins) and *Thick Face, Black Heart* (Warner).

We all have had the experience at some point. Maybe it's a blind date...or an interview for the position of a lifetime. You psych yourself up and resolve to make an unforgettable impression. But you try so hard that you wind up falling flat on your face.

Why, when a situation seems particularly important, do people so often fail? Psychologists theorize that we sabotage ourselves because we believe we are not worthy of our highest aspirations.

I see it much more simply. When we feel self-conscious, we try to control behaviors that are best left on automatic pilot.

EASE UP

Making an effort and being at ease are *not* polar opposites. They are complementary.

Example: An Olympic runner must put forth a heroic effort to win a medal. At the same time, he/she must "let go" intellectually. If he thinks too much, his stride loses its natural fluidity…and the race is lost.

There is a fine line between persistence and obsession. I know of a talented entrepreneur who couldn't stop selling even after prospective clients indicated they were ready to buy. As a result, he literally talked himself out of deals. When he learned to stop running frantically after success, success came to him.

Sometimes, you just have to let the success happen. It's like water. It won't boil if you don't light the fire. But if you keep taking the lid off to check every 10 seconds, it will take much longer to boil.

FORGET THE CLOCK

For all the hoopla about time management—studies, courses, self-help books—"successful" time management is largely illusory. Instead of thinking of time as an external reality, think of it as internal. How you experience it depends entirely on you. Five minutes spent listening to a boring sales pitch can seem like an eternity…five hours focused on a productive task can seem like five minutes.

Know yourself: If you prefer to think long and hard about each problem that confronts you, it is probably unwise to try to manage several tasks at once.

If you are action-oriented, on the other hand, you will be less effective if you focus on just one task.

Understand how you work best by observing yourself as you perform your tasks. Learn to manage yourself so you use time efficiently.

Delegate whenever it's possible. The biggest time-waster is the belief that no one else can do what you can do. No one is equally talented at every task. Give up the things that someone else can do better—or at least just as well. You even may have to accept slightly lower quality in order to focus on what you do best.

HAVE NO REGRETS

At the end of the day, congratulate yourself for what you accomplished—whatever it was. Do not put yourself down for what you have left undone.

BE RUTHLESS WITH PAPER

Once you touch a piece of paper, act on it …file it…or throw it away. Paper that clutters your desk sends a subconscious message that you're swamped or disorganized.

Larry Wong, the former president of Ford Motor Company of Taiwan, has a foolproof paper-management method. He has three drawers—one labeled *relatively important*…one labeled *less important*…and one labeled *least important*. Every week, any papers remaining in the first drawer are relegated to the second drawer…second-drawer leftovers to the third drawer. Whatever is left in the third drawer gets thrown away.

LOSE YOUR WORST FEAR

Paradoxically, the thing we cling to most fiercely is the thing that limits us the most.

I am talking about *fear*. Until you embrace the possibility of your worst fear coming true, you can't really be free from it.

Helpful: Imagine that you have one year to live. Write a description of what your life would be like. Then write the description of what your life would be like if you carried on with business as usual *without* the constraint of only one more year. Why are the two lists so different? Because one is governed by fear and the other is not.

Review the two lists, and you will understand why so many people who have had a near-death experience report a new willingness to embrace challenges as well as a new sense of freedom and peace.

Fear is not always bad. If you never experience fear, you are probably living too safely, beneath your capacity and avoiding challenges. Do what you have to do in spite of your fear.

If You're a Perfectionist...

Being a perfectionist can be exhausting. *To control perfectionist tendencies...*

•**Realize that you always will have critics** and everyone fails at times.

•**Start every morning by giving yourself permission to be imperfect.**

•**Go easy on criticizing yourself and other people.**

•**Occasionally admit out loud that you were wrong.**

•**Don't take on too much at once.** Set realistic goals.

•**Try to develop optimism**—instead of thinking about what went wrong during the day, think of things that went right.

•**Don't carry grudges.**

Kevin Leman, PhD, psychologist in Tucson, AZ, and author of *The New Birth Order Book* (Fleming H. Revell).

How to Get Much More Done with Much Less Stress

David Allen, president, David Allen Company, management consultants and executive coaches, 1674 McNell Rd., Ojai, CA 93023, www.davidco.com. He is author of *Getting Things Done: The Art of Stress-Free Productivity* (Penguin).

Is it possible to be more relaxed *and* more productive? Absolutely. But first, you have to be organized.

Strategies for greater productivity...

•**Clear the distractions.** If there is something on your mind other than the job at hand, you won't do your best. *When a problem distracts you from your work, it is often for one of three reasons...*

•You have not yet figured out what you want the outcome to be. *Example:* You receive a premium increase notice from your auto-insurance company. Do you want to look for a lower rate? Just pay the extra? Buy a car that would be cheaper to insure? Or ditch the car and take the train to work?

Until you decide what you want to do, the problem will kick around in the back of your mind, taking up precious space—and you won't make any progress. This adds to your stress.

•You haven't decided on your next action. If you want to clear your mind of the problem, plan your next move. *Example:* Perhaps you have decided to find a better insurance rate. Your next action might be to ask a friend where he/she gets his insurance, since you know that person is happy with his rate. Or you might go online to compare quotes.

•You do not have a follow-up plan. Whether you use a simple calendar or a handheld computer, you must have a fail-safe system to remind yourself of what you need to do and when. Otherwise, you are forced to hold all of these responsibilities in your mind, and this can be a major distraction.

•**Manage your in-box efficiently.** Most of us have E-mail, voice mail and papers competing for our attention throughout the day. But few people have an effective plan for controlling it all.

Dilemma: If you try to cope with everything as it rolls in, you will be distracted from other projects. But if things pile up, you might miss important opportunities or have to search to find what you need.

Strategy: Clear the stacks at least once a day. For each item in your in-box or any other "collection bucket," start by asking if it requires action. If the answer is *no,* it belongs in one of three places—the trash...a reference file...or a "tickler" file, which kicks the idea back to you at some point in the future.

If action is required: If you can accomplish the task in less than two minutes, do it immediately—it would take longer than two minutes just to file the item and retrieve it later. If it is a larger task, who should handle it? If it is someone else, pass it on. If it is you, decide on your next action. Then file any backup in the appropriate spot.

Do not get sidetracked by trying to complete tasks that will take longer than two minutes.

Important: *A well-planned filing system...*

- Filing cabinets should be at arm's reach of your swivel chair.
- Cabinets should never become more than three-quarters full. When they get crowded, add more filing cabinets or toss old files.
- Use a simple alphabetical filing system. People who use complicated filing systems, with subsections or categories, tend to lose track of where things should go. Make sure labels are easy to read.

- **Follow the *Natural Planning Model*.** This is a five-step way in which all decisions should be made—decide on a *purpose*...clarify the *vision*...brainstorm *ideas*...organize *the plan*...take *action*.

We all use this process for small decisions without thinking about it.

Example: *Let's say the "project" is dinner with an important contact...*

- Your purpose might be a good meal and an opportunity to network.
- You clarify your vision, perhaps picturing a trendy French café.
- You quickly brainstorm the options. Is it warm enough to eat outdoors? Would we need to dress up? Is the restaurant even open tonight?
- To organize, you decide whether to call the restaurant for reservations first...or ask your dining partner to confirm his interest.
- Finally, you settle on the proper plan and take action.

Unfortunately, it is easy to lose sight of this five-step model on major projects. When things get busy in the workplace, the inclination is to work harder—that is, step five, taking action—rather than start at step one and work through the problem.

When companies hold brainstorming sessions, they are prone to settle on one path too soon, jumping ahead to step four and perhaps missing a better option.

Better brainstorming: Do not judge or critique. Go for quantity, not quality. Consider the options later when you organize the plan.

- **Sort your next action list by context.** Most of us have dozens of items as *next actions*—things we need to do to keep our various projects moving along.

To use your time most effectively, sort your projects into next actions according to where you need to be to get them done.

Categories might include...

- Call list for calls you can make from any telephone.
- Computer list for things you can do only at your computer.
- Home list for jobs around the house.
- Office list for things you must be in the office to do.
- Errands list for tasks that need to be done while you are out and about.
- "With assistant" or "with partner" list for tasks that require you to be in contact with someone else.

- **Establish satellite offices for home and road.** To work effectively at home—for both off-hours office work and personal household responsibilities—you need a designated location. Finding and clearing a space every time you need to get something done is inefficient.

To handle personal business efficiently, one spouse must take the lead on any given job—even if his/her next action is simply "discuss with spouse."

Road work: Organize your briefcase, personal digital assistant, calendar and whatever tools you use so that you can complete a task whenever you have a little spare time—for example, while waiting at the airport or doctor's office. Every idle minute used effectively is one less minute you will need later.

- **Don't let long-term projects languish.** Sometimes, important goals suffer because daily activities keep us occupied.

When big projects remain big projects—and not a series of distinct actions—they can drag on.

Self-defense: Keep the ball rolling on major projects by pinpointing the next section of the major goal and scheduling it—or doing it right away if it takes less than two minutes.

■ *Your Leisure* ■ ■ ■

Example: Lots of executives return from seminars determined to change their corporate cultures—but few ever get around to actually doing anything. Changing a corporate culture is such an abstract idea that the day-to-day concerns of running a business inevitably push it to the back burner.

Although the task itself is complex, the first step is probably simple. Perhaps it is E-mailing an assistant to ask him/her to schedule a meeting.

Bottom line: To get the big projects under way, complete the small things quickly.

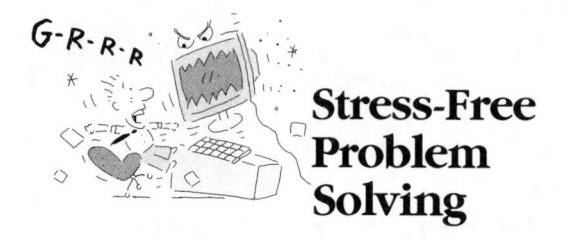

Stress-Free Problem Solving

Overwhelmed by a particular problem—or maybe several? *Try these helpful tips…*

• **Concentrate on one problem at a time.**

• **Define it clearly in writing.**

• **See the problem as an opportunity** for positive change.

• **List all possible causes of the problem.**

• **Identify all conceivable solutions.**

• **Decide which solution is your first priority,** assign responsibility for implementing it and set a deadline for accomplishing it.

C. Norman Shealy, MD, PhD, founder of the American Holistic Medical Association, and author of *90 Days to Stress-Free Living* (HarperCollins).

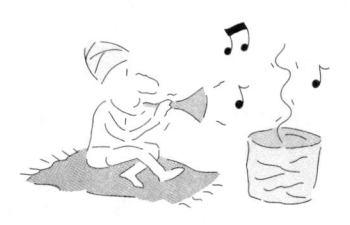

How to Handle Difficult Conversations

Sheila Heen, Esq., coauthor of *Difficult Conversations: How to Discuss What Matters Most* (Penguin). She is a lecturer on negotiation at Harvard Law School and a partner at the Triad Consulting Group, both in Cambridge, MA.

Imagine sitting down to talk to your family about how you plan to finance your retirement years…about the lack of structure and discipline in your grandchildren's lives…about your fears that your elderly parent may harm herself—or someone else—if she continues to drive…about your concerns over the direction your child's career is taking.

Don't *avoid* these and other difficult conversations. Just learn how to have them in a constructive manner.

Begin by identifying your purpose in bringing up the uncomfortable matter. Your goal should be to share your point of view, learn the other person's perspective and brainstorm to reach a resolution.

Beware: If your purpose in initiating the conversation is to change the other person's behavior and/or attitudes simply because you don't like them—or just to vent your feelings without regard for his/hers—keep your concerns to yourself. You are likely to do more harm than good.

THREE MINI-CONVERSATIONS

Every difficult conversation is made up of three underlying mini-conversations. Understanding beforehand how you feel about *each* of these will reduce your dread of uncomfortable discussions and ensure that, when you do have them, they're more productive.

• **The "What Happened?" conversation** is about what has already taken place (or what should take place)—who said what and did what…who is right and who is wrong…and who is to blame.

• **The "Feelings" conversation** is about whose feelings are valid and appropriate, and to what extent feelings can be openly shared.

• **The "Identity" conversation** is an internal monologue that defines what the difficult situation means to you. *Does it mean you are competent or incompetent...good or bad...worthy of love or unlovable?*

The answers you give yourself during the course of this internal debate determine how stable and confident—or anxious and unsure—you feel going into the larger conversation.

A BETTER WAY

After you've thought through the three mini-conversations, approach the discussion as an opportunity to exchange information and learn from—and connect with—the other person involved. *Here's how...*

•**Begin the discussion from the "Third Story."** The third story isn't yours or the other person's. It's the story a keen observer would tell about what's going on—someone with no stake in the discussion at hand.

The third story removes judgment, accusations and blame from the conversation and, instead, describes the problem as a difference of opinion or perception between people.

Example: Your father has just died, and your sibling feels that the will is unfair to her. *Your story:* "If you contest Dad's will, it's going to tear our family apart." *The third story:* "I want to talk about Dad's will. You and I have different ideas about what Dad intended, and what's fair to each of us. I want to understand why you see things the way you do, and share with you my perspective. I also have concerns about what a court fight would mean for our family. I suspect you do, too."

How to lead off with the third story: Say, "My sense is that you and I perceive this situation differently. I'd like to share how I see it and learn more about how you see it."

•**Reframe to move the conversation forward.** "Reframing" means taking the essence of what the other person says and translating it into concepts that are more constructive.

Example: Your spouse has just recovered from a heart attack and the doctor has advised him to lose weight. For what seems like the umpteenth time, the two of you are sitting in a restaurant arguing over what to order, and you're reminding him of what the doctor said. "We're all going to die someday," he says. "I should eat what I like and enjoy myself while I'm alive."

Reframe what he's said this way: "It's true that no one lives forever, and I understand your wanting to take pleasure in your life. However, both of us might live longer and enjoy traveling and spending time with our family if we make healthful eating a priority."

•**Really listen to what the other person is saying.** You can't move the conversation in a positive direction until the other person feels understood.

Example: Your elderly mother refuses to stop driving despite the fact that she has crippling arthritis and has had several fender benders in recent months. She says, "I can't give up my car. How would I get to the bank, the grocery store and the hairdresser?"

When you set aside your concerns that her next accident may harm or kill her—or someone else—and you really listen to what she's saying, you hear that she fears losing her independence. She wants to be able to do exactly what she wants to do when she wants to do it—as she does now.

•**Begin to problem-solve.** Problem-solving consists of gathering information and creating options that meet both sides' primary concerns.

Example: Once you can understand your mother's wish to retain her independence—and you reframe what she's said in that context, so you are both on the same page—you begin problem-solving. Your goal is to find a solution that is both safe and convenient for her.

After ruling out buses (their schedules are too rigid) and taxis (they are too expensive), you decide to contract with a car service she can phone when she wants to go somewhere, and prepay for the first year of service with the proceeds from the sale of her car.

•**Accept that not every difficult conversation will end with everybody happy.** Not every conflict can be resolved. Sometimes you must agree to disagree...or go your separate ways.

Example: You and your spouse are concerned about the lack of discipline in your grandchildren's lives—they seem to get whatever they want.

■ *Your Leisure* ■ ■ ■

Every time you discuss your concerns with your daughter and her husband, they become defensive and tell you that "things are different today than when you were raising children."

As long as your daughter feels defensive, she'll resist *any* advice. Your job is to support her, understand why she's making the choices she's making and offer your view if and when doing so is helpful. But she gets to decide. Accepting that will help both of you enjoy the time you spend together.

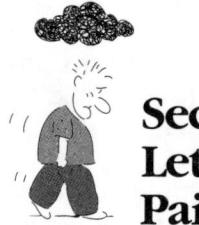

Secrets to Letting Go of Painful Memories

Martin G. Groder, MD, psychiatrist and business consultant in Chapel Hill, NC.

A lover who proved untrue...the parent whose death remains vividly painful even years later...the aspiration that you realize will never come to fruition. Sometimes it seems impossible to say good-bye.

Let go of it...get on with your life. Sound advice, but often impossible to put into practice. Instead, you watch helplessly as your fixation slowly takes over your existence, leaving little room for pleasure or fulfillment.

This is not about normal grief. This is an inability to resume your daily life after a period of normal grief—a year or two.

THE SURVIVAL BRAIN

Undying memories and passions that we can't let go of resemble the compulsive behavior patterns we call addictions. These thoughts recur throughout the day and are often your last before falling asleep.

There is a biological reason for the intensity of the hold these thoughts have on you. The human brain has a special biochemical "circuitry" geared for survival. It is what drives you to eat when you are hungry, quickens your steps toward water when you are thirsty and makes it impossible to hold your breath until you pass out.

A vital circuit, for sure. But the same pathway in the brain can be hooked by alcohol, nicotine or surges of adrenaline. In fact, it can really be hot-wired by *anything* that we have invested with supreme importance. The pining lover who says, "I can't live without her," is simply under the spell of his nervous system's survival mode.

DIAGNOSIS

Before you can cure yourself of this problem, you must be willing to accept the gravity of the condition. Has this memory/obsession taken over your life?

Example I: You wrestle every day with the urge to get in touch with a former lover. Or you simply withdraw, stop trying to connect with other people and spend more and more time alone and depressed.

Example II: It has been more than a year, and you miss a deceased loved one more than ever. Friends and family seem unimportant.

Example III: You always looked forward to retirement. Now that you are retired, however, you don't do much of anything. You used to feel important, active and engaged with a career. Now you feel like a nothing.

CEREMONIES OF RIDDANCE

Rituals play a major role in life passages. We have ceremonies for marking coming of age, marriage and death. These events have great power to move us from one stage of life to the next.

Harness that power to free yourself from painful memories. Design a ritual that acknowledges the importance of what you have lost... and then take steps to act out the process of letting go.

Such a ritual could involve expressing everything that you have to say to a person—out loud, if possible—in a place that has some symbolic importance to you.

Example: A woman had a stormy relationship with her deceased mother. She made an early morning visit to her mother's grave to express her regrets for what didn't happen...

her resentments about things that did happen...and her gratitude for all that her mother had done for her. The woman returned to the grave several times until she felt there was nothing left unsaid.

Important: Determine in advance what you want to say, and also choose with care where you will say it. The better the preparation, the more "cleansing" the ritual.

The rituals of release are especially effective when they involve destroying or burying something that symbolizes the lost person or unrealized dream.

Examples: A man could not stop pining for a woman who had jilted him. He gathered her love letters and a ring she had given him. He went to the beach where they had spent countless hours together and read the letters aloud. Then he burned the letters and threw the ring into the sea.

A retiree who can't let go of his old identity might do the same thing with a cherished letter from the president of his company or a gold watch he received for his years of service.

To be effective, the sacrifice must be real. Ask yourself, *If everything else were taken from me, what is the one precious keepsake related to the loss that I would hold on to?* Then destroy it.

MOVING ON

Before performing the ritual of riddance, give some thought to the new life that awaits you. What activities would you do if you were free? Plan how your reinvigorated self will go back out into the world and recover your life.

Do something to mark the new beginning. Buy a lovely painting or a piece of furniture. Schedule a get-together with friends. Or just open your eyes, and go about your ordinary life with a new zest and a conscious appreciation of all that you have.

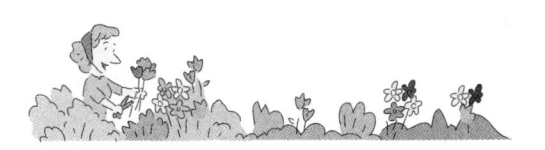

Cures for Common Phobias

Edmund Bourne, MD, therapist in private practice in Kona, HI, who has specialized in anxiety disorders for two decades. He is author of *The Anxiety & Phobia Workbook* (New Harbinger).

Fifteen percent of the adult population suffers from a phobia severe enough that it restricts their behavior.

Fear of public speaking is the most common phobia, followed by fear of flying. Other types include fear of enclosed spaces...public places...fire...heights...water...and social situations, such as dating or using public rest rooms.

Symptoms range from mild anxiety to full-fledged panic, including rapid heartbeat and breathing...lightheadedness...nausea...chills...tingling or numbness...trembling...sweating...and feelings of unreality, detachment, terror or lack of control.

CAUSES

Phobias may have been started by a specific event, often during childhood—a bumpy plane ride might trigger a fear of flying, for example. Phobias sometimes develop over time. If you see enough plane crashes on the evening news, you might develop the fear of air travel even if you have never been afraid to fly before.

Phobias may run in families. Certain ones have a genetic component—a person may be born with the tendency to panic. Other fears are learned.

Example: If a child repeatedly sees that his/her parent is afraid of water, he might develop this phobia as well.

FACE YOUR FEAR...SLOWLY

Exposure therapy is often the best way to curb a phobia. The person with the phobia confronts the fear incrementally with the help of a supportive friend or relative or a therapist. *Let's say you're afraid of elevators...*

•**Step 1.** Stand with a support person in front of an elevator, and watch other people get on and off. To relax, take slow abdominal breaths and focus on reassuring thoughts.

Examples: *I've handled this before... this is an opportunity for me to confront my fears...*or *it's just anxiety—it will pass.*

Keep a list of these affirmations with you to pull out in difficult situations. Your support person should remind you to breathe slowly from the abdomen and focus on your affirmation statements.

•**Step 2.** Once the sight of an elevator no longer causes anxiety, you and your support person might practice stepping on an elevator when it has stopped. When that is no longer anxiety producing, you could then try riding it together for just one floor, then two, etc. until you feel relaxed.

•**Step 3.** Take a ride all by yourself—with the support person waiting where the doors open. When you are comfortable with that, take a ride in the elevator without having your support person nearby.

This entire process could take weeks, months or, in some cases, longer.

Some phobias are harder to address. If you are afraid to fly, you can't beat the phobia just by walking on and off a plane several times. Instead, sit in a quiet room and visualize every aspect of taking a flight. Imagine what you would see, hear, smell and feel. Next, go to the airport and watch planes take off and land. Picture yourself in the plane. Finally, take a flight with a support person.

COPING WITH PANIC

What if a panic attack hits during exposure therapy? Some experts recommend *flooding*—pushing on despite the attack. Flooding works for some people, but in most cases, it just exacerbates the phobia.

I encourage my phobic patients to temporarily retreat. When you think you are about to lose control, pull back, take some abdominal breaths, wait a few minutes until the panic has passed and then try again.

DRUG THERAPY

When phobias are so severe that they significantly affect daily life, taking an antidepressant, such as *fluvoxamine* (Luvox), *paroxetine* (Paxil) or *sertraline* (Zoloft), often can be helpful.

Usually, the patient also meets regularly with a therapist who specializes in anxiety disorders. After 12 to 18 months, about half the people on antidepressants are able to taper off. The other half may need to go back on the medication intermittently or take a lower dose long-term to maintain quality of life.

Another group of drugs known as the beta-blockers, including *propranolol* (Inderal) and *metoprolol* (Lopressor), are helpful for cases of severe performance anxiety. These typically are taken 20 minutes before performing in public to control heart palpitations, shakiness, sweating, blushing and stomach upset. A pianist I treat takes Inderal for the shaky hands she suffers before performances.

Tranquilizers, such as *alprazolam* (Xanax) and *clonazepam* (Klonopin), can be appropriate for phobias that do not need to be confronted very often, such as fear of flying or heights. But tranquilizers can be addictive if taken more than twice a week.

Note: Klonopin is less addictive than Xanax.

DO HERBAL REMEDIES WORK?

Herbs may help control mild to moderate anxiety. But generally, I recommend exposure therapy for that level of anxiety.

If a patient still wants to try herbs, valerian is a mild tranquilizer. But it is important not to exceed the recommended dosage. In rare cases, valerian causes depression or even, paradoxically, anxiety. Check with your doctor before taking valerian.

To find a therapist who specializes in anxiety, contact the Anxiety Disorders Association of America at 240-485-1001 or *www.adaa.org*.

How to Defuse an Angry Confrontation

When anger is directed toward you, consider these actions to defuse it...

•**Acknowledge or agree with at least part of the complaint—**"I can understand why that bothers you."

- **Step back emotionally,** and look at the other person as if he/she were an actor on a TV screen.
- **Take a break if the anger gets too intense** to permit a constructive discussion.
- **Don't accuse with the word "you"**—instead, use "I" to explain your feelings and reactions.
- **Encourage him to give details about his complaint**—"Can you tell me more?"

Rachelle Zukerman, PhD, professor of social welfare, University of California at Los Angeles, and author of Young at Heart: The Mature Woman's Guide to Finding and Keeping Romance *(McGraw-Hill/Contemporary).*

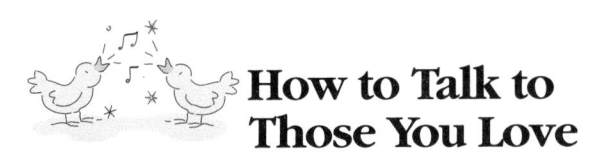

How to Talk to Those You Love

Deborah Tannen, PhD, professor of linguistics, Georgetown University, Washington, DC, and best-selling author. Her most recent book is I Only Say This Because I Love You: Talking to Your Parents, Partners, Sibs, and Kids When You're All Adults *(Ballantine).*

To escape from today's ever more complicated, impersonal and overwhelming world, most of us turn to our families for comfort and a sense of belonging. But, all too often, we find ourselves frustrated instead of comforted by the contact we look for with those closest to us.

When we talk to family members, we sometimes are met with criticism and judgment rather than approval and acceptance. Searching for love, we find disapproval instead.

By studying the ways family members talk to each other, we can understand how these conflicts develop. We can learn how to work things out, rather than continue to work each other over.

MESSAGES AND METAMESSAGES

When we talk to someone, our conversation echoes with meanings from our past experience with each other and with other people. Nowhere is this more true than within the family. We react not only to the meaning of the words spoken (the *message*), but also to what those words say about the relationship (the *metamessage*).

Metamessages are the unstated meanings we glean based on how someone spoke...tone of voice...phrasing...old associations we brought to the conversation. The message communicates *word* meaning, but the metamessage yields *heart* meaning. A crucial step in breaking the gridlock of frustrating conversations is separating messages from metamessages.

Example: Whenever Esther's mother tells her, "I only say this because I love you," Esther knows that the next statement will be a remark about her weight. The message that's delivered is simply an observation about Esther's weight, but each party hears a different metamessage. To Esther's mother, the metamessage is, "I want you to improve because I care about you." But Esther interprets it as, "My mother is criticizing me again."

One of the most powerful ways to improve conversations and the relationships they reflect is to *reframe* the message—to interpret it in a different way.

Example: When her mother makes comments about her weight, Esther can decide to view it as her mother's way of showing caring and trying to help, rather than considering it criticism. Or her mother, realizing the remark will sound like criticism, can decide to refrain from offering such advice.

CONTROL, CONNECTION AND CONSIDERATION

Being part of a family means being closely connected with the other members of the family. When you are close to others, you care what they think, and so you have to act and speak in a way that considers their needs and desires. This controls your actions, which then limits your independence.

The way we talk to each other reflects both of these constant struggles for connection and for control.

Within the family, our close feelings often allow us to relax the rules we apply when dealing with outsiders. This can lead to problems in communication.

Example: Radio talk show host Diane Rehm was with her husband, John, at a meeting when one of the attendees made a good

▪ *Your Leisure* ▪ ▪ ▪ ▪

suggestion. John told Diane, "Write that down." She responded, "I'm not your secretary, but I'll be happy to make a note of it."

When they left the meeting, Diane told John, "You know, I felt that you were talking to me as if I were a secretary."

John replied, "I think you're overly sensitive about that."

Diane, who in reality had been a secretary before they married 40 years earlier, responded: "You're right. I am overly sensitive, and I would appreciate it if you kept that in mind. If you had asked me, 'Would you be kind enough to write that down?' I would have reacted differently."

Later that evening, at their dinner table, Diane stood up and said, "Well, I'm finished."

John said, "You just did the same thing I did to you this afternoon. I'm sensitive to the fact that I wasn't finished with my dinner yet."

Both Diane and John wanted their partner to have sensitivity to the other's feelings and give the same courtesy they would show to a stranger they respected. Because they were able to talk calmly to each other about their feelings, they learned from the experience and resolved to be more careful in the future.

PARENTS AND ADULT CHILDREN

As adults, we feel we should be free from our parents' judgment. At the same time we still crave their approval. Meanwhile, parents often still feel impelled to judge their children's behavior as adults the same way they did when they were young. Having children who grow up well puts a stamp of approval on their performance as parents.

Example: When my father was a young married man, he once visited an older female cousin he did not know well. After a short time, the cousin remarked, "Your mother did a good job," crediting his mother instead of him.

Flip side for parents: If their adult children have problems, parents believe that their life's work of parenting has been a failure and fear that those around them will think the same way. This gives an extra intensity to parents' desire to set their children straight, but it may blind them to the emotional impact their corrections and suggestions have on their children. When parents and their adult children live far apart, as they often do today, their brief visits often turn into replays of childhood or adolescent parent–child relationships.

Common result: Explosive conflict.

How to defuse the adult parent–child conflict: Bite your tongue. An older woman I know enjoys an excellent relationship with her two married-with-children daughters.

Her secret for success: "When my daughters tell me they plan to do something that I think is not a good idea, I don't comment on it unless they ask my advice. And whenever I visit one of my daughters' homes, I behave like a guest."

As a parent, you will always have a special power over your children. Remember to wield it with discretion.

Are Your Good Friends Good for You?

Jan Yager, PhD, Stamford, CT–based sociologist who has studied friendship for 20 years. She is author of three books on friendship, including *When Friendship Hurts: How to Deal with Friends Who Betray, Abandon, or Wound You* (Fireside), *www.whenfriendshiphurts.com.*

We know that good friends enrich our lives in numerous ways. They make the good times better and the bad times bearable. They give us support and keep us connected. They are stress-reducing as well as energizing.

But not all of our friendships are good. We all have had friends who drained our energy, eroded our self-esteem…who have upset, disappointed or betrayed us.

HOW FRIENDS GO BAD

A good friend is honest without being cruel. He/she is reliable—promises are kept, phone calls returned, support offered when you need it. A real friend is empathetic, not judgmental, a good listener and someone you have fun with.

Toxic friends lack some or all of these traits. Why do we make or keep such friendships? For one thing, no one comes into our lives bearing a label that says "promise breaker" or "fault finder." It takes some time for true colors to emerge.

Also, friendship is fluid, and people change. A friend's desire to talk about himself may become overwhelming when he is under stress—or when new responsibilities limit the amount of time and energy you have for listening.

Most people are a mixture of positive and negative. A friend may be so supportive that you are willing to overlook his tendency to break dates.

It is useful to identify potentially harmful traits, though, so you can decide whether to cease a developing friendship, terminate an established one or continue cautiously, taking steps to minimize the harm. *Learn to recognize the common types of negative friendships...*

PROMISE BREAKER

The Promise Breaker cancels get-togethers, doesn't do what he promises and generally lets you down. This trait may surface early or later.

Strategy: If "something comes up" the first three times you plan to meet for lunch or a movie, it's a signal to consider putting your energy elsewhere.

If your friend has enough other virtues that you want to maintain the relationship, make your disappointment clear. You may also need to lower your expectations or have backup plans so you're not always left alone.

COMPETITOR

Competition between friends motivates both to achieve their best. But a friend should celebrate your accomplishments. If your triumphs trigger put-downs or jealousy, it can sabotage your drive to do your best.

Strategy: Consider making this friendship casual rather than close. Be selective in sharing information. You may not want to share your success with him until it has already happened.

INTERLOPER

You expect a friend to be interested in your life, but the interloper takes this too far. For example, he might make phone calls on your behalf without being asked, such as calling an acquaintance at a company at which you have interviewed "to find out how it went."

Such behavior violates boundaries and privacy, undermines your independence and self-esteem and may cause problems in personal or professional relationships.

Strategy: Make it clear to your friend that you don't want his help unless you ask for it. If he persists, you may have to put an end to the friendship.

THERAPIST

He listens sympathetically to your problems. Then he will tell why you acted as you did, explaining the hidden motives of others and offering advice, even if you don't ask for it.

Unless your friend actually is a therapist, his advice may lead you seriously astray, particularly if you are upset and vulnerable. Your friend is also failing to honor your need to simply vent your problems.

Strategy: State bluntly, "Please don't analyze what I'm sharing with you unless I ask you to." Be cautious about confiding experiences.

SELF-ABSORBED

This friend dominates every conversation with talk about himself. When you manage to switch topics, he adeptly switches back. If you start to talk about yourself, he will look at his watch or say that he has to go.

This can eat away at your self-esteem. You end up feeling used and ignored.

Strategy: Many people are not aware that they are self-absorbed. Gently bring to your friend's attention that the give-and-take of most of your conversations is unequal. If he doesn't change and you still want to remain friends, plan activities where the trait will be less annoying, such as playing tennis or going to a movie.

REJECTOR

When you first get to know him, he's supportive. But when you start getting closer, he becomes critical, even hostile. He pulls away and rejects you instead of getting closer. Intimate information starts to be withheld. He cancels get-togethers for no reason. This person usually has a deep fear of intimacy, possibly because he was rejected during his childhood.

Strategy: If you've decided to maintain the friendship, accept that you may never be close unless your friend gets help. If the opportunity

■ *Your Leisure* ■ ■ ■ ■

arises, you could encourage your friend to consider therapy.

DOWNER

When a friend is discouraged or demoralized, you want to be there for him. But if low spirits are continual, you have to think about their effects on you.

Strategy: Make your get-togethers positive—go to see a fun movie or have dinner with a group of friends.

When your friend ruminates about his griefs and grievances, suggest he get it all out and then try to have a good time. Explain that his bad mood brings you down.

If you feel his depression requires expert help, you may be doing him a favor by encouraging him to seek therapy.

DANGEROUS FRIENDS

Avoid a physically or emotionally abusive friend—someone who abuses others or himself with alcohol or drugs, for example.

ENDING A FRIENDSHIP

To end a friendship gracefully, avoid a dramatic confrontation. Wind down the friendship by being "busy" when your friend wants to get together.

Don't bad-mouth the person. Don't do, say or write anything that could come back and haunt you.

If you do discuss your decision to end the friendship, make it very clear that you are not rejecting the friend, just the way in which the two of you interacted.

How to Stay Open-Minded

When you have an immediate negative reaction to something or someone, ask yourself why. Then ask whether the reason is really important.

Example: Having poor table manners does not make someone a bad person.

Also: Boosting your own self-esteem makes it easier to keep an open mind about those who are different from you.

Herbert Fensterheim, PhD, clinical professor of psychology, Joan and Sanford I. Weill Medical College of Cornell University, New York City.

Boost Your Self-Esteem

To feel better about yourself, try practicing these helpful strategies...

• **Raise others' self-esteem** by supporting them and giving them the benefit of the doubt.

• **Ask for help** when you need it.

• **Thank someone who helps you out**—promptly and sincerely.

• **When you notice that someone else could use help,** offer it immediately.

• **Forgive and forget after you are hurt**—then move on with your life.

• **Recognize and apologize for your own mistakes.**

• **Congratulate others on their achievements** and good fortune.

Mark Goulston, MD, psychiatrist and senior vice president at Sherwood Partners, a business consulting firm in Los Angeles, *www.shrwood.com*. He is author of *The 6 Secrets of a Lasting Relationship* (Perigee).

How to Make People Like You in 90 Seconds or Less

Nicholas Boothman, licensed practitioner of neurolinguistic programming, a branch of applied psychology devoted to the improvement of communications skills, *www.nicholasboothman.com*. He first developed an interest in the field when he was a photographer and needed to establish instant rapport with his subjects. Based in Ontario, Canada, he is author of *How to Make People Like You in 90 Seconds or Less* (Workman).

People decide if they like you within two seconds of meeting you. *Here is how to make sure that your first impression is a good one...*

- **Smile.** If you are worried that your smile doesn't look natural, try standing six inches from a mirror and saying the word "great" in funny voices. This will almost certainly make you smile. The next time you meet someone, think *great*. A natural smile will form.

- **Notice eye color.** This ensures that you are meeting the other person's gaze. Poor eye contact suggests you have something to hide. But don't stare—it may make him/her uncomfortable. Oddly enough, occasionally looking down at your hands conveys the impression of active listening.

- **Use "open" body language.** Keep your arms uncrossed and hands unclenched. If you are unsure of what to do with your hands, put them in your back pockets or at your sides.

Point your heart toward the heart of the person you are talking to.

- **Mirror the other person's arm gestures and body language.** People take an instant liking to those who are similar to themselves. If you meet someone who is loud and talks with his hands, be equally loud and use the same gestures. If the person laughs a lot, do the same.

This technique can even defuse a hostile situation. A corporate student of mine was one of three people berated by an important client, the intimidating owner of a large grocery store chain. The bully's other two targets meekly apologized. That only made the client angrier.

My student "matched" the client. Using similar arm gestures and a similarly raised voice, he told the man that he was absolutely right—that they had let him down. Within minutes, the client had his arm around my student's shoulder.

Helpful: After a few moments of matching, change your movements. If the other person follows suit, he feels in sync with you. If not, continue matching movements and try again. If you are dealing with an angry person, gradually lower your voice and open your body language. If you are speaking with someone who seems bored, lean forward and see if he becomes more animated.

- **Ask open-ended questions.** Who, what, where, when, why and how questions are conversation starters. Questions beginning with "Have you...?," "Are you...?" and "Do you...?" are conversation killers. They can be answered with one word—"yes" or "no."

- **Relax.** A Princeton University study found that trying too hard to be liked is a big turnoff in first encounters. Before meeting someone, take a few deep abdominal breaths to relax. When you are nervous, you will take shallow breaths. This makes your voice high-pitched and shaky. Deeper breaths make your voice richer and more confident.

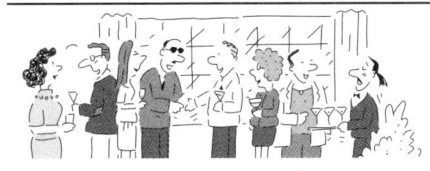

How to Feel More Comfortable at Parties

To overcome shyness at parties, ask people about their interests, work and travels—people love talking about themselves. Compliment them on something they're wearing or a piece of jewelry—or a recent accomplishment if they've just told you of one. If crowds make you uncomfortable, single someone out, talk with him/her for a while, then move around the room together. Also, ask the host or hostess to introduce you to a few people.

Lara Shriftman, partner, Harrison & Shriftman, a public relations, special events and marketing company in New York City.

Rekindle Your Creative Spark at Work and Home

Alan Gregerman, PhD, president and chief innovation officer of the consulting firm Venture Works, 1210 Woodside Pkwy., Silver Spring, MD 20910, www.venture-works.com. He is author of Lessons from the Sandbox: Using the 13 Gifts of Childhood to Rediscover the Keys to Business Success (McGraw-Hill).

As kids, most of us were more creative and enthusiastic than we are as adults. But somewhere, we lost the knack for generating new ideas and getting excited about things. As a result, we miss much of life's magic.

I help organizations to be innovative and passionate about their work. For inspiration, I spent countless hours studying small children. I visited museums, parks, playgrounds, preschools and school gym classes. Whenever I saw youngsters in their "natural habitat," I recorded my observations of their behavior.

I realized that the gifts of childhood are all there for us to rediscover as the keys to success and happiness...

THE GIFT OF WONDER

To kids, almost *everything* is amazing. When small children walk through a park, they are captivated by the big and little things around them. They pick up leaves and branches... investigate tree stumps where worlds of creatures live...and pick up worms and bugs with delight. Other than noticing a colorful flower or the sound of a woodpecker, most adults just walk past a universe of miracles.

To create wonder: Spend 15 minutes a day thinking like a child. Walk around with the eyes of a five-year-old. Note anything with "wonder potential."

Example: I urged executives at a telecommunications company to study insects for clues to improving the effectiveness of their procedures. They were amazed at how ants work together to create networks and move incredible amounts of material.

THE GIFT OF INNOVATION

To adults, everything has a specific purpose. Kids have no preconceived notions and are open to many possibilities. They rarely say, "That's a dumb idea."

To think more imaginatively: Broaden your sense of what is possible. Attend a lecture or seminar on a topic of interest that you know little about. New ideas spark creativity.

Example: An adult with a ball will probably throw or kick it. A child with a ball will throw it, kick it, hide it, balance it on his/her head, sit on it or slip it under his shirt.

Museums are a wonderful laboratory for creating innovation...

- **History museum.** Imagine living in a different civilization. Think about how someone from another era would have resolved a challenge you face now.
- **Art museum.** Look at paintings as a source of inspiration on how to put more energy and enthusiasm into your activities. If you are planning a civic event or a big party, for example, look at paintings of festive occasions from the Renaissance or Impressionist era.

Ask a child to be your museum guide, and let him tell you what is "cool."

THE GIFT OF PLAY

Kids naturally inject play into whatever they do. In fact, their "job" is to play—so at the end of the day, they do not want to stop "working." Not so with adults. Most of us cannot wait for the end of the workweek so we can finally play. We do not realize that we can be more fulfilled and successful by injecting play into our work lives.

To make play part of your routine: Rather than wait for time off, look for ways to have more fun. I urge companies to create playful *innovation rooms,* with toys and floor-to-ceiling dry-erase boards—even sandboxes.

You can start by bringing things into your workplace that inspire laughter and playfulness. During lunchtime, take a walk with your imagination wide open.

THE GIFT OF TRYING

Children see the world as a place filled with new skills to master. If something is worth knowing how to do, such as learning to ride a bike, kids will keep trying until they get it right. For guidance, they study older children and ask for help.

As adults, we often ask ourselves, *Is it easy to do?* We become cautious, reluctant to stretch to our full potential. Too often, we find reasons *not* to do something new—such as learn a foreign language or take up a new sport. We are unwilling or even embarrassed to ask others for some help.

Don't stop trying: Try something new that you would love to master. Let yourself make mistakes. You don't have to be great at something to enjoy it. Provide encouragement to others when they try something new.

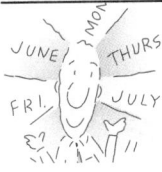

How to Keep Your Mind Sharp at Any Age

Guy McKhann, MD, professor of neurology and neuroscience at Johns Hopkins School of Medicine, and director of the Zanvyl Krieger Mind/Brain Institute at Johns Hopkins, both in Baltimore. He is coauthor, with his wife, Marilyn Albert, PhD, of *Keep Your Brain Young: The Complete Guide to Physical and Emotional Health and Longevity* (Wiley).

Who hasn't had a "senior moment"—when you find yourself groping for the name of an acquaintance—and worry that it may be a sign of mental decline, or even Alzheimer's?

While the majority of healthy older people can have changes in brain and memory function, it doesn't mean you're losing your faculties. *Here are seven ways to keep your brain functioning well...*

ADAPT TO CHANGES

Older people often take longer to learn and also have more trouble remembering, especially when they're tired or under stress.

The good news: Studies show that older people take in and retain new information just as well as those decades younger—provided they take enough time to learn it well. In other words, though older people may think they're forgetting things more easily, the reality is that they are just not learning them as well in the first place.

Names and phone numbers are among the most difficult things to learn and remember because they tend to be entirely arbitrary.

To improve your memory for new pieces of information...

- **Concentrate** completely on the new information as you are taking it in. Reinforce it by repeating it aloud.
- **Write down** key information as you get it.
- **Break up any long lists** of names, numbers or grocery items into chunks of five to seven items.
- **Create a mental picture** of what you're trying to remember.
- **Make associations.** Attach a name with a rhyming word or phrase or action, or join it to a color or important occasion.

Example: If you want to remember to call someone when you get home, imagine that you are inserting your door key into a telephone instead of a lock.

Or try this trick. When meeting new people, mentally link their name to their state and profession—so that John becomes *John the automobile dealer from Colorado.*

This strategy will work because memory is embedded within many different connections in the brain. The more associations you make to new information, the more brain pathways are involved, and the more likely you are to retrieve the information later.

STAY MENTALLY ACTIVE

In one study, our research group selected 1,200 high-performing individuals between the ages of 70 and 80 and tracked them for 10 years. *Those who maintained all of their mental abilities exercised their brains daily in challenging ways, including...*

- **Reading books.**
- **Doing crossword puzzles.**
- **Using a computer.**
- **Playing a musical instrument.**
- **Attending lectures or concerts.**

You can also do specific exercises (dubbed "neurobics") to stimulate your brain. One of the best books on this subject is *Keep Your Brain Alive: 83 Neurobic Exercises* by Lawrence Katz, a noted brain scientist.

MINIMIZE TV TIME

The group whose minds stayed sharpest also spent the least time watching television. Watching TV puts the brain in a passive mode, which is less stimulating than active thinking.

STAY PHYSICALLY ACTIVE

Another common factor among the group who maintained their mental capacity is that they did some physical activity every day—walking a mile, riding a bicycle or stationary bike, swimming laps, lifting light weights at home or walking up and down stairs.

Other research has found that daily exercise helps to sharpen cognitive skills, lift depression

■ *Your Leisure* ■ ■ ■

and ward off changes in memory due to age. Daily exercise has also been linked to lower incidence of dementia and Alzheimer's.

STAY INVOLVED

The final factor common to the people in our study who maintained their mental abilities was a sense of effectiveness. They felt in control of their lives and that they had something to contribute to their family and society.

Supportive relationships provide proven neurological benefits. For example, studies with rats have indicated that an enriched environment, including interaction with other rats, strengthens connections between existing nerve cells in the hippocampus and increases production of new nerve cells.

TAKE VITAMIN E DAILY

Vitamin E is a powerful antioxidant. It mops up "free radicals" formed in the brain by the oxidation process, which otherwise stick to the brain's nerve cells, damaging and even killing them off.

Studies show that taking vitamin E delays the onset of Alzheimer's disease, and may even slow its progression. It also may lower the risk for Parkinson's disease and other types of degenerative ailments.

It's not clear yet whether vitamin E can actually prevent such diseases or how it may benefit healthy people. Studies are now under way on these questions. Despite this uncertainty, I tell my patients to take 800 international units of vitamin E supplements per day. This amount is effective and safe.

CONSIDER OTHER SUPPLEMENTS

There is no strong evidence for the benefits of these substances, but more studies are currently being conducted with each...

•**Vitamin C** is another powerful antioxidant, with similar benefits to vitamin E.

Recommended dose: 300 milligrams.

•**Co-enzyme Q10** helps maintain healthy mitochondria, the small packets of enzymes that produce energy in all cells, including the brain's. It also may prevent or slow the progression of Parkinson's.

•**Ginkgo biloba** seems to have a modest benefit for people with moderate-to-severe Alzheimer's. Because ginkgo thins the blood, it should not be taken with other blood thinners, such as aspirin or *warfarin* (Coumadin), or before undergoing surgery.

Recommended: Talk with your physician before adding any supplement to your diet.

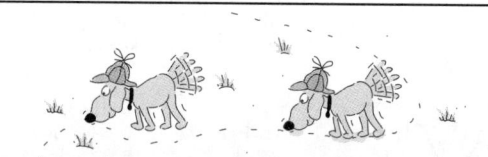

Stop Misplacing Things

Throughout a lifetime, the average American wastes three years searching for lost things. *To keep better track...*

•**Keys.** Install a key hook near the door. Hang up keys as soon as you walk in.

Also: Keep keys on a *large* key ring that's not easily misplaced.

•**Reading glasses.** Attach a strip of Velcro to your glasses case and the corresponding strip to your reading chair or nightstand.

Also: Wear your glasses attached to a chain or cord hung around your neck. When you take them off, hang them on a hook you've installed near your desk or reading chair.

Sherri Brennen, Emmy award–winning broadcaster and author of *Better Living: Tips for Saving Time and Money* (Council Oak Distribution).

More from Sherri Brennen...

How to Keep Track of Kids in Crowds

Keep tabs on children in shopping malls, amusement parks and other crowded areas by dressing everyone in the same bright color.

For toddlers, tie a helium balloon to a belt loop so you can find him/her instantly if he wanders off.

Smart Business Moves

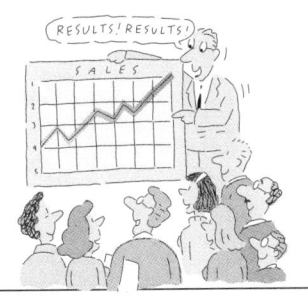

How to Succeed in Business Without Working So Hard

People work much harder than they need to. The average workweek is now 60 hours and getting longer. In some professions, employees are expected to put in 100-hour weeks.

This marathon approach to working creates stress and limits quality of life. It also hinders performance, productivity and creativity.

Working a lot harder is not the only way to achieve your goals and dreams. *Here's how to succeed in business without working so hard...*

SLOW DOWN

One reason people work so hard is because they try to work too fast. When you hurry, you make 25% more mistakes, according to research by Quality College in Atlanta.

Rushing just ruins quality, communication and innovation.

Ask yourself if something *needs* to be done. Many people will try to do things faster and cheaper that shouldn't be done at all.

TRY EASIER

The sports cliché is to give 110%. But this causes people to try too hard, which creates tension and impedes performance. Many successful coaches tell players to give 90%. The best players always seem to perform effortlessly because they're not *over*trying.

In experiments with sales groups, I tell half the group to make as many calls as they can. I tell the other half to make fewer calls than they normally would. Without fail, results from the group that makes fewer calls are at least 20% better. Why? Quality and communication increased when they were not rushed.

Robert J. Kriegel, PhD, expert on human performance and the psychology of change who has coached both Olympic and professional athletes, 16344 Sharon Way, Grass Valley, CA 95949, www.kriegel.com. He has taught at Stanford University's Executive Management Program, was a commentator for National Public Radio's Marketplace and is author of How to Succeed in Business Without Working So Damn Hard (Warner Business).

■ *Your Life* ■ ■ ■ ■

Strategy: Don't go all out. A passionate 90% effort is more productive than a panicked 110%.

TAKE THINKING TIME

Businesspeople have grown accustomed to always being available. Some won't play golf or even go on vacation without a cell phone.

As an athletic coach, I've learned that you can't get maximum efficiency from a muscle without a recovery cycle. The same is true for mental muscles. Without a rest, your brain will fatigue and you'll make more mistakes.

For peak performance, you should take *at least* one 15-minute break from work each day in addition to lunch.

Some people listen to music. Some exercise. The idea is to take a temporary respite from your most pressing work concerns. This doesn't mean goofing off. Downtime often produces many new ideas.

Have a really tough problem? Learn everything you can about the problem. Then stop thinking about it. Focus on something else. When the problem unconsciously pops back into your mind, chances are you will think about it in a new, more creative way.

AVOID THE E-MAIL EPIDEMIC

E-mail is a great communication tool, but it is overused.

•**Don't use E-mail if phoning or talking to someone in person would be better.** Personal meetings or phone calls are more effective for inspiring and motivating. Don't e-mail people who sit nearby. Go see them.

•**Keep it vital.** Limit E-mails to one screen, and stick to critical points. Send the message in the subject line if possible. Don't send jokes.

•**Don't reply unless you absolutely must.** Some people send more E-mails thanking people for their E-mails than they do saying anything of substance.

Also: Don't leave a voice mail to confirm that someone has received your E-mail.

MEET LESS

•**Bring people up to speed before a meeting.** Distribute an agenda and any back-up material in advance—and stick to it during the meeting.

•**Calculate time costs for the meeting.** Is it really worth it? One major firm was holding weekly hour-long teleconferences until management figured out that it was costing the company $1.5 million a month in lost time.

•**Cut the duration and frequency in half.** Remove chairs. If people can't sit, they will leave sooner and get back to the real work.

•**Don't tolerate lateness.** It wastes everyone's time. Lock the conference-room doors. Start on time and charge tardy attendees $1 for every minute they are late. Give the money to charity.

•**Make sure there is a good reason for the meeting.** If not, cancel it.

WORK SMART, NOT HARD

•**Eliminate performance reviews.** People should know on a daily basis how they are doing. The best feedback isn't a piece of paper every three months. It's a pat on the back after they do something right or a word of advice when they haven't. Telling someone what he/she has done wrong months after he's done it doesn't help him do it better.

•**Keep memos, reports, proposals, etc. to one page.** Everyone will appreciate it. If you can't say it on one page, you don't know what you're writing about.

•**If you really want new ideas or to find out what's not working in your organization, ask.** Talk to the people who have been with the company for the least amount of time. Recent hires may have better ideas than longer-term employees about new products, systems and services and about what is not working.

•**Think like a beginner.** Experts tend to rely on yesterday's solutions to solve today's problems. Beginners don't have such preconceived notions. They approach new situations with curiosity and open minds.

•**Restart your business.** Imagine it's your first day on the job. What would you do differently? Question everything.

Example: When Hewlett-Packard tried this on an assembly line in one plant in the early 1990s, the company cut material costs by half, got rid of 90% of its paperwork and reduced labor by 75%.

- **Focus on success.** Fixating on mistakes will shatter confidence. Instead, focus on past successes. This is a great motivator and confidence builder.

Keep a victory log: Jot down a quick line or a few words to evoke a past triumph. Read the log before a big event. This will give you insights into your particular strengths and help you appreciate your potential.

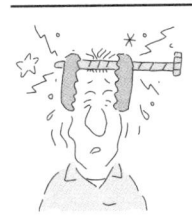

Stress Self-Defense

Stress could become the leading cause of disability within the next 20 years. Stress-related workers' compensation claims are rising dramatically. People stay at home "sick" because of worries about the pace of work and fears of layoffs, workplace violence and, since September 11, 2001, working in high-rise buildings. Our culture believes that every ailment can be treated...and many medications are effective against stress symptoms.

Better: Accept stress as normal, but don't let it rule your life. Take steps to relieve it.

Examples: Exercise, massage, a hobby, deep breathing.

Arnold Brown, chairman of Weiner, Edrich, Brown, Inc., consultants in strategic planning and management of change for businesses and nonprofit organizations, New York City.

Better Hiring

When interviewing, ask candidates how they have handled workplace problems, such as a conflict with a coworker or a difficult boss. Focus on specific projects or transactions, not just the work in general. Listen as the applicant talks about past workplace problems. Does he/she still seem angry or irritated? Does he talk disparagingly about coworkers?

You should also know the stressors inherent in the position for which the candidate is interviewing, and look for someone who has handled these successfully in the past.

Ask the candidate to sign a waiver allowing you to talk to his former employer and waiving any liability as a result of the conversation. Fax it to the reference prior to your conversation. Ask the employer for names of vendors or clients with whom you can talk.

Joni E. Johnston, PsyD, president and CEO of Work-Relationships, Inc., a training and consulting firm that helps companies increase productivity and eliminate unnecessary legal risks, San Diego, *www.workrelationships.com.*

Resolving Personality Conflicts at Work

David J. Lieberman, PhD, behavior therapist in private practice in New York City. He is author of four books, including *Make Peace with Anyone* (St. Martin's).

Sooner or later, everyone has interpersonal conflicts with colleagues. Such rifts can drag on for years. *With the right technique, most can be resolved quickly...*

UNDERSTAND THE CAUSE

Sometimes it's clear why a person doesn't like you or why you don't like him/her. Perhaps you said or did something the other person objected to—or vice versa.

If you have no idea why someone dislikes you, the animosity probably has more to do with him than with you...

- **He thinks you dislike *him*.** It doesn't take much for a person with low self-esteem to jump to this conclusion. In his mind, his dislike is simply reciprocal.

- **He feels threatened by you.** You may be more successful at work or happier at home. He may envy you and imbue you with negative traits to justify his dislike.

- **He sees characteristics in you that he dislikes in himself.**

Example: A stubborn person may react negatively to someone who is close-minded because he recognizes that trait in himself—consciously or not.

MAKE PEACE

No matter what the cause may be, you can resolve the conflict in the same way...

•**Establish respect.** Confide in a mutual friend something that you like about the person who is holding the grudge. Usually, the mutual friend will relay the compliment. This is more effective than a face-to-face compliment, which may seem insincere to someone who dislikes you.

•**Allow the person to do something for you.** It would seem that the way to get someone to like you is for you to do something for him. In truth, it is more effective to let *him* do something for *you*. This gets him invested in you. It allows him to feel better about himself for doing a good deed.

It also makes use of a psychological phenomenon called *cognitive dissonance*. A person feels that he needs to have a favorable impression of someone for whom he has done a favor, or else why would he have done the good deed in the first place?

Best: Try to combine these first two steps. When passing along the compliment, include the request for a favor.

Example: You might say to the mutual friend, "Sally is great in sales meetings. Do you think she would be willing to give me some tips? Would you mind asking her? She may not say yes if I ask." This way, the third party is sure to relay your compliment along with your request.

•**Be self-deprecating.** Most people boast a bit when trying to boost others' opinions of them. This only makes someone with a grudge more annoyed. Self-deprecation is more effective. It shows humility, honesty and trust.

Example: Tell an embarrassing story about yourself and laugh along with others.

DAMAGE CONTROL

When you know you have said or done the wrong thing, it is vital to react quickly to prevent a full-fledged conflict from developing. *To limit the damage...*

•**Depersonalize it.** If the sales staff just heard you yelling at Bob, dilute the insult by dispersing it over a larger group. If you blurted out, "Bob, you really screwed up," follow up with, "We have all been off our games lately," or "There has been too much of this sort of thing from the whole company."

•**Apologize.** Say that you regret blowing up, especially in front of the staff. Don't do this until *after* you have depersonalized the comment. If you jump right to the apology, the impression is that Bob really did blow it, which won't make Bob feel any better.

•**Follow up.** Once the situation has cooled down, speak to the person in private. Apologize again for "losing it." You might add, "I just need a vacation." This places the blame on you.

Get People to Want What You Want

Rick Maurer, organizational consultant, 5653 N. Eighth St., Arlington, VA 22205, www.beyondresistance.com. He consults with such companies as AOL Time Warner, Deloitte Touche Tohmatsu, IBM and Lockheed Martin. He is author of Why Don't You Want What I Want? How to Win Support for Your Ideas Without Hard Sell, Manipulation or Power Plays *(Bard).*

Say you dream up an innovative product or advertising strategy. Or you have devised a better system for paying bills at home. But when you present the idea to your colleagues, boss, spouse—whomever—you are met with resistance.

Here's how to head off opposition, before it gathers steam, by addressing the three types of resistance...

"I DON'T GET IT"

The individual or group simply doesn't understand your idea. Perhaps you used the wrong language. Jargon may work in your department, but to those down the hall, it may sound like you come from another country.

Or your audience lacks the background to understand the concept. When my accountant reviews my retirement plan, my mind wanders. It isn't because I'm not interested. I just don't have the financial background he has.

Signs of resistance: The listener looks confused. He/she has a furrowed brow or vacant stare. He doesn't ask questions or asks questions that are simplistic or have little to do with what you said.

Remedy: Figure out the best way to explain the idea so anyone can grasp it. Put yourself in your listeners' shoes. Think about the background they have and the information they need to understand. Periodically ask if anything needs clarification.

"I DON'T LIKE IT"

This response usually arises out of fear—of change, loss of status, loss of control or that the idea is going to make life more difficult. Instead of listening to you, your audience is listening to the internal message, *How am I going to stop this?*

Signs of resistance: The listener grows quiet...fidgets...looks worried...argues...finds holes in your idea.

Remedy: Try to avoid knee-jerk reactions, such as...

- **Repeating**—explaining the sticking point over and over again.
- **Deal making**—"Lunch is on me if we can move on this."
- **Sidestepping**—"Once we implement this, he will come around."
- **Attacking**—getting angry or belittling the questioner.

Instead, really *listen*. That means listening with a willingness to be influenced, not just to offer a rebuttal. Ask questions and leave time for the other person to respond.

Ask, "Is there some part of this that needs more thought?"..."How does this look to you?"..."If you were going to propose this, how would you present it?"..."What are your concerns about this plan?"

"I DON'T TRUST YOU"

The listener is thinking, *I'm not confident that you can pull off this idea*. Or he doesn't trust you because of what you represent—union or management...a different generation...an outside consultant.

Signs of resistance: The listener shoots down your suggestions but seems to listen when ideas come from someone else...ignores your calls, E-mails and memos...responds sarcastically...harps on previous failures.

Remedy: Demonstrate that you are not what he thinks you are. If the listener thinks you are unreliable, show him that you honor commitments, deadlines and promises. If he thinks you don't have the skill or knowledge to complete a task, prove otherwise.

Example: Your wife doesn't want you to fix the leaky kitchen faucet because the last time you worked on a plumbing project, you flooded the bathroom. Show her exactly what you plan to do, how you plan to do it and the tools you plan to use. Explain your backup plan if Plan A doesn't work.

How to Be a Successful Leader

Oren Harari, PhD, professor of management, Graduate School of Business and Management, University of San Francisco. He is author of *The Leadership Secrets of Colin Powell* (McGraw-Hill) and *Leapfrogging the Competition* (American Century).

Military leader Colin Powell rose from humble beginnings in New York City's impoverished South Bronx. Raised by immigrant Jamaican parents, he went to public schools and attended City College of New York (CCNY), where he joined the Reserve Officer Training Corps (ROTC).

There he began a military career that ultimately led to his appointment as chairman of the Joint Chiefs of Staff under two presidents, George H.W. Bush and Bill Clinton. Of course, he is now secretary of state.

Whether you are a corporate manager, a small-business owner or a PTA president, the "Powell Principles" can help you to achieve excellence...

STATE YOUR MISSION IN A FEW WORDS

In the military, to "close with the enemy" means to identify your opponent, then organize your resources to fight.

■ *Your Life* ■ ■ ■ ■

In more general terms, it means identifying goals, then taking steps to achieve them. Most business or personal goals can be expressed in just a few words.

Examples: *We will reduce production costs by 10% in the next three years...I will pay off my mortgage by the time I'm 55.*

Company executives often spend months composing elaborate mission statements that few employees can understand.

Powell believes the most effective goals are the simplest. He relays the story of Napoleon Bonaparte, who occasionally mingled with the troops and asked the lowest-level soldier to explain the army's overall mission. Bonaparte felt that if the lowest soldier could understand it, the mission was clear.

Once you have a sense of direction, you can select strategies that will help you reach your goals. Without this guiding vision, you are wasting your time.

YOUR MISSION IS MORE IMPORTANT THAN BEING NICE

Powell learned this lesson in college. As company commander of the Pershing Rifles, an ROTC military society at CCNY, he had responsibility for the group performing in a drill competition at an ROTC meet.

As the competition approached, he heard complaints about the student he had selected to lead the trick drill routine. The cadet, a friend, was distracted by relationship problems.

Powell talked to the cadet but didn't relieve him of his command. The Pershing Rifles lost, and Powell realized that his being nice had cost them the medal. As he later said, "An individual's hurt feelings run a distant second to the good of the service."

Achieving your mission might also mean challenging the pros. On a Vietnam War flight, Powell saw unfamiliar terrain from his plane window, but the pilot repeatedly insisted that they were in safe territory. Powell wasn't convinced. He ordered the pilot to turn around. Later, Powell learned that they *had* been over enemy territory.

WORK AROUND THE RULES

This is key for employees of large, bureaucratic organizations.

In 1976, Powell was at the elite National War College (NWC), which trains top officers. He learned that after graduation he would get the plum assignment of commanding the Second Brigade of the 101st Airborne Division at Fort Campbell, KY.

When the brigade commander of the 101st left early, Powell still had two months until graduation. The NWC had a policy of not allowing students to leave before the end of the program. Powell had to choose between turning down the assignment and giving up his degree.

Instead, he developed a solution that satisfied both organizations. He used the NWC's traditional field trip to travel to Fort Campbell. The 101st would not let him assume temporary command while still attached to the NWC, so he arranged *temporary duty at the NWC* and took command of the brigade that way.

TRUST THOSE IN THE TRENCHES

"The people in the field are closest to the problem, closest to the situation. Therefore, that is where real wisdom is," said Powell.

Innovations arise from small laboratories, district divisions and areas where the actual work of a company is accomplished. Your front-line employees should be encouraged to pass along information and recommendations. Powell has said, "The day soldiers stop bringing you their problems is the day you have stopped leading them."

As people rise in the hierarchy, they tend to talk more, listen less and surround themselves with yes-men.

Managers should spend at least half of their time managing people. Most executives don't do this because managing people is messy. They are more comfortable dealing with facts and figures than wrestling with the personality conflicts, egos and underachievers. Executives should emphasize people-oriented tasks, such as recruiting, performance assessments, improving work environments, etc.

MAKE WORK FUN

Powell once told a group of newly appointed US ambassadors to take their jobs seriously—but still have great fun. "The two are not mutually exclusive," he said.

Example: When Powell and Soviet General Mikhail Moiseyev were making a ceremonial tour of a US warship in 1990, they saw a sack of potatoes and some potato peelers in the galley. Powell and Moiseyev laughingly decided to see who could peel a potato faster. Moiseyev won.

TAKE TIME OFF

In Powell's first major speech to State Department personnel, he said, "Do your work, then go home to your families. Unless the mission demands it, I have no intention of being here on Saturday and Sunday."

Six Special Ways to Reward Employees

John Putzier, president of FirStep, Inc., a consulting firm that strategizes with companies to improve workplace performance, One Prospect Place, 223 Oakview Dr., Prospect, PA 16052, www.getweird.net. He is author of Get Weird! 101 Innovative Ways to Make Your Company a Great Place to Work *(Amacom).*

A lack of recognition is the number one cause of employee dissatisfaction. Give creatively to employees, and they will give back productivity, loyalty and team spirit. *Here are low-cost ways to reward employees...*

- **Name it.** If Kelly was drinking coffee while working on a report until 2 am, post a sign on the coffeemaker dedicating it to her. Name the conference room after the employee who scored a big account. Change the names as the people who deserve recognition change.

- **Bribe the spouse.** Show appreciation to the support person behind the star employee. A simple note works. Flowers, wine or dinner is even better.

- **Give discounts.** Macy's employees enjoy discounted store purchases, but how do you give discounts to employees at a plastics factory? If your plastics company sells to a toy manufacturer, ask the manufacturer to give your employees a discount on its merchandise in December. Or if you're buying bulk coffee at discounted prices for the office, buy extra cases that employees can purchase at the same rate.

- **Encourage employees to applaud one another.** One way is to take turns awarding a special coin or trophy at monthly meetings. The reigning champion could make a short speech praising the person that he/she felt contributed the most over the past month and then present the award to the new winner.

- **Create a Wall of Fame** in a public space to showcase employee accomplishments. Display awards employees have won...or simply post a letter from a satisfied customer.

- **Put on a one-minute parade.** To celebrate a star employee, march around his desk wearing newspaper hats and blowing kazoos.

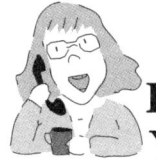

If Asked to Evaluate Your Boss...

Be very careful when evaluating your boss—an increasingly common practice in many companies. Assume that he/she will find out who said what, even if comments are supposed to be kept confidential. Also, give facts—not opinions—and do not repeat hearsay. Only mention things you personally heard or saw. Avoid making recommendations even if asked what the boss could do to improve performance. Most bosses prefer to believe subordinates like and respect them. Anything negative you say could become a problem for you later.

Marilyn Moats Kennedy, editor of Kennedy's Career Strategist, *1150 Wilmette Ave., Wilmette, IL 60091.*

More from Marilyn Moats Kennedy...

Are You a Layoff Candidate?

The most likely layoff candidates are employees who resist new technology or are not interested in upgrading their skills...ones who demonstrate little or no emotional commitment to the company...those disliked by peers and subordinates...and finally, those who made any major mistakes—even many years ago.

■ *Your Life* ■ ■ ■ ■

Make Time for Networking

Even during busy days, take a few minutes to talk to someone who calls. Be encouraging even if you can't help him/her. Refer the caller to other people who can help. Confirm his phone number and E-mail address so you can get back to him—and to show you really want to stay in touch. When unemployment rises, you may get more calls from people wanting help. It is good business to have them think well of you.

Alice Bredin, founder and president, Bredin Business Information Inc., marketing consultants to large corporations, Cambridge, MA.

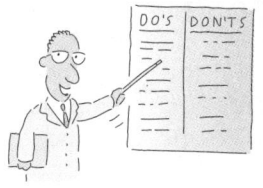

Business Card Dos and Don'ts

When creating business cards, be aware of these dos and don'ts...

•**Do** use a white background, not colored. List a home number only if you have a phone line dedicated to business. Present the card at the end of a conversation, when both parties have an interest in staying in touch.

•**Don't** list an unbusinesslike E-mail address ...have a photo of yourself on the card...mention a degree, unless it is necessary for your specific field.

Helpful: Keep cards in a place that you can reach easily so you never have to search for them in a purse or pocket.

Consensus of career counselors, reported in The Wall Street Journal.

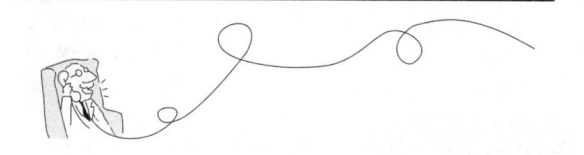

What to Do When Your Computer Screen Freezes

When a computer screen freezes and the cursor won't move...

•**PC users**—hold down the Ctrl, Alt and Delete buttons together to call up Windows *Task Manager*...use arrow keys to find the option that says "not responding"...click on "end task." Reboot.

•**Mac users**—press the Command (Apple), Option and Escape keys simultaneously.

If these strategies fail: Reboot the computer and run repair software, such as *ScanDisk* for PCs or *Disk First Aid* for Macs.

Dana Blankenhorn, Internet consultant and writer at a-clue.com in Atlanta.

Easy Ways to Control E-Mail Overload

Jan Jasper, productivity consultant in New York City, www.janjasper.com. Ms. Jasper is the author of Take Back Your Time: How to Regain Control of Work, Information, and Technology *(Griffin Trade).*

The average office worker sends and receives more than 200 E-mail messages per day.* But there are ways to manage the deluge.

If you're not sure how to set up any of the following timesaving features in your E-mail program, click on "Help."

•**Set up E-mail folders.** Drag and drop messages worth saving into client- or project-specific folders.

Some E-mail programs allow automatic filing through filters that route E-mail from specific senders to the appropriate folders. Do this only if you check the folders daily. Otherwise, you might miss important messages.

•**Don't print out messages.** Printing wastes time and makes information harder to find.

*According to the information-management company Pitney Bowes.

Exceptions: Print out a message if you will need the information outside of the office—for example, travel directions...or if you have hard copy on file on the subject and might overlook a computer file.

•**Use detailed subject headings.** When you send an E-mail, be specific in the subject box—for example, "7/22/02 Market Trends Report." This makes it easier to find important messages. Also, when the recipient clicks on "Reply," related information will be returned under the same heading.

•**Delete E-mail immediately,** unless you wish to save it. Every month, go through your in and out boxes to delete what you can. Purgings will alert you to any messages that require follow-up.

•**Develop custom templates for quick replies**—especially if you repeatedly type the same messages. This function is available in most E-mail programs.

If your E-mail program doesn't allow custom templates, save the text in a word-processing file. Then copy and paste it when necessary.

•**Adopt a smart spam strategy.** Use the "Block Sender" feature when you receive any unwanted E-mail to block additional E-mails from the same source.

In addition, create message rules that route E-mail containing common spam phrases—such as *preapproved, valuable offer* and *100% satisfied*—directly to the trash or a deleted-items folder. Set up the program so the trash is automatically emptied daily.

Caution: Do *not* respond to the spam message, *To be removed from this list, respond to this E-mail address.* This simply confirms that your E-mail address is active. Those who reply often receive even more spam.

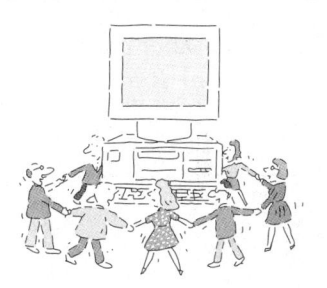

Customer Service Via E-mail

Mike Johnson, journalist and business owner, Cody, WY, *www.mikeleejohnson.com,* and author of *101 Ways to Provide Exceptional Customer Service Today* (available from the author).

When using E-mail for customer service purposes, be sure to follow this helpful advice...

•**Answer quickly**—customers using E-mail expect a prompt response, usually within the same business day.

•**Use the "Reply" key** in your E-mail program so that the customer's note is part of your response.

•**Avoid slang,** jargon and anything else that could be considered insulting, such as writing in all capital letters.

•**Don't send attachments**—not everyone can open them, and some users are afraid to open them because of the threat of viruses. Instead, paste the contents of the attachment directly into the body of the E-mail.

•**Treat E-mail as you would paper documents**—assume it will be kept somewhere indefinitely.

How to Win a Business Award

Business awards attract media attention and raise your profile. *Here's how to increase your chances of winning...*

•**Inquire about awards and nominations** through your local chamber of commerce and trade groups.

•**Complete applications for awards carefully.** Profile your business...describe major challenges you have faced and overcome...explain your solutions.

•**Submit your entries well in advance of the deadline.**

■ *Your Life* ■ ■ ■ ■

•**When you win**—and even when you are just nominated—write press releases about the awards and send them to local media.

Debbie Allen, Scottsdale, AZ, marketing expert and author of Confessions of Shameless Self Promoters *(Success Showcase). www.academyofmarketing.net.*

Seven Steps to Increase Business In Tough Times

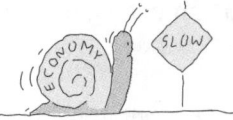

Paul Lemberg, director, Stratamax Research Institute, an executive coaching and consulting firm for entrepreneurs, Box 676173, Rancho Santa Fe, CA 92067, www.lemberg.com. He is author of Faster Than the Speed of Change *(Akiba).*

When sales are slower, it doesn't mean that you have to slow down the business or settle for diminished returns. Any economic downturn is a wake-up call for you to look for new opportunities.

Seven steps to improving business and getting ahead in slow times...

RESHAPE YOUR VISION

Redefine your original business vision and start projects so dynamic that you'll be eager to get to work each morning. Take a few days off, and ponder the direction you want to follow. Recognize that you will have to work smarter and possibly harder.

ANALYZE NEW MARKET CONDITIONS

Which parts of the market are most profitable? How large are these parts, and who is there already?

Say you're a CPA. Your hectic tax season is over, but clients are worried about the shrunken value of their investment portfolios. Maybe they would pay for some sound retirement planning help. Pretend that you're one of those clients. What services would you need? Better yet, interview some of your clients to discover any new and pressing needs. Then incorporate those solutions into your service.

BE MORE EFFICIENT

Tighten standards in your existing business. Make quick assessments of who is likely to buy, and don't waste time on those who probably won't. Redirect that time and energy to growth projects.

SET NEW GOALS

What do you want from the business? If you're a carpenter, perhaps you want to grow tenfold over the next five years and focus on the booming home-improvement market instead of seasonal construction. If so, concentrate on getting those types of jobs and gradually hiring your crew.

Or perhaps you want to go it alone in cabinetmaking and increase your profit margin—finding a niche where you can charge 30% more—and do it with less overhead and a smaller staff.

SET ACTION GOALS

What will you do every week to achieve results—15 cold calls to prospective clients...a mailing to past customers...handing out 25 business cards...sending 200 copies of a press release and making five follow-up calls a day to recipients?

CREATE A MEASUREMENT SYSTEM

This will allow you to see if you are meeting your action goals.

Example: I like to use a graph that contrasts my goals with my results—for example, planned phone calls against actual calls made. By doing this, I can see whether I am above or below my planned target and can make continuous adjustments.

REVIEW

After six months or a year of following your plan, step back and take a fresh look. Is it working? Are you having fun? You may want to focus on the part of the business that you enjoy and taper off other parts.

The real bottom line: Find the balance that will produce the income you want with the effort you want to invest.

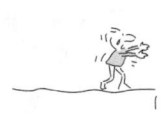

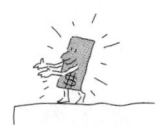

How to Create a Simple Web Site to Boost Your Business

Larry Chase, New York City–based publisher of the *Web Digest for Marketers,* a free E-mail newsletter that reviews marketing-oriented Web sites, *www.wdfm.com*. He is coauthor of *Essential Business Tactics for the Net* (Wiley).

It's not too late to put your business on the Web. Virtually any size company can create a simple Web site. I know a massage therapist who brings in three or four clients a week with hers.

GETTING STARTED

Your site needn't be fancy. One that functions as a digital business card can boost business profits and generate sales.

• **Get a domain name from a Web hosting company.** The least expensive options ($35 or less) are available from the company you already use for Internet service, whether it is a dial-up or a broadband account from your local cable-TV or phone company. In most cases, the hosting company will keep your site's content on its central computer as part of your monthly service arrangement.

• **Design your site.** You probably already have the software. For example, some versions of *Microsoft Office* include *Front Page* Web-design software. Using this is almost as simple as creating and managing *Microsoft Word* document files. The software shows you how to post your site on the Web and create a "mail-to" tag so customers can e-mail you.

• **Post only three or four pages at first.** See how many hits or sales the site generates before adding to it.

• **Go light on the photos and graphics.** Designers want to load up sites with bells and whistles. They make for nice pages in their portfolios but can interfere with your message and slow its display.

USING PROFESSIONALS

To find a Web designer, get referrals or search for "Web designer" at *www.google.com*. Check the candidate's references and previous work. Have him/her handle everything, from creation to uploading the site to the Web.

Cost: Between $200 and $300 for a no-frills site. Elaborate sites can cost thousands of dollars or more.

Making the Most of Fringe Benefits

Edward Mendlowitz, CPA, partner, Mendlowitz Weitsen, LLP, CPAs, K2 Brier Hill Ct., East Brunswick, NJ 08816.

A fat paycheck isn't the only way to take money out of your company and it's not always the most sensible tax-wise. Fringe benefits often accomplish more in the way of tax savings. *Review these possibilities with your tax adviser...*

FOR COMPANY OWNERS

Loophole: **Have your company buy a hefty group term life insurance policy on your life.** The premiums will be fully deductible by the company as long as the plan coverage does not discriminate against lower-income employees. Through a quirk in the tax law, this strategy creates tax savings for you.

How it works: Say your company pays the premium on a $1 million insurance policy on your life. The "taxable cost" of the premium must be included in your taxable income. Depending on your age, this taxable cost, which is figured according to an IRS table (in Publication 15-B, *Employer's Tax Guide to Fringe Benefits*), could be substantially less than what the policy would cost you if you bought it yourself.

Benefit to you: You get $1 million of life insurance for a small amount of extra tax.

Loophole: **Have your company pay for your medical insurance.** Premiums for the insurance are deductible by your company and are not considered income to an owner/employee.

Caution: Because all eligible employees must be covered by the plan, this strategy is cost effective only in companies with few or

■ *Your Life* ■ ■ ■ ■

no employees. Also, it can't be used by those owning more than 2% of S corporations.

Loophole: **Set up an educational assistance program.** Such a plan, set up under Section 127 of the Tax Code, can pay up to $5,250 a year of your college or graduate school education expenses (or your child's expenses if your child is an employee)—tax free. The company can deduct the payments it makes under the plan.

Note: The education need not be job related to qualify for favorable tax treatment.

Caution: Such a plan can't discriminate in favor of "highly compensated individuals"—employees who own more than 5% of the business or earn more than $90,000 a year.

Additional benefit: If the courses are job related and maintain or improve your current job skills, there is no dollar limitation.

Loophole: **Take out a disability insurance policy in your name.** At the end of the year, when you know that you will not collect any money on the policy, ask your company to reimburse you for the premiums you paid.

Reason: When your company pays the premiums on a disability insurance policy, they are deductible. But if you subsequently collect disability insurance, you will owe tax on the amounts you receive. If you pay the premiums yourself, however, the money that you collect under the policy is not taxable.

Caution: This plan is subject to nondiscrimination rules similar to those that apply to health insurance plans.

Loophole: **Adopt qualified retirement plans that benefit you more than other employees.** Amounts contributed to a retirement plan can be deducted by the company. They aren't treated as income until you begin taking money out.

If you are more than 20 years older than other company employees, consider setting up a defined-benefit pension plan instead of a defined-contribution plan.

Reason: The amounts put away on your behalf will be much larger than with a defined-contribution plan because you are funding a specific retirement benefit (rather than taking a percentage of eligible salaries) and you have fewer years to do so because of your age.

FOR EMPLOYEES

Loophole: **Motivate and retain employees with these fringes...**

●**Tax-free retirement planning.** Companies with retirement plans (including pension plans, Simplified Employee Pensions and IRAs) can now offer tax-free retirement planning services to employees.

How it works: The tax-free services are not limited to information about the company retirement plan. They also apply to advice about retirement income and how the company plan fits into the employee's retirement plan. However, the related accounting, brokerage or tax preparation services can't be given tax free.

●**Frequent-flier miles.** Employees are not taxed on the value of frequent-flier miles or similar promotional benefits (earned through hotels or rental cars) accumulated during business travel.

Caution: Travel/promotional benefits that are converted to cash are not eligible for tax-free treatment.

●**No-additional-cost services.** You can motivate employees by providing, at a reduced price, "services" which would remain unused otherwise—and no tax would need to be paid on the services.

Examples: Hotel rooms, airline or cruise line tickets.

Ineligible services—those that cannot be totally tax free—can be offered at employee discounts of up to 20% of the value of the service.

Example: Providing legal services for law firm employees.

●**Working condition fringe benefits.** These products or services help employees to perform their jobs.

Examples: Business magazine subscriptions, professional dues, outplacement services, reimbursements of business-related employee automobile expenses.

These benefits are tax free to the extent that employees could deduct the cost as business expenses on their tax returns.

- **Company car.** The value is tax free to the extent the car is used for business. The cost of the portion not applicable to business use is taxable as compensation.

Note: Using the car for commuting is not a deductible use.

- **Adoption assistance.** Employees having modified adjusted gross income of no more than $155,860 can receive up to $10,390 tax free for 2004 under an adoption assistance plan that meets the requirements of Section 137 of the Tax Code. The cost is deductible by the company. While the benefit is not subject to income tax withholding, it is still subject to FICA and FUTA taxes.

- **Nontraditional benefits.** In recent years, more companies have started offering benefits that have a minimal direct cost but that are highly valued by employees. These benefits may actually save the employer money by increasing morale and reducing absenteeism and turnover. The benefits also improve your ability to recruit new employees. *Examples...*

- Flextime—working a full schedule with hours and days selected by employees on an individual basis.

- Telecommuting—working entirely or partially from home.

- Job sharing—two employees sharing one full-time position.

New Tax Deductions For Business...and Often Overlooked Old Deductions

Barbara Weltman, attorney in Millwood, NY. She is editor and publisher of the on-line newsletter *Barbara Weltman's Big Ideas for Small Business, www.bwideas.com.* Ms. Weltman is author of numerous books, including *J.K. Lasser's Small Business Taxes* (Wiley) and *Bottom Line's Very Shrewd Money Book* (Bottom Line Books).

New deductions spring out of legislation, court decisions and IRS rulings. *Here are several recent developments affecting deductions that you won't want to miss on your business return...*

- **Deduct restorative contributions made to a retirement plan.** You may have been forced by the down market to put money into the company retirement plan to make up for its lost value. The payment might have been required to avoid a lawsuit by employees for breaching your fiduciary duty.

Such a "restorative payment" is *not* necessarily treated as a contribution to the plan and is not subject to the dollar limitation on annual contributions. It can, instead, be deducted as an ordinary and necessary business expense—an expense required to avoid liability for breach of fiduciary duty. [Revenue Ruling 2002-45, IRB 2002-29, 1.]

- **Deduct home-office expenses for part of a room.** A new Tax Court case says that if you use a portion of a room as your principal place of business, you can deduct the expenses allocated to that portion.

Example: A music teacher could deduct expenses for the part of his bedroom in which he gave lessons. [*Jack C.C. Huang,* TC Summary Opinion 2002-93.]

- **Claim an additional deduction for the cost of laundry,** cleaning, lodging taxes and telephone calls while on business trips. If you substantiate your business travel using the government's per diem allowance, you can claim this allowance *and* a separate deduction for these items.

Caution: Be sure to keep receipts and other records to back up your deduction. [Revenue Procedure 2002-63, IRB 2002-41, 691.]

THE TIMING OF ITEMS

Most expenses incurred in the course of running a business are deductible. Usually, the key question for business owners is *when* to claim the write-off. *Taking deductions at the right time can improve after-tax profits...*

- **Equipment and real estate.** It's best to elect to expense equipment in the year it is placed in service rather than depreciating it over several years (usually five or seven years, depending on the type of equipment).

For 2003 and 2004, the dollar limit on expensing is $100,000.

Caution: Don't make the election to expense if you're not making a profit—the deduction will be worth nothing to you. Instead, depreciate the equipment over its recovery period. In the future, when you're profitable, the depreciation deductions will be more valuable.

Consider using "bonus depreciation." This is an additional first-year write-off of 30% of the property's basis, after subtracting the amounts expensed (50% for any property acquired after May 5, 2003).

Note: Bonus depreciation will automatically apply unless you decide not to use it. If you had a bad year and can't benefit from the extra write-off, waive the deduction. You'll then have larger depreciation deductions to claim in coming years when you have profits to offset.

Segregate certain building components to qualify for more rapid depreciation. For example, special wiring may be depreciated over seven years rather than as part of the building itself, which is depreciated over 39 years (for nonresidential realty).

Other separately depreciable items: Air-conditioning systems, light fixtures, partitions and plumbing especially for some machinery.

If you abandon or retire equipment that has not yet been fully depreciated, don't overlook a final deduction for the remaining undepreciated cost basis.

Expense the cost of a new roof for your office building or factory (instead of depreciating its cost) if it merely fixes a leak and doesn't make structural changes or add to the value of the property. [*Nevia Campbell,* TC Summary Opinion 2002-17.]

•**Buy the right car.** The size of the car you buy determines the size of your write-off. Generally, there is a dollar limit on depreciation for cars. But this dollar limit doesn't apply to vehicles weighing more than 6,000 pounds, which includes many SUVs.

Such cars can be depreciated using regular expensing and depreciation rules, which currently enable you to write off more than 70% of the cost of a $50,000 vehicle in the first year. Congress may close the SUV loophole.

•**Review net operating losses.** If you have a net operating loss in 2003, you can carry it back for two years and obtain an immediate refund. But you aren't required to use this carryback. You can opt to carry the loss forward for up to 20 years.

Consider waiving the carryback if you expect to be in a higher tax bracket in future years compared with your bracket in potential carryback years.

•**Expiring carryovers.** Make sure you can use carryovers that are about to expire. These include net operating losses, foreign tax credits and corporate capital losses. To use the carryovers, you need to generate offsetting income.

Example: Say you sold property in 2003 on the installment basis. To produce income needed to offset an expiring capital loss carryover, you can elect out of installment reporting and claim the entire gain on the sale for 2003 when you file your 2003 return.

TAX CREDITS

Increasingly, businesses have the opportunity to write off certain expenses as tax credits rather than as ordinary deductions. As you know, tax credits produce a dollar-for-dollar tax savings for the business.

•**Small-employer retirement plan start-up credit.** If you start a retirement plan this year, you can claim a credit of up to $500 on your return for setup costs, including expenses to educate employees about plan participation.

Caution: You can claim this credit only if the plan covers at least one employee who is not a highly compensated employee. You can't claim the credit if you, as the owner of the business, are the only participant in the plan.

•**Credit for child-care facilities and referrals.** If you build a child-care facility (say you convert office space into an employee day care center) or you pay to help employees find reliable child care, you can claim a tax credit of 25% for facilities and 10% for referral services. The maximum credit is $150,000 annually.

OTHER OVERLOOKED DEDUCTIONS

•**Bad debts.** Review your accounts or notes receivable. Look for items that will never be collected, even in part. The business can claim a deduction for uncollected bad debts.

If you turn bad accounts over to a collection agency that bases its fee on a percentage of the amount they collect, say 30%, you can immediately deduct that percentage of the debt as a bad debt.

Past returns: Review all outstanding debts for the previous seven years. You can file an amended return for this period to claim a bad-debt deduction and obtain a tax refund.

Caution: Cash-basis businesses cannot claim bad-debt deductions for uncollected fees for labor (since these fees were never included as income in the first place).

•**Excess inventory.** Check to see whether your inventory has decreased in value or if there are items that will probably never be sold. To nail down the change in value, offer items for sale and use this lowered price as your new inventory value.

By reducing the inventory carried on your books, you'll be able to reduce your closing inventory, thereby increasing your cost of goods sold. This minimizes the income you report from sales.

•**Interest on below-market loans.** If you lent money to your corporation at no interest, or at a rate below the IRS interest rate for the term of the loan, the corporation can deduct this "phantom" interest payment (which you must report as income).

What's the IRS interest rate? It's the applicable federal rate (AFR), which is set monthly by the IRS. An index of these rates is available at *www.irs.gov* (in "Search" box enter "Applicable Federal Rates").

More from Barbara Weltman...

How to Deduct a Home Office

You can deduct the space in your home that you use regularly and exclusively for your business. Your home office must be your primary place of business. This can be a separate room or a corner of the basement. The deduction is the proportion of the rent or depreciation and mortgage interest for that space on a square-footage basis. You can also deduct utilities, repairs, painting, etc.

Under new tax rules, claiming home-office deductions won't limit your ability to exclude up to $250,000 ($500,000 jointly) of gain when you sell the home. But you will have to pay tax at a 25% rate on all depreciation that is claimed after May 6, 1997.

For more information, see IRS Publication 587, *Business Use of Your Home,* available by calling 800-829-3676 or at *www.irs.gov.*

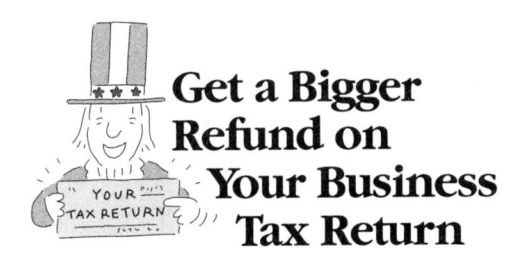

Get a Bigger Refund on Your Business Tax Return

Martin S. Kaplan, CPA, PC, 11 Penn Plaza, New York City 10001. He is author of What the IRS Doesn't Want You to Know *(Wiley).*

Don't miss these smart filing strategies that will help you save taxes and generate valuable cash flow on the business's tax return...

•**Claim a carryback refund if the business suffered a loss in 2003.** You can carry the loss back to the prior two tax years and obtain a refund.

To claim a quick refund from a loss carryback, corporations file IRS Form 1139, *Corporation Application for Tentative Refund.* Individuals claiming business losses on their personal returns can file IRS Form 1045, *Application for Tentative Refund.* The IRS will respond within 90 days.

•**Get back overpaid estimated taxes.** A corporation that overpaid estimated taxes during the past year doesn't have to wait until it files its return to get them refunded. Instead, it can get a quick refund by filing IRS Form 4466, *Corporation Application for Quick Refund of Overpayment of Estimated Tax,* as soon as possible after year-end, before it files its tax return.

The IRS will respond within 45 days—even if the company obtains a filing extension and doesn't file its tax return for another six months.

It's safer to claim a refund of overpaid taxes for 2003 and then just pay any tax due for 2004 quarter by quarter.

■ *Your Life* ■ ■ ■ ■

Trap: Don't apply the estimated tax overpayment to 2004 taxes. If a sudden need for cash arises, the company won't be able to get the overpayment back from the IRS. Even if business conditions worsen so the company runs a loss and doesn't owe any tax at all for the year, it still won't be able to get the overpayment back until the year is over—and the overpayment will be out-of-pocket cash that it is entitled to have for the entire year.

Unincorporated businesses: If your business is a pass-through entity (S corporation, partnership or limited liability company) or proprietorship, it can't use Form 4466. Instead, overpaid taxes must be reported on your personal return.

Again, if you made a large tax overpayment for 2003, it's better to claim a refund of it on your personal return than to apply the refund to 2004 taxes, for the same reasons.

●**Use increased depreciation deductions.** Congress increased the 30% bonus depreciation to 50% for depreciable equipment purchased after May 5, 2003. This allows 50% of the expense of the equipment to be deducted immediately, before applying normal depreciation rules to the rest of its cost.

Note: The 50% extra depreciation is automatic. If you do not wish to take it, you must attach to your tax return a statement that indicates that you have elected not to take it.

More depreciation strategies...

●Accelerate deductions for equipment that has been retired. For tax purposes, many kinds of equipment are used for shorter periods than their depreciable lives. *For example:* Computing and telecommunications equipment with five-year depreciation schedules may be replaced by a business after only two years.

Many firms overlook the fact that when equipment is abandoned or retired, all of the firm's remaining undepreciated cost basis in it becomes deductible immediately.

Be aware that many firms that carefully record when they place depreciable items in service do not similarly record when the items are retired from service—with the result that the items then continue to be carried forward on the books as if still in use.

A careful review of the business's listing of all items that are currently being depreciated may turn up items that have been retired—and, as a result, extra deductions have been lost.

●Examine real estate acquisitions and improvements. Commercial real estate generally is written off over 39 years for nonresidential and 27.5 years for residential—but many component parts of a real estate project may qualify as personal property that is deductible over a much shorter period, such as five years.

Items that seem to be part of a building may in fact qualify as personal property. *Examples:* Air-conditioning systems, light fixtures, partitions, plumbing installed to service machinery, even foundations installed to support heavy equipment.

A careful allocation of items to their appropriate categories—instead of lumping everything together as a "real estate addition"—may significantly accelerate depreciation deductions. Consider consulting a real estate depreciation specialist for help.

●Use Section 179 expensing. Up to $100,000 of equipment placed in service during 2003 and 2004 can be "expensed"—written off in full immediately, rather than depreciated over several years.

The election to do so must be made on the first return filed for the year. Pick the best items to expense (generally those with the longer recovery periods).

●**Fund retirement plan contributions with a refund.** Deductible contributions to qualified retirement plans—such as simplified employee pension (SEP) and self-employed plans—can generally be made up until the extended due date of the tax return, even if the return is actually filed before then.

Cash flow tactic: File an extension, then file the tax return to claim a refund—deducting plan contributions on the return to help generate the refund. When the refund arrives, use this to help finance the retirement plan contributions.

●**Take inventory write-downs.** Especially after a recession, a business is likely to have excess inventory that has lost some or all of its value. Reducing the reported value of the inventory on the company's books to its true value can provide another cash-saving deduction.

Document evidence of inventory value in the company's records. Best is a bona fide offer to sell some of the inventory at a lowered price, even if the offer is not accepted. Such an offer made within 30 days after year-end may document the inventory's new value—but check with the firm's tax adviser for details and specific requirements.

• Identify bad debts. The weak economy may have increased the number of debts owed to your company that have become uncollectible. These may be deductible—but their amount cannot be estimated. Only the specific debts that are identified as having gone bad can be deducted.

Strategy: Carefully examine the business's accounts receivable. By doing so, the company may obtain not only an increased deduction for identified bad debts but also a better picture of its cash flow that will help it improve its cash management.

• Meet the deadline for paying accrued expenses. When a corporation that is using accrual accounting accrues deductible items (such as employee bonuses, charitable contributions or other payments to cash-basis taxpayers) by year-end, it must actually pay them within 2½ months after year-end to get a current deduction for them. Thus, a calendar-year business must make such payments by March 15, 2004, to deduct them on its 2003 tax return. Don't miss the deadline or deductions will be delayed a year.

Note: Deductions paid to owner-employees of a firm may be restricted by special provisions of this rule.

• File amended tax returns to get tax refunds. Remember that when a new tax-saving strategy is found for the 2003 return that was overlooked in prior years, it's possible to file amended tax returns to also claim it for up to three prior years. So one newly found deduction may save up to four years of taxes.

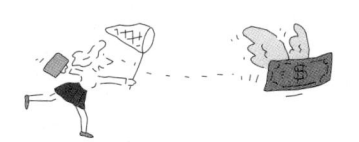

More from Martin Kaplan...
How Your Children Can Help the Family Business Cut Taxes

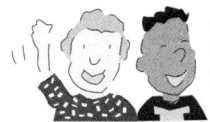

Tax planning involving your children can cut taxes on your business's income and give children a financial leg up.

SHIFTING INCOME

The simplest tax-saving tactic is to pay children for working in the business. Their pay is taxed at their low tax rate—which may be zero—and deductible at the higher tax rate of the business or parent, creating a tax savings.

Additional tax breaks: Wages of children under 18 are not subject to federal employment taxes (such as Social Security tax) when paid by a parent's unincorporated business. And the earned income of children is not subject to the so-called kiddie tax, which taxes only the investment income of children under age 14 at the tax rate of their parents.

Opportunity: Each child can take the standard deduction of $4,750 in 2003 ($4,850 in 2004) tax free. Each child can also use his/her salary to make a deductible IRA contribution of up to $3,000. This means each child can receive a total of up to $7,750 tax free in 2003 ($7,850 in 2004).

Beyond that, the following $7,000 ($7,150 in 2004) of earned income is taxed at only 10%, and the $21,400 ($21,900 in 2004) after that is taxed at only 15%—which will probably still be lower than the rate at which the salary can be deducted by the family business.

Example: A child is employed by a parent's unincorporated business. It deducts the child's salary at the parent's personal tax rate, which may be as high as 35%. The child can receive up to...

...$7,850, while owing no federal income tax in 2004. The parent's tax deduction for that pay may be worth as much as $2,747.50—saving almost $3,000 for the family.

...$15,000, while owing only $715 of tax. The parent's tax deduction may be worth as much as $5,250—saving more than $4,500 for the family.

▪ *Your Life* ▪ ▪ ▪ ▪

These tax savings can be multiplied if the business employs more than one of your children. *More...*

• **Tax savings may be even larger** when state and local income taxes are considered.

• **The IRA contributions can provide a child with a great start on lifetime financial security,** due to the pretax compound growth that will occur in the IRA over the decades.

Deduction key: The child must perform real work for the business, and be paid a reasonable amount for it.

Good news: The Tax Court has permitted deductible salaries for children as young as seven years old who performed tasks for the family business, such as answering the phone, taking messages and doing cleanup chores. [*Walt E. Eller,* 77 TC 934, and *James A. Moriarty,* TC Memo 1984-249.]

And such deductions are not a priority audit target of the IRS.

Corporations: If the business is organized as a corporation, wages it pays to children will be subject to federal employment taxes. But the same income tax savings described above will be realized. Also, the employment taxes are deductible by the corporation. If a nonfamily member were employed to perform the same work as the family member, these taxes would have been incurred.

Note: Before hiring your child, check to see if state or local labor laws apply.

RENTAL INCOME

A second way to cut the tax bill on a family business's income is to have the children own assets that are used by the business—such as real estate—and lease them to it.

Lease payments made by the business are deductible by it, while payments received by the children are taxed to them at their lower personal tax rates—and may also be sheltered from tax by depreciation deductions.

Result: The children receive income from the business that is either free of income tax or taxed at a lower rate, and not subject to employment taxes. The business deducts the payments to the children at a higher rate—again producing cash tax savings.

How it's done: A pass-through entity, such as a family limited partnership or limited liability company, is created to own the assets and lease them to the business. The entity's income and deductions are reported on the personal tax returns of its owners.

Ownership shares in the entity then are given to the children.

A note on gift tax: Gifts may be made each year free of gift tax, using the annual gift tax exclusion ($11,000 in 2003 and 2004 per recipient). And gifts of ownership shares in a pass-through entity may qualify for some substantial valuation discounts—such as 35%—due to their lack of marketability and status as "minority interests."

With a 35% discount, shares allocable to $16,900 of assets may be transferred with an $11,000 gift. Joint gifts made by a married couple can transfer twice as much—to each child, each year.

Lease income received will pass through to the children in proportion to their ownership interests. The owners can take depreciation deductions for the leased assets and they will offset some of the lease income, so no tax is due on it.

The kiddie tax *does* apply to taxable lease income, so major tax savings result only to children over age 13. They receive the benefit of the 10% and 15% tax brackets as described above—while the business takes an expense deduction for the payments at its own higher tax rate.

Separate ownership of the assets outside the business creates extra benefits as well...

• **The owners can finance or sell the assets** for their own account without the proceeds going to the business, and with any gain on a sale being tax-favored capital gain for them.

• **Assets are removed from the estate of the business's primary owner**—possibly reducing future estate tax.

SHIFTING OWNERSHIP

A third way to reduce the taxes of a family business is by giving children ownership in the business itself.

The method here is to organize the business as a pass-through entity and give children ownership interests in it. Again, children over age 13 can utilize the 10% and 15% tax brackets to lower the tax rate on their share of the business's income.

A series of annual gifts made over a period of years using the gift tax exclusion combined with valuation discounts may transfer a large portion—or even most—of a business's value, decreasing the taxable estate of the original owner as well as reducing the family's annual income tax bill.

The original owner can retain management control over the business even after giving away majority ownership in it.

How: If the business is organized as an S corporation, the original owner can retain its voting stock while giving nonvoting shares to the children. If the business is organized as a partnership or limited liability company, the original owner can act as the managing partner while making the children limited partners.

Key: Begin making gifts of interests in a growing business early so they transfer future appreciation in the business's value as well.

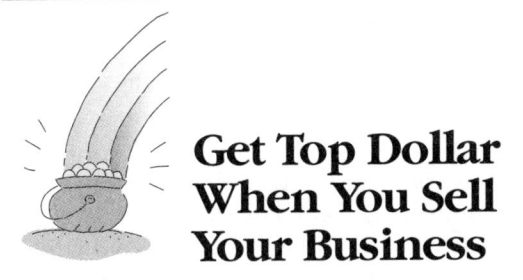

Get Top Dollar When You Sell Your Business

Joel Getzler, president of Getzler & Company, Inc., longtime turnaround specialists for troubled small businesses, 295 Madison Ave., New York City 10017.

When the time comes to sell a business, most entrepreneurs overestimate its value. How do you put a price tag on something to which you have devoted decades of hard work?

Result: The process drags on, and the business is neglected to the point that it sells at a price far below what was initially offered. Or the business declines so much that interest from buyers dries up.

Here's what entrepreneurs need to know before selling a business...

WHAT IT IS WORTH

- **Find out what similar firms have sold for in the recent past.** Consult with bankers, trade associations or long-term suppliers to get information on recent sales.
- **Determine the market capitalizations** (number of outstanding shares times share price) of small public companies in the field.
- **Hire a business appraiser.** Get a referral from your banker.

GET THE PRICE YOU WANT

To fetch a higher price, begin "primping" your business at least three years before you plan to sell.

- **Cut costs.** Instead of focusing on reducing your tax liability, try to maximize profits.
  - Accurately evaluate inventory. Write off excess items to clean up your books.
  - Trim unnecessary expenses—fancy leased cars, travel that is only partly for business purposes, costly entertainment, little-used business and country club memberships that are paid for by the business.
  - Eliminate nonessential employees, even family members. Help them find other employment. The new owners will surely let them go.
- **Once you start shopping the company,** offer to remain onboard for a few years after the sale to maintain relationships with key customers. In exchange, ask for a premium—15% to 20% over the sale price—if higher revenues and/or profits are achieved within a specified time period, say, three years.

When the Company You Work for Is in Trouble

If a big scandal hits the company you work for, decide if the company has a future. Evaluate if it has been honest with the public and employees. Don't leave immediately—a potential new employer might suspect you of being involved in, and trying to escape, the scandal.

Helpful: Step up networking activities at associations and professional groups. Work with a professional résumé service to put your career in the best possible light. Think about approaching your company's competitor—it may be looking to hire people from your firm who are not involved in the scandal.

Terri Levine, personal and business coach, North Wales, PA, and author of *Coaching for an Extraordinary Life* (Lahaska).

How to Make the Most of a Job Loss

Avery E. Neumark, Esq., CPA, partner in charge of employee benefits and executive compensation at the accounting firm of Rosen Seymour Shapss Martin & Co. LLP, 757 Third Ave., New York City 10017.

More than two million Americans have lost jobs since the economy began a downward spiral in March 2000. And despite recent economic improvements, companies are still laying people off. Anyone, it seems, can suddenly find himself/herself negotiating a severance package with his employer. *Here is what you need to know to negotiate wisely...*

SEVERANCE PAY

The law doesn't require companies to give severance pay to terminated employees. Unless specified in an employment contract or collective bargaining agreement, severance is given at the company's discretion. *Most companies, however, do offer something to laid-off employees, giving it in one of two ways...*

•**Continuation of salary**—for a number of weeks or months, but usually not more than a year.

•**A lump-sum payment**—typically geared to the length of employment.

Example: A month's pay for each year of employment.

No matter how it's paid, severance is taxable to you as income, and is subject to Social Security and Medicare (FICA) taxes. Payment for unused vacation days is also fully taxable.

Severance vs. pension: If your company has a pension plan, it may give you a choice between severance pay and additional pension credits. Your decision will depend on several factors—your age, your immediate need for cash and how much is being offered.

To make a fair comparison between the cash severance and credits, multiply the pension credits by 100 (a rule of thumb) and weigh this number against the severance payment.

Example: XYZ Corp. offers to make a $30,000 severance payment or a $400 additional pension credit. In this example, the pension credit ($400 x 100 = $40,000) proves to be the larger benefit. *Tax break:* The pension credit isn't subject to FICA.

If the choice is between severance pay and additional credits for years of service or some other additional benefit, the comparison becomes more complex. Consult a tax adviser.

HEALTH AND LIFE INSURANCE

If the company continues to pay for some or all of your medical insurance, this is a tax-free benefit...

•**COBRA.** If the company regularly employs 20 or more workers and there's a health plan, you're entitled under federal law (COBRA) to continue the same coverage at your own expense for up to 18 months. You can reduce the coverage—for example by eliminating dental benefits—to save on premiums, but you can't increase coverage.

Important: Even if your company isn't subject to federal COBRA law, state law (referred to as "mini-COBRA") may entitle you to continuation of coverage. To determine your eligibility and the length of mini-COBRA coverage, check with your state's insurance department or visit Insure.com (*http://info.insure.com/health/cobra3.html*).

•**Life insurance.** Some companies continue to pay for life insurance following forced retirement. This benefit is tax free up to $50,000 of coverage. Excess coverage is taxed.

STOCK OPTIONS

Be sure you understand the terms and tax implications of stock options you hold.

•**Incentive stock options (ISOs).** These options must be exercised within three months of termination. While there's no regular income tax on the exercise of ISOs, the spread between the stock's fair market value at the time of exercise and the amount paid for the stock is an adjustment item that's included in alternative minimum tax (AMT) calculations. This could trigger the AMT for you, or increase the amount of AMT you owe.

- **Nonqualified stock options.** ISOs that are not exercised within three months of termination automatically become nonqualified stock options.

If the exercise of nonqualified options occurs within the same calendar year as the termination of employment, the resulting income is subject to regular withholding taxes, as if the income were additional salary. If the exercise occurs in a subsequent year, the income will then be taxed at the supplemental withholding rate of 25%.

DEFERRED COMPENSATION

If you deferred a year-end bonus or other compensation under the company's deferred-compensation plan, termination generally entitles you to receive the deferred amount, plus any earnings on it. The receipt of deferred compensation is fully taxable. However, it is *not* subject to FICA taxes. FICA was already deducted from your pay the year you earned the deferred compensation.

OUTPLACEMENT SERVICES

Résumé writing, office space, interview assistance and other job placement services or job retraining paid for by the company are considered tax-free fringe benefits to you. This is so even though you are no longer an employee.

RETIREMENT PLAN BENEFITS

Upon termination you may be able to take your pension, 401(k) or retirement plan benefits with you. *Assuming your plan allows you to take benefits, you can...*

- **Roll over the benefits to your IRA.** Under new law you no longer have to set up a separate IRA to receive a rollover—you can add the rollover to an existing IRA.

- **Roll over the benefits to your new employer's plan.** Retirement plans are not required to accept rollovers, but they may be permitted under the company's plan documents. Check with the plan's administrator.

- **Leave the benefits in the plan.** This may be advisable if you like the investment options offered by the plan. Another reason to leave benefits within the plan is that federal law provides complete protection of retirement plan benefits from creditors' claims, whereas state law may provide only limited or no protection for benefits rolled into an IRA.

- **Take a distribution.** A distribution is subject to automatic 20% withholding—you'll pay any additional tax on the distribution when you file your return. (If you were born before 1936, you may be eligible for 10-year averaging to reduce the tax on the distribution.) If you're under age 55, you'll also be subject to a 10% early distribution penalty.

Distribution is advisable only if you have an immediate need for cash. Taking a distribution ends the tax deferral on the plan's earnings.

Of course, if you take a distribution, you can make a rollover of benefits to an IRA to avoid immediate tax if you act within 60 days. But you'll have to add the 20% withholding to the IRA and wait until you file your return to recoup it.

Plan loans: If you have any outstanding plan loans at the time of termination, they must be repaid in full. If not, they're treated as a taxable distribution.

UNEMPLOYMENT

If you are terminated, you generally are eligible for unemployment compensation. This may be so even if the termination is labeled as early retirement. Unemployment compensation includes benefits paid by states as well as supplemental benefits paid by the company or through a union.

Unemployment compensation is fully taxable. You can opt to have income taxes withheld from benefits at the rate of 10%. Withholding is an easier way to pay tax than having to make estimated payments.

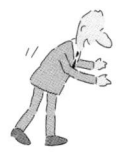

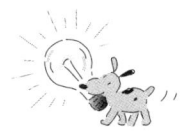

■ *Your Life* ■ ■ ■ ■

Losing Your Job Can Be Good for Your Health

The rates of death, smoking, obesity, heavy drinking, heart disease as well as some back problems decline when unemployment rises. The number of fatal car accidents is also reduced. There are various reasons for these declines.

Examples: Heavy drinking and obesity decline because unemployed people have less money to spend on liquor and more time to exercise…fatal car crashes drop because people drive less often when times are bad…and heart disease falls because lifestyles become healthier.

Christopher Ruhm, PhD, professor of economics at the University of North Carolina, Greensboro.

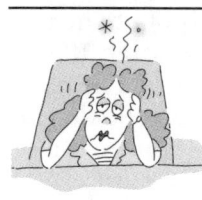

Finding a Job in Tough Times

Bob Dilenschneider, chairman of The Dilenschneider Group, a strategic counseling/public relations company at 200 Park Ave., New York City 10166. He is author of *50 Plus! Critical Career Decisions for the Rest of Your Life* (Citadel).

With the uncertain economy and many retirement accounts hit by the stock market crash, more and more seniors are trying to get back into the workplace. If you're among them, be prepared for lots of competition.

Good news: Employers are more eager than they have been in many years to hire older workers. In these tough times, employers place a high value on the experience and judgment of mature employees. Gone are the days of the technology boom, when the main emphasis was on youth.

These changes in employer values mean that people over age 50 need to adapt their strategies for landing a position.

EXAMINE YOUR MOTIVES

Unless your financial situation is dire, look for a job you truly enjoy. If you don't, you risk performing poorly, burning out early and missing better opportunities.

Take a hard look at your motives. Do you want to resume work just because some colleagues have done it—or do you sincerely long for professional achievement? Talk over your situation with your family, friends and, if appropriate, your financial adviser.

If you don't have a deep longing for professional achievement, getting back into the workforce could create frustration for you and your family.

Helpful test: When you hear the news about businesses today, do you get angry at the mistakes they're making? Do you say to yourself, *If I were at that company, I could do something about those problems?* If so, you probably miss the challenges of a career.

If not, there are many alternatives, such as working part-time or working at home.

USE YOUR NETWORK

One of maturity's many advantages is that many of your younger former colleagues are now in positions of influence. Ideally, you have stayed in touch with these people as well as other business contacts. Even if you have not spoken with someone in years, that person may still want to help you now as a job seeker.

Don't be afraid to ask. Start by making a list of six friends who hold positions of influence in companies you might be interested in working for. Tell them you intend to get back into the job market.

Be straightforward. Remind him/her that you once assisted him. Then ask if he would be willing to help you now. The most persuasive strategy is to point out diplomatically that he'll benefit by helping you.

Example: You might say to a friend, "Help me find a position with your company, and I'll introduce those advertising ideas that you developed a while back."

PLAY TO YOUR STRENGTHS

Your track record and accomplishments are important, of course, but do not rely only on your curriculum vitae. Many aspects of business have changed drastically in the last few years.

Examples: New marketing concepts, attitudes toward technology, workplace rules.

Employers today want to hear less about your track record and more about your ability to be creative in helping the company solve its problems and develop its opportunities.

Before applying to a company, find out as much as you can about it. In interviews, don't hesitate to offer ideas. If the company isn't reaching as many customers as you think it could, for example, suggest ways in which you could help broaden its appeal.

That type of suggestion might sound brash coming from a 25-year-old applicant, but not from someone who is over 50. Your ideas will also show an interviewer that you have done your homework.

GOOD PROSPECTS

•**Sales.** Five years ago, companies were hiring 22-year-old salespeople who spoke in Internet jargon. Today, an increasing number of employers are looking for mature salespeople who have credibility with customers and an understanding of human behavior.

If you apply for a sales position, give examples of how your understanding of people has resulted in closing a deal.

•**Teaching.** Because credibility is so important in the positions that require teaching and training, mature job applicants often have an immediate advantage over younger ones.

Today, you can take that advantage one step further by emphasizing not just your ability as a teacher but also your ability to help employees learn on their own. Employers are especially eager to find that skill because it saves companies money and builds morale.

•**Jobs requiring knowledge of the community.** Young people simply haven't had the time to develop a knowledge of the community that's valuable to many businesses—from the marketing departments of nationally known retailers to the personnel offices of local law firms.

Knowledge of your community is particularly important to companies that are engaged in niche marketing.

Examples: Residents of specific neighborhoods or those with children in school.

Make sure the interviewers know that you are informed about your community. Tell them where you have lived, and mention the social and civic clubs that you belong to. Without blatantly name-dropping, talk about community leaders you know.

•**Front-office work.** Depending, of course, on the type of business a company is in, it may be eager to hire front-office workers who will give the workplace an image of maturity and stability.

Examples: Insurance companies, doctor's offices, investment advisory services.

•**Personal assistant.** This is a large job category that is often overlooked by mature job seekers.

Executives are eager to find an assistant who can help set priorities, deal with executives at other firms and help with meeting preparation. Nearly always, those skills are the product of good judgment and many years of business experience.

During job interviews, describe achievements that illustrate your good judgment and, if possible, your ability to deal with people who are in positions of power.

Check Your Credit Before a Job Search

Your credit may be checked out when you apply for a job. Businesses must get your permission to do so—but if you refuse, a company may think you have something to hide.

Self-defense: Check your credit with major credit bureaus before starting a job search. Correct any errors.

Major credit bureaus: Equifax (800-685-1111 or *www.equifax.com*)...Experian (888-397-3742 or *www.experian.com*)...TransUnion (800-888-4213 or *www.transunion.com*).

Bettye Banks, senior vice president for education at the Consumer Credit Counseling Service, Dallas.

■ *Your Life* ■ ■ ■ ■

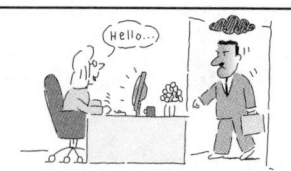

Secrets for Getting Past the Receptionist

To get past a gatekeeper, such as a secretary, assistant or receptionist, and reach the decision maker...

- **Treat the gatekeeper well.**
- **Use his/her first name.**
- **Ask for his help.**
- **Send him his own set** of promotional materials when you send a set to the boss.
- **Think how you would like to be treated** if the roles were reversed.

Bob Burg, president, Burg Communications, which provides business networking and positive-persuasion consulting services, Jupiter, FL, *www.burg.com*. He is also author of *Endless Referrals* (McGraw-Hill).

More Effective On-Line Résumés

When sending a résumé on-line, send it as an attachment in *Microsoft Word*—the business standard. Name the attachment with your name—last name first—and the word *résumé*. In addition, cut and paste your résumé into the body of the E-mail, below your introduction—some recruiters will not open attachments because of a fear of viruses. Use the subject line to get attention—try something like *Results-oriented business leader*. Use standard fonts, such as Arial and Times Roman. Avoid graphics, pictures and Web addresses.

Daniel Abramson, president, Staffdynamics, business consultants, St. James, NY, *www.staffdynamics.biz*.

Negotiating Know-How

When negotiating a new contract or starting a job, it is still smart to ask about stock options and awards. Valuable options and awards can still be had. Companies that acknowledge their options are worthless may be willing to grant new options at attractive exercise prices. Others may award stock, now that options are frequently treated as a company expense.

Background: The value of an option is the spread between a low exercise price and a higher price for the publicly traded stock. Many stock options are worthless because they were issued at an exercise price above the stock's current price.

Alan Johnson, managing director of Johnson Associates, Inc., compensation consultants, New York City.

310

20

Planning for College

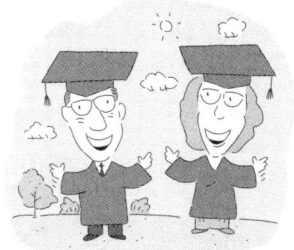

How to Write a Winning College Essay

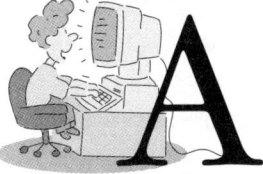

A college application essay can help clinch an acceptance. But many students will waste the opportunity by writing predictable or poorly thought-out essays. *How to help your child write a winning essay...*

•**Strive for an emotional response,** not an intellectual argument. Some applicants feel they must write essays that sound "serious." When an applicant writes about the environment, civil rights or presidential politics, it can sound like he/she is lecturing the reader.

Unless the essay question specifically asks you to do otherwise, focus instead on personal matters that tell the reader more about you. Your goal should be to have the admissions officer finish the essay and say, "I really like this kid."

•**Be original.** College essays hit on the same themes again and again—wrestling taught me to concentrate…Grandma's death helped me to appreciate life…I like to give to others, etc. Instead, focus on something more original.

Example: Rather than write about what you have learned from playing soccer, write about a hobby, perhaps pitching horseshoes or grooming dogs. That is more likely to give the essay reader something he hasn't read numerous times before.

•**Be positive.** Choose an upbeat topic. The very best essays are about passions, not doubts or failures.

Example: If a student intends to write about the strained relations within his family, I would suggest he instead focus on the great relationship he has with one particular relative or friend, set against the backdrop of his family troubles.

Sanford Kreisberg, JD, former teacher of expository writing at Harvard University and director of communications at MIT's Sloan School of Business. He currently runs Cambridge Essay Service, an undergraduate and business school essay consultancy, 40 Tierney St., Cambridge, MA 02138, http://world.std.com/~edit.

Your Life

- **Use dialogue.** Few applicants do this, but dialogue is a great way to convey the personality of a character and make an essay more entertaining and readable.

  Instead of: "Mrs. Von Crabbe, my piano teacher, taught me more than just how to play the piano. Her lessons were filled with advice that one could use in life. Even though her English was often just a little off and her manner seemed odd, she will always be memorable to me…"

  Try: "*Alex,* Mrs. Von Crabbe would say, *the concert is starting even so before you sit down on the bench.* She told us the first day never to call her Mrs. Von Crabbe Apple *even with my back in the behind.* But how could we? We loved and feared her too much." The dialogue brings the character to life.

- **Be reflective.** When asked to write about a person or an event that deeply affected them, many applicants reenact rather than reflect. A good trick is to briefly explain what affected you, then write the phrase, "Looking back, I now realize…" and see where it leads you.

  When you're finished with the essay, remove the phrase, "Looking back, I now realize…" It's a cliché—but a useful tool to get you started.

- **Polish your work.** I recommend at least three drafts. Leave enough time—at least one day—between drafts so that you can read it with a fresh eye each time.

Don't Be Put Off by College Costs

Many high-priced private colleges now provide generous financial aid to students—making their actual cost competitive with the cost of public colleges. Up to two-thirds of college students now receive such financial aid as scholarships, grants and loans.

Frank Burtnett, EdD, president, Education Now, education and career consultants in Springfield, VA, www.ednow.org.

Get the Inside Scoop On Colleges

Kenneth Hartman, PhD, director of the National Technology Institute for School Counselors in Cherry Hill, NJ, www.techcounselor.org. He is former director of admissions and guidance services at The College Board and is author of Internet Guide for College-Bound Students *(The College Board).*

College Web sites are helpful for finding general information, but don't stop there. *The following "unofficial" resources can show your child what a school is really like…*

UNOFFICIAL INFORMATION

Speak with students and faculty members during a visit to find out about the school's ambience and academic rigor and what students do for fun. *Then, go deeper…*

- **Student newspaper.** Most are now on-line and allow you to search archives.

  Example: A minority student who wants to know the racial climate can do a search for coverage of any issues.

- **Virtual visits to student organizations.** Encourage your child to send E-mail to clubs that reflect his/her interests—athletic, religious or cultural. Links to their Web sites are usually on the school's home page. Many clubs post meeting dates and announcements.

- **Research on specific courses.** To gauge the difficulty of a program, look at professors' Web sites. They list course requirements, syllabi, schedules, etc.

OFF-LINE RESOURCES

- **Alumni in your child's area of interest.** Alumni groups and college newspapers have names of graduates, their majors and contact information. If you can't find E-mail addresses for these groups, use an Internet search engine, such as *www.google.com.*

- **Contact professional associations.** Ask which schools are held in high esteem and if you can get in touch with the members who attended them.

  Resource: Encyclopedia of Associations, available in most public libraries.

•**Students from your hometown.** Ask the college or your child's high school guidance counselor for a list of student contacts.

More from Kenneth Hartman...

Web Sites That Help Kids Choose Colleges

The specialized search engines help students to narrow their lists of desirable colleges. *www.petersons.com...www.collegeboard.com* and *www.princetonreview.com* allow students to input their preferences. The engines search selected lists of more than 4,300 institutions in the US and generate a list of schools that fit the criteria, which can be based on tuition, the student/faculty ratio, location, curriculum, etc.

Sample criteria: A school in the Northeast with a strong biology program for less than $15,000 a year.

If Your Child Doesn't Want to Start College Right Away...

Frank Leana, PhD, educational consultant located in New York City.

A high school graduate who doesn't want to start college immediately should use the year off to further his/her college and future prospects—engaging in an activity that has some academic value, such as assistant teaching. He also should take a course or two at a local college in his area of interest. If his high school career did not include community service activities, he should participate in some during his year off. Any outdoor activities should include an academic component, as do some Outward Bound or National Outdoor Leadership Schools (NOLS) programs.

If he wants to earn money, he should aim for jobs in areas he might be interested in pursuing later. Work experience is particularly valuable for students planning to major in business or communications.

Important: A year of travel will not improve his chances of college admission unless the time is put to some educational purpose, such as learning a foreign language.

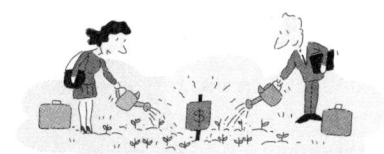

College Savings Plans: Some Are Much Better Than Others

Joseph Hurley, CPA, CEO of Savingforcollege.com, which offers guidance on financial planning to families of college-bound students. The Web site rates the performance of 529 plans of all states on a scale of one cap (weak) to five caps (excellent). He is also a partner in Bonadio & Co., an accounting firm in Pittsford, NY.

Don't let a volatile stock market cause you to snub the college savings plans. The markets will recover—and perhaps even bounce back to historic rates of return if you have a long-term horizon. If not, you can invest in bonds within the plan to reduce risk.

College savings plans—also known simply as 529s (after Section 529 of the Internal Revenue Code)—are a great deal for almost anyone trying to fund an education for a child, grandchild, friend's child, etc.

Exceptions: Families who expect to qualify for financial aid...couples earning up to $83,000 in 2003 ($85,000 in 2004) who qualify for a full tax credit on their federal income tax returns to help cover college costs. You may not use 529 plans on a tax-free basis for the same college expenses covered by the credit.

For everyone else, 529 plans allow years of tax-free savings. Withdrawals before 2011 are free of federal income tax when used to pay college-related expenses. Later withdrawals will be taxable to the student.

CHOOSING THE RIGHT PLAN

Look at your own state's plan first to see if it offers special tax benefits to residents. Almost every state offers a 529 plan, but only 24 of the states currently provide a state tax deduction for

■ *Your Life* ■ ■ ■ ■

some or all of your contributions.* Also, check with your state's plan to see if withdrawals are free from state taxes.

If your state plan provides significant tax advantages, you should seriously consider it.

My Web site, *www.savingforcollege.com,* offers free comparative information on 529 plans, including expenses and links to related Web sites.

Caution: Many employers now allow employees to contribute to the company's choice of 529 plans through a payroll-deduction program. However, your state's 529 plan may be a better choice.

COMPARE INVESTMENT OPTIONS

After evaluating any state tax advantages, narrow your 529 plan options to the state plans that offer the best investment choices. A typical 529 plan uses a *fund-of-funds approach*—different portfolios, each built around an array of mutual funds.

• Number of options. Plans should offer at least four portfolios—aggressive...balanced... conservative...and one with investment selections based on the age of the participant.

With age-based portfolios, you designate the year in which the money will likely be needed. As college nears, the asset allocation changes automatically from aggressive to conservative by shifting gradually from equities to fixed income.

Most plans offer choices from a single fund family. Of course, those with different families give you more investment options.

• Investment performance. Savingforcollege.com shows quarterly performance for all plans. But not every savings plan has been established long enough to have produced meaningful long-term results.

Since most plans invest in existing mutual funds, it is best to research those funds' 10-year performance figures by contacting the fund families directly and asking for prospectuses or by checking *www.morningstar.com.*

• Plan expenses. Expenses should be no more than 1% of assets per year, including expenses of the underlying mutual funds. Information is included in the enrollment materials.

Trap: Most plans are managed by mutual funds, but some are sold by brokerages. Brokerage-sold plans tend to levy higher fees.

Note: Even states that sell their plans primarily through brokers may allow you to bypass the commission if you enroll with the state directly.

Low-cost leaders: TIAA-CREF (800-842-2776 or *www.tiaa-cref.org*), whose core business is managing funds for teachers, provides 529 programs in California, Connecticut, Georgia, Idaho, Kentucky, Michigan, Minnesota, Mississippi, Missouri, New York, Oklahoma, Tennessee and Vermont. Low-cost plans using Vanguard funds (800-523-7731 or *www.vanguard.com*) are offered in Iowa and Utah.

COMPARE OTHER FEATURES

Gauge a plan's flexibility in terms of...

• Transfers. You should be able to make at least one shift per year within the plan and to transfer ownership of the account.

Example: Grandparents who start an account for a grandchild should be able to transfer ownership to the child's parents.

• Time or age restrictions. Some states require that the account be used before the beneficiary reaches a specified age—otherwise, the account will be terminated and paid out as a nonqualified taxable distribution.

• Withdrawal procedures. Some programs insist that you prove the money is being used to pay college costs. Other plans put you on your honor to use the money only for higher-education bills. If you're caught using distributions for another purpose, they will be taxed.

• Creditor protection. Unless state law says otherwise, assets in a 529 plan could be seized by the contributors' creditors in case of bankruptcy or a court judgment. Some states simply say that all 529 assets are protected from creditors. Elsewhere, the laws can be more complicated.

Example: In New York's plan, the entire amount is protected from creditors if the plan was set up with a transfer of funds from a child's *Uniform Gifts to Minors Act/Uniform*

---

*Those states are Colorado, Georgia, Idaho, Illinois, Iowa, Kansas, Louisiana, Maryland, Michigan, Mississippi, Missouri, Montana, Nebraska, New Mexico, New York, Ohio, Oklahoma, Oregon, Rhode Island, South Carolina, Utah, Virginia, West Virginia, Wisconsin.

Planning for College

Transfers to Minors Act account. Only a limited amount of assets is protected if the plan was created directly by a parent or grandparent.

More from Joseph Hurley...

Look Beyond 529 Plans

There are two other education savings plans you might want to consider in addition to 529 plans...

•**Coverdell Education Savings Accounts (ESAs).** There is no tax deduction for contributions to ESAs. Once you contribute, money in the account builds up tax free until you withdraw it. Provided all the money goes to pay school bills, withdrawals are tax free as well. The maximum annual contribution is $2,000. You can contribute if taxable income is less than $220,000 for married couples filing jointly...$110,000 for singles.

ESAs are not limited to paying college bills. They can pay *any* school bills, starting with kindergarten. Ask your financial institution if it offers ESAs.

ESAs also are not limited to a few investment options, as in 529 plans. You can invest the money any way you like—including in a self-directed brokerage account.

Note: The beneficiary will retain control of the money after the age of majority. ESAs *do* count against you for purposes of determining financial aid eligibility.

•**Prepaid college tuition plans.** These plans, available in 16 states, let you pay future college tuition at today's rates. You pay the bill today, no matter how much college costs when your child starts school. Most plans are only for residents attending school in that state. Ask your child's school guidance office or board of education if your state has a plan and how to apply.

Such plans make the most sense if your youngster plans to go to college in-state and you don't expect to be eligible for financial aid. Benefits usually can be transferred to an out-of-state college.

Strategy: You may also use a prepaid tuition plan for tuition and a 529 plan to cover other college expenses.

Also from Joseph Hurley...

College Savings to Use First

If your child is a high school junior and you are hoping to qualify for financial aid, spend money from custodial accounts and Coverdell Education Savings Accounts before applying for financial aid. They are considered student assets. Financial aid offices expect at least 35% of student assets to go toward college. Custodial money can be used for anything that benefits your child, such as a car and summer school expenses. Coverdell accounts can be spent on education-related expenses, such as school trips and a home computer.

Tax Breaks to Help Pay For College

Lisa N. Collins, CPA/PFS, vice president and director of tax services, Harding, Shymanski & Co., PC, Evansville, IN. She is author of an authoritative book on tax deductions.

A four-year college education at a public institution now costs around $50,000. It's more than $105,000 for a private school. Fortunately, the tax law provides special tax breaks—exclusions, deductions and credits—for education expenses. Don't miss any that apply to you or your family.

EMPLOYER AID

You can exclude from taxable income up to $5,250 of employer-provided tuition reimbursement each year—even if the courses are not job related.

This break now applies to college courses *and* graduate school. In the past, only college-level courses were covered. *Special rules...*

•**Job-related courses.** There's no annual dollar restriction on the exclusion when your employer pays the cost of job-related courses. The benefit is fully excludable from your taxable income (it is treated as a "working condition" fringe benefit).

•**Out-of-pocket expenses.** When you take courses to maintain or improve job skills—or

315

Your Life

as a condition of your employment—you can deduct your out-of-pocket expenses (including transportation to and from school). This write-off is a miscellaneous itemized expense and is deductible to the extent it exceeds 2% of adjusted gross income (AGI).

- **Tuition reduction.** If you work for an educational institution, you, your spouse and even your children may be eligible for reduced tuition for undergraduate courses. This benefit is tax free to you.

This exclusion applies to tuition reduction at your employer's institution or at another institution under a reciprocal agreement. Ask your employer whether tuition at another institution is covered by such an agreement.

STUDENT LOAN INTEREST

Personal interest (other than home mortgage interest) generally is *not* deductible. However, a special rule applies to interest on student loans.

Up to $2,500 of interest you pay on loans for higher education is deductible each year —if your income falls within limits (outlined below). The deduction is taken above the line, meaning you can claim it whether or not you itemize your deductions.

Income limits: Deductibility of education interest depends on your AGI. Higher income limits than in the past now apply.

You can take the full deduction so long as your AGI doesn't exceed $50,000 ($100,000 on a joint return). The deduction phases out for singles with AGI between $50,000 and $65,000. For married couples filing jointly, the phaseout range is AGI between $100,000 and $130,000.

You get no deduction if your AGI exceeds $65,000 ($130,000 on a joint return).

In the past, only interest paid within the first 60 months of the loan was deductible. Now, there is no time limit.

EDUCATION EXPENSES

Through 2005, you can deduct some of your tuition and fees (although not room and board) —if your income isn't too high. The deduction is taken above the line, as is the student loan interest deduction.

For 2003: The maximum deduction is $3,000. You can take the maximum as long as your AGI is not more than $65,000 for a single return ($130,000 on a joint return).

Caution: Even one dollar of excess AGI means no deduction. There's no phaseout for this, as with student loan interest.

For 2004 and 2005: The deduction cap is $4,000. The same AGI limit mentioned above applies. However, for those with AGI between $65,000 and $80,000 (over $130,000 but not over $160,000 on a joint return), a deduction of $2,000 can be claimed.

Caution: You can't claim this deduction in a year in which you take an education credit (see below). Also, a dependent cannot claim this deduction. For example, your college-age child who pays some of his/her tuition cannot claim a deduction if you claim the child as a dependent.

US SAVINGS BONDS

Interest on Series EE or I bonds that are redeemed to pay higher college tuition and fees can be excluded from income. *The following requirements must be met...*

- **The bonds must have been purchased after 1989.**
- **The bond owner must have been at least age 24** when the bonds were purchased.
- **The redemption proceeds must be used to pay tuition and fees for yourself,** your spouse or dependent. (A grandparent cannot use this exclusion unless he claims the grandchild as a dependent.)
- **The bond owner's AGI cannot exceed set limits** in the year the bonds are redeemed. For 2003, the AGI limits are $58,500 ($87,750 on a joint return). The exclusion phases out for AGI between $58,500 and $73,500 ($87,750 and $117,750 on a joint return). You can't claim an exclusion if AGI exceeds $73,500 ($117,750 on a joint return).

For 2004, the AGI limits are $59,850 ($89,750 on a joint return). The phaseout is between $59,850 and $74,850 ($89,750 and $119,750 on a joint return). You can't claim an exclusion if AGI exceeds $74,850 ($119,750 on a joint return).

SCHOLARSHIPS, ETC.

If you are a degree candidate, scholarship, fellowship and grant money covering tuition, fees and supplies is tax free. But payments for room and board (and all payments for nondegree candidates) are fully taxable.

EDUCATION CREDITS

You can reduce your tax bill dollar for dollar if you qualify for an education credit.

•**Hope credit.** This tax credit applies only to tuition and fees for the first two years of schooling after high school. It is limited to $1,500 per year per student (100% of the first $1,000 of eligible expenses, plus 50% of the next $1,000 of eligible expenses).

•**Lifetime Learning credit.** This credit is 20% of the first $10,000 of tuition and fees, or $2,000. It applies *per return* (regardless of the number of people in the family attending college or graduate school).

Limits: The same AGI limits apply to both of these credits. For 2003, you can take the full credit only if your AGI does not go over $41,000 ($83,000 on a joint return). The credit phases out for AGI between $41,000 and $51,000 ($83,000 and $103,000 on a joint return). No credit can be claimed if your AGI exceeds $51,000 ($103,000 on a joint return).

For 2004, the full credit applies if AGI doesn't go over $42,000 ($85,000 on a joint return). The phase out is between $42,000 and $52,000 ($85,000 and $105,000 on a joint return). No credit can be claimed when your AGI exceeds $52,000 ($105,000 on a joint return).

Important: The credit can be claimed by either parent or child—regardless of which person actually pays the expenses. But the parent must waive the dependency exemption for the child to enable the child to claim the credit.

GIFTS OF TUITION PAYMENTS

Payments made directly to an educational institution for someone else's tuition are treated as a tax-free gift.

In addition to these amounts, you can give that person up to $11,000 in 2003 and 2004 completely free of gift tax.

This "directly paid" break applies not only to college tuition, but also to tuition for any level of schooling, from preschool on.

HELP FROM THE IRS

See IRS Publication 508, *Tax Benefits for Work-Related Education;* IRS Publication 520, *Scholarships and Fellowships;* and IRS Publication 970, *Tax Benefits for Higher Education* at *www.irs.gov.*

When Education Expenses Are Deductible

Education expenses are deductible if they help in your current line of work—but not if they qualify you for a new one.

Recent case: A woman with 25 years' experience as a law school librarian obtained a law degree. She deducted the degree as a business expense, saying that it helped her work as a legal librarian.

Tax Court: Deduction disallowed. The degree was not required for the job. It also qualified her for a new line of work as a lawyer—and education that qualifies one for a new line of work is not deductible.

Stephen Galligan, et ux., TC Memo 2002-150.

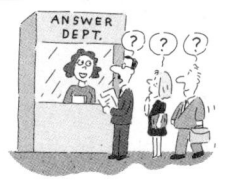

Financial Aid Basics

Need-based college financial aid packages are awarded for one academic year at a time. The student must reapply each year.

To maximize aid: Control your income. While you shouldn't turn down a salary raise, avoid transactions that could inflate discretionary income, such as taking capital gains or early withdrawals from retirement plans. If a parent is divorced or widowed, remarriage could affect a student's future eligibility.

Also: Schools require a minimum grade point average for eligibility.

Kalman Chany, president, Campus Consultants, Inc., 1202 Lexington Ave., New York City 10028.

■ *Your Life* ■ ■ ■ ■

Where to Find Financial Aid for Adult Students

Raymond D. Loewe, CLU, ChFC, Financial Resources Network, a financial planning firm, and president, College Money, which provides financial aid solutions for higher education, both are located at 112-B Centre Blvd., Marlton, NJ 08053.

Getting sufficient financial aid for graduate school is tough—tuition and other costs are as much as $45,000 a year, and most aid is awarded based on merit, not need.

MERIT-BASED AID

There is more than $1 billion available annually in aid, but much of it is never even tapped. *Consider...*

• **Grants and fellowships.** They will often cover full tuition, plus a stipend. *Resources...*

• *Peterson's Grants for Graduate & Postdoctoral Study* (Peterson's Guides).

• *Yale Daily News Guide to Fellowships and Grants,* by Justin Cohen (Kaplan).

• *www.career.cornell.edu/students/grad/fellowships/fellowshipTOC.html,* Cornell University's career services Web site.

• The National Association of Graduate and Professional Students, 209 Pennsylvania Ave. SE, Washington, DC 20003, 888-886-2477, *www.nagps.org.*

• **Scholarships are usually annual awards.** Avoid fee-based scholarship matching services. You can obtain the same information from the Internet or the library.

Resource: The Graduate Student's Complete Scholarship Book (SourceBooks).

• **Graduate assistantships.** Stipends and/or tuition rebates for teaching or research.

Resource: The searchable job bank at *www.ujobbank.com/index.html.*

NEED-BASED AID

You are most likely to qualify for grants and loans if you are single, unemployed and returning as a full-time student. You will need to fill out the *Free Application for Federal Student Aid* (FAFSA) form, plus any other forms the schools require. If you work part-time or you and your spouse have amassed significant savings, you probably won't qualify for aid.

Resource: For information on how graduate financial need is calculated as well as Web links to financial aid offices—check out the Web site, *www.finaid.org.*

GOVERNMENT LOANS

These loans have better terms than private loans for graduate school...

• **Stafford Loan Program.** Up to $18,500 annually is available to graduate students.

Information: Federal Student Aid Information Center, Box 84, Washington, DC 20044, 800-433-3243, *www.studentaid.ed.gov.*

• **Sallie Mae.** Federally guaranteed student loans for more than seven million borrowers. 888-272-5543, *www.salliemae.com.*

• **The Education Resources Institute.** This nonprofit organization provides loans for part-time students. *www.teri.org.*

More from Raymond Loewe...

How to Use Life Insurance To Pay for College

Life insurance can pay for college—if the policy is properly structured. The savings component of a variable life policy allows a portion of the premiums to be invested tax-deferred. The value built up through this investment can be tapped by a tax-free loan to pay for college costs. The death benefit, which is free of income tax, repays the loans.

Caution: The investment value can go up or down based on market conditions. Consult an insurance agent or financial adviser to be sure the policy is set up correctly.

Also from Raymond Loewe...

Better Investing for College

Invest at least 80% of money earmarked for college expenses in stocks until your child reaches age 15. At that point, reallocate 25% to cash and short- and intermediate-term bond funds...leave 75% in stocks. Each subsequent year, move another 25%, so that by age 18, all these funds are in short- and intermediate-term bond funds.

Planning for College

Finally from Raymond Loewe...

If You're Falling Behind On Tuition...

If you're behind on tuition payments, be sure to take the following measures...

•**Contact the school's financial aid officer immediately.** Schools don't want students to drop out for lack of money. They will work to find solutions. *Examples...*

•Switch from annual to monthly payments to spread out the charges. Do this through the financial aid officer or an outside service, such as Academic Management Services (888-664-6082 or *www.tuitionpay.com*), which charges an average annual enrollment fee of $55.*

•Arrange for extensions on your tuition bills.

•**Seek tuition assistance from federal loan programs** (800-433-3243 or *www.fafsa.ed.gov*). Federal Plus loans are unsubsidized loans to parents that may be used to refinance existing loans.

•**Turn to a home-equity loan only after you have exhausted all options,** since it puts your home at risk.

*Fee varies by college.

education expenses. The 529 plan's assets also become subject to the claims of the successor owner's creditors in all but eight states (Colorado, Louisiana, Maine, Nebraska, Ohio, Pennsylvania, Virginia and Wisconsin). Consult your financial adviser for more information.

Jane King, financial adviser, Fairfield Financial Advisors, Wellesley, MA.

What You Should Know About College Insurance

College-withdrawal insurance usually is not worth the cost. It will refund tuition payments if a student leaves school—but *only* if he/she withdraws because of injury or physical illness. Mental illness is covered at 60%. There is no coverage for dropping out because of bad grades or a change of mind. The insurance is offered by around 170 colleges.

Cost: About $200 to $300 a year.

Best for: Athletes and students suffering from chronic illnesses.

Judy C. Miller, CFP, financial planner and principal, College Solutions, Alameda, CA, *www.4collegesolutions.com*.

Protect College Savings

A trust should own your 529 college savings plan if your state allows it. Currently, several states do—including Alaska, California, Connecticut, Idaho, Missouri, Montana, Rhode Island, Vermont and Virginia. More states are planning to allow it.

If a trust owns the 529, the donor has full control over the timing and purpose of any distributions even after he/she dies. If a trust does *not* own the plan and the plan owner dies, the assets pass to a successor owner, who is usually designated by the original owner. The successor owner then can withdraw funds at any time for any purpose, subject to a 10% penalty if the funds are not used for the beneficiary's

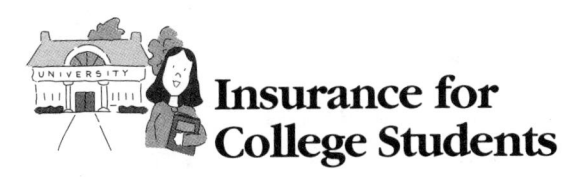

Insurance for College Students

If you have a child in college, be sure he/she has adequate insurance coverage...

•**Renter's insurance** protects personal property in a dorm room or off-campus residence. Some parents' homeowner's policies cover students in college housing but not off-campus.

•**Health insurance.** Parents' policies usually cover a child until age 23 if he qualifies as a dependent. But they may cover only emergency care if the student no longer lives in the local network area. Many colleges now offer insurance for students.

■ *Your Life* ■ ■ ■ ■

●**Auto insurance** varies based on where a student attends school and whether he drives his own or a family car. Ask your insurance agent for specifics.

Christina M. Povenmire, CFP, principal, CMP Financial Planning, 3960 Lytham Ct., Columbus, OH 43220.

Save on College Textbooks

Before classes start, find out from the instructor which textbooks are required. If a book is a new printing but not a new edition, look for a used copy. Ask the instructor for names of last year's students...or use an on-line search engine to find sources of second-hand textbooks. If a book is a new edition with minimal updates, ask the instructor if he/she would be willing to create and hand out a synopsis of the new material for students who own older editions. If you must buy the book, check prices on-line at such Web sites as *www.amazon.com...www.studentmarket.com ...*and *www.barnesandnoble.com.*

Edward Fischer, PhD, psychologist in private practice, Jersey City.

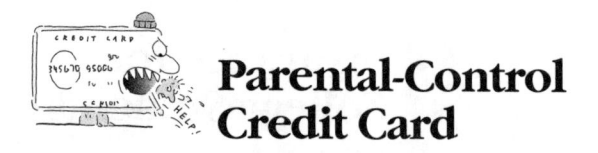

Parental-Control Credit Card

A parental-control credit card can help a college student learn to handle credit responsibly. With a MasterCard offered by College Parents of America and MBNA, parents set a credit limit and then can use the Internet or a toll-free phone number to watch their student's use of the card. They also can choose to receive the bill. The card has no annual fee and charges 11.99%* interest. It is sent directly to parents, so they can discuss credit issues before handing it over.

More information: 800-932-2775 or *www. collegeparents.org.*

Nancy Deevers, director of education and community relations at Consumer Credit Counseling Service of Northeastern Ohio, Cleveland.

*At press time.

Smart Financial Aid Strategies

Nancy Dunnan, financial adviser and author in New York City. Her latest book is *How to Invest $50–$5,000* (HarperCollins).

Most colleges use a standard financial aid formula that requires parents to contribute 5.6% of their assets per year (while their child is actually in college) toward tuition. The child, on the other hand, is required to fork over a whopping 35% of assets held in his/her name.

So if you are planning to apply for financial aid, you will want to minimize the amount of money held in your child's name. Keep in mind that money in a Coverdell education savings account (once known as the education IRA) is counted as the student's asset. Money in a *state* 529 college savings plan, on the other hand, is treated as the parents' asset.

If your parents want to help pay for your child's college tuition, they should pay the school directly or gift you the money. Check with your accountant first.

More information: *www.collegeboard.com.*

■■■■■ Your Life ■

21

Self-Defense for Tricky Times

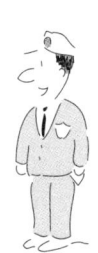

The Best Way to Protect Your Family Against Terrorism

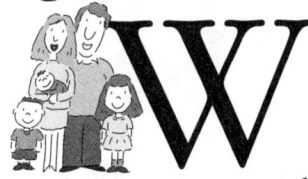

With the continuing threat of terrorism, many Americans are unsure how to prepare for a possible attack. *Terrorism specialist Michael Shannon, MD, gives his advice...*

If disaster does strike, tune in to the radio or TV to learn whether it's safe to evacuate and what routes to take. The authorities will alert the public if a nuclear, chemical or biological attack has been waged.

All families should have an agreed-upon meeting place near their home, in case it's not reachable...and an out-of-state contact whom family members can phone to find out each other's location. (Local phone lines are often jammed in an emergency, while long-distance lines are likely to remain open.)

Keep an "evacuation kit" packed and ready to go. Store it in your home in a secure and accessible place, such as a closet or under a bed. It should include prescription medications ...flashlight and battery-powered radio, plus extra batteries...first-aid kit...bottled water...a change of clothes and a sleeping bag and pillow for each household member—preferably in airtight plastic bags...and key family documents, such as photo identification and Social Security cards.

If evacuation is impossible, you'll be forced to seek shelter in your home or office. *In addition to your "evacuation kit," keep the following "shelter kit" items on hand in your home and office...*

A three-day supply of water in plastic containers (one gallon of water per person per day) ...a three-day supply of canned or other nonperishable foods, utensils and a nonelectric can

---

Michael Shannon, MD, member of the American Academy of Pediatrics Task Force on Terrorism. He is also associate professor of pediatrics at Harvard Medical School, and the acting chief of emergency medicine at Children's Hospital, both in Boston.

■ *Your Life* ■ ■ ■ ■

opener...duct tape and plastic sheeting...and prescription and nonprescription medicines, including aspirin or other pain relievers, antidiarrhea medication and antacids.

Here are the specific steps for different types of terrorist attacks...

NUCLEAR ATTACK

The American Thyroid Association recommends keeping a supply of potassium iodide on hand if your community is within 50 miles of a nuclear power plant. Potassium iodide is an antidote to the radioactive iodine that is released in a nuclear disaster. Without this antidote, anyone exposed to radiation will be at high risk for thyroid cancer.

Some on-line pharmacies offer potassium iodide pills over the counter for about $10 per 14 pills. (Be wary of so-called "crisis kits," which can cost three times this amount.) Pills should be taken within three hours after radiation exposure.

In the instance of a nuclear emergency, brick or stone buildings provide better shelter than wood. Get into a basement, if possible, or an interior room. Stay away from windows.

If you are exposed to radiation, get out of your clothes right away and seal them in a plastic bag. Discard the clothing outside your home. Removing clothing typically reduces contamination levels by more than 90%. Be sure to take a shower. Then change into some clean clothes.

What won't help: A home Geiger counter.

Reason: Many smoke detectors and other household devices emit low levels of radiation that activate Geiger counters.

CHEMICAL ATTACK

If you have been exposed to some chemical agent, such as nerve gas, mustard gas or chlorine, quickly undress, wash and change your clothes, if you are able. Many chemical agents are absorbed through the skin within minutes. If you're unable to wash your skin with water, wipe or blot it thoroughly with a clean cloth.

When seeking shelter from a chemical attack, do *not* go to a basement. Many chemical agents are heavier than air and will collect in the lower floors. Retreat to a windowless interior room, on the second story, or higher, if possible.

To protect your respiratory tract, put a wet towel under the door of your interior room and seal the edges of the door with duct tape. If you're in a bathroom, close the sink and bathtub drains.

Seek medical attention as soon as possible. Unlike radiation poisoning, the toxic effects of chemical exposure start causing damage immediately. If you can leave your home safely, go to the closest health care facility.

What won't help: Gas masks.

Reason: Gas masks are effective only when they are put on *before* exposure occurs—meaning you would have to carry one with you at all times.

BIOLOGICAL ATTACK

An attack with a biological agent, such as anthrax, smallpox or plague, is the most difficult to protect against. That's because there's typically an incubation period, ranging from hours to days, between exposure and the emergence of symptoms.

If you suspect that you or a family member has been exposed to a biological agent, seek medical care promptly. Since the medical community is the main line of defense against bioterrorism, your local hospital should have a plan for disseminating appropriate medication in case of emergency. Ask the safety officer at your local hospital what plans are in place to deal with a bioterrorism attack.

What won't help: Unless you are a health care worker or a member of the military, the Centers for Disease Control and Prevention recommends against smallpox vaccination.

Reason: For the average citizen, the current level of risk does not warrant exposure to the vaccine's potential for side effects.

Do *not* stockpile antibiotics in your home. Not all biological agents respond to the same antibiotic, so the chances of your choosing exactly the right one are slim. Antibiotics also have a limited shelf life.

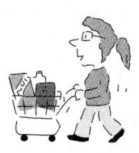

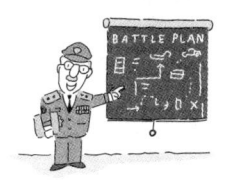

How to Cope With the Threat of Terrorism

Gavin de Becker, CEO, Gavin de Becker and Associates, a consulting firm that advises such clients as the US Supreme Court and Central Intelligence Agency on how to assess threats and deal with violent behavior, Studio City, CA. He is author of the best-selling *The Gift of Fear* (Dell) and *Fear Less* (Little Brown).

Don't let the continued threat of terrorism cheat you out of the daily pleasures of living your life.

You take all sorts of risks when you drive. If you focused only on the risks, you would never leave home. Instead, you compartmentalize the danger so that you can drive when you need to.

Do the same thing with the risk of terrorism. Could someone launch a nuclear attack on the US? Sure. Could an asteroid hit Earth? Absolutely. But the odds are overwhelming that neither will happen anytime soon.

Here's how to feel safe in an unsafe world...

•**Don't believe you are powerless.** Before September 11, 2001, Americans were under the illusion that we were safe from all of our foreign enemies.

We have replaced that illusion with another one—*powerlessness*.

We fear that our enemies can attack us at any time, in any place, and there is nothing our government can do to stop them.

The reality is that our government continues to be on high alert against terrorists. So are 250 million Americans.

Examples: Passengers intervened to stop attacks on four different Greyhound buses. In addition, a terrorist transporting a bomb in his shoe on an international flight was seized by other passengers.

When we act like victims, we give in to our imaginations.

•**Put the risk of terrorist violence in perspective.** It is natural to see the latest risk as the greatest risk. Putting things in perspective helps us see that the newest risk—while threatening—is just one of many risks we face each day.

The violence unleashed against the US was shocking because it was so unexpected and killed so many people at one time.

But our lives are filled with dangers. During the next 24 hours, 400 Americans will be killed or wounded by gunfire. That statistic is not meant to instill alarm—only to put things into perspective.

Smoking kills more people every day than lightning does in a decade. But there are people who ease their fear of being struck by lightning during a storm by smoking a cigarette. It isn't logical—but anxieties rarely are.

I have friends who were afraid to visit Egypt because of the threat of terrorism. So they stayed home in Detroit, where the homicide rate is many times higher than in Cairo.

•**Turn off the news.** TV news presents us with alarming images that take our worst fears a step further than we had imagined. When you turn off the tube, you'll quickly find out, as I have, that you're not missing anything.

Get your information from the print media. Even though articles and photos can paint vivid pictures, they are usually less alarming than video images.

TV connects you to nothing except the illusion that you "know" the news anchors and reporters. Establish real connections and reduce anxiety by talking with friends, family members, neighbors and coworkers.

•**Recognize the power of your natural survival instinct.** Each of us has an astonishing innate defense system. It is built around our intuition, which can protect us more effectively than any other force on earth.

Thanks to intuition, we know when we're in danger even when we don't know why. It may not be immediately clear where the danger lies. But intuition lets us know that there *is* danger and we need to protect ourselves.

Example: The intuition of just one man helped defeat one of the most serious terrorist threats the US has ever faced. In 1942, German saboteurs landed on Long Island, New York. They planned to panic Americans by bombing department stores and bridges. When John

■ *Your Life* ■ ■ ■ ■

Cullen, a local Coast Guardsman, was strolling on the beach and saw the men, his intuition told him something wasn't right. He alerted the authorities. The German agents were arrested before they could carry out their plans.

The tragedy of September 11 alerted Americans to pay attention to their intuition. That alone will make our nation safer—not only from terrorism, but from all types of crime.

In Case of a Terrorist Attack...

In the event of a terrorist attack, the average American needs enough cash on hand to cover a few days' worth of expenses. Withdrawing large amounts from the bank is unnecessary. Even after the September 11 terrorist attacks, electronic payment systems and banks functioned normally. For extra security, also carry a major credit card.

Steve Rhode, president and cofounder of Myvesta.org, a financial management organization in Rockville, MD.

Protect Yourself From Terrorist Bombs

William F. McCarthy, PhD, president, Threat Research Inc., an Alexandria, VA–based international security consulting firm that provides threat analysis and disaster recovery planning. When he was commander of the New York Police Department (NYPD) Bomb Squad, he implemented bomb security plans for anniversary celebrations at the United Nations and Statue of Liberty.

Small bombs are most terrorists' weapon of choice around the world. They are cheap and easy to hide, and their damage draws media attention. As a former commander of the NYPD Bomb Squad—the largest civilian bomb unit in the US—I assure you that your chances of being a victim are tiny.

This does not mean you should be complacent. *Here are measures to increase safety...*

• **Be vigilant about unattended bags**—even if the person just seems to step away for a moment. In Israel, people aggressively confront anyone who tries to leave a bag. I don't suggest that, but distance yourself from a suspicious package. An attaché case can hold 10 to 25 pounds of explosives with a fragmentation radius of several hundred feet. If you are waiting on a train platform, walk to the far end of the platform.

• **Alert law enforcement immediately.** Many people are afraid or embarrassed to create false alarms. The truth is, law-enforcement officers need your help to watch for threats. Be specific. Tell the closest officer, "Excuse me, I noticed an unattended bag there. It's a green duffel bag, and I am suspicious."

• **Put a solid structure between you and the suspected bomb/bomber.** Most victims of bombings die or are injured from flying debris —not the blast. As you move away quickly, try to turn a corner or walk behind a concrete pillar. Don't stand near windows.

• **Avoid rush hour.** The hours from 7 am to 10 am and 4 pm to 7 pm provide a maximum amount of victims for bombings and suicide bombers. Law enforcement's ability to watch so many people is strained, so the likelihood of detection drops.

If you have a long wait for a train or public transportation, stay away from the crowds and areas of congestion. Sit in a nearby coffee shop if possible.

New Security Measures in Apartment Buildings

Building landlords are stepping up security measures in light of recent antiterrorism warnings. The FBI is advising that landlords screen apartment applicants more carefully by requiring original identification (not photocopies), passports and/or visas and Social Security numbers. Landlords are advised to closely monitor boiler rooms, maintenance areas and other spots that are off-limits to the tenants... inspect packages brought in by nonresidents ...and not allow food deliveries directly to apartments. Tenants will be asked to alert the building security or police about any suspicious activity they see.

Jay Harris, vice president of property management, National Multi Housing Council, Washington, DC.

The Smallpox Threat: What You Need to Know

Joanne Cono, MD, medical epidemiologist with the Bioterrorism Preparedness and Response Program of the Centers for Disease Control and Prevention in Atlanta.

Almost one-half million emergency and military personnel in the US have been vaccinated for smallpox. The complication rate has been relatively low, but dozens of people have suffered serious side effects, including heart problems.

The vaccine is not yet available to the general public, but it may be in 2004.

Smallpox expert Dr. Joanne Cono answers the most pressing questions...

•**How deadly is smallpox?** Smallpox kills about one-third of the people who contract it.

•**How is it spread?** The disease is transmitted via airborne droplets when an infected person coughs, sneezes or talks. It also may be spread by contaminated clothing or bedding.

Smallpox becomes contagious only after the appearance of its symptoms—high fever, body aches, vomiting—which occur seven to 17 days after exposure.

The sufferer is most contagious when he/she has a rash, which first appears as flat, red spots. Within two days, these lesions become filled with clear fluid and then with pus. The pustules leave severe, pitted scars.

•**How would the government deal with a smallpox terrorist attack?** In the event of an attack, anyone exposed to the virus or in contact with victims would be vaccinated.

Vaccination within three days after exposure prevents the illness or greatly diminishes its severity. The vaccine probably still offers some protection if taken within seven days after exposure. This "ring vaccination" approach eradicated smallpox outbreaks worldwide.

Large-scale vaccination also might be initiated in the event of an attack. There is enough vaccine to immunize the entire US population.

If there is an outbreak of smallpox, public health authorities will inform the public about the necessary actions to take, including if vaccination is necessary. There would be many official announcements and updates. People who contract smallpox would be isolated in hospital rooms so they would get health care without infecting others.

•**Can you tell us more about the vaccination program that is now under way?** One vaccination program is for members of emergency "smallpox response" teams. These teams would care for patients and provide other critical services should an attack occur. Military personnel also are being vaccinated. Emergency workers, such as firefighters and police, will be the next group vaccinated.

•**Can I get vaccinated if I'm not in one of these groups?** Only if you wish to participate in clinical trials of the next generation of the vaccine. To find these trials, visit *www.clinicaltrials.gov.*

•**Is the vaccine that is used today the same as the original vaccine?** The vaccine today is a variant of the original, which was developed at the end of the 18th century by an English country physician Edward Jenner. He noticed that milkmaids who contracted a related but mild disease called cowpox were immune to smallpox. Using blood from people who had had cowpox, Jenner developed the vaccine.

Today's vaccine contains the live *vaccinia* virus, which is similar to the cowpox virus. It is administered through small punctures in the skin and provides nearly 100% protection against smallpox.

•**Is the vaccine safe? What about side effects?** Most people have a sore arm, slight fever and body aches after smallpox vaccination. About one-third are sick enough to miss a day or two of work or school. An estimated one in 1,000 people vaccinated will have serious reactions, such as encephalitis, which could

■ *Your Life* ■ ■ ■ ■

require medical attention. Between 14 and 52 people per million may have potentially life-threatening reactions, such as tissue destruction by the virus, that require immediate medical care. One or two will die.

•**Can I get smallpox from the vaccine?** The vaccine does not contain the actual virus that causes smallpox, therefore it cannot give you the disease.

•**After I am vaccinated, can I spread the *vaccinia* virus to others?** Because the vaccine contains live virus, it potentially can be transmitted for two to three weeks after vaccination. Someone would have to come into physical contact with the virus—touch it—in order to catch it.

To prevent spreading the *vaccinia* virus, keep the site of vaccination covered with a gauze bandage, which needs to be changed every one or two days. Wash your hands with soap and warm water after contact with the vaccination site. Maintain these precautions until the scab forms and falls off—usually in two to three weeks.

If someone does pick up the *vaccinia* virus from someone who was vaccinated—and if that person develops a *vaccinia* mark that forms a scab—it is presumed that person has become protected from smallpox as well.

•**I was vaccinated against smallpox years ago and had chicken pox as a child. Am I immune?** If you were vaccinated as a child or later, you have little, if any, immunity left. Chicken pox is unrelated to smallpox and so confers no protection.

•**Is vaccination especially dangerous for some people?** The risk of serious harm is increased if you are being treated—or live with someone being treated—with immune-suppressing drugs, such as those used in cancer chemotherapy...for autoimmune diseases like rheumatoid arthritis...or as part of organ-transplant care.

Vaccination is dangerous if you—or someone you live with—have had eczema (atopic dermatitis), even if it hasn't come back since you were a child...an *active* skin condition, such as shingles, impetigo, severe acne or psoriasis...an immune system weakened by HIV infection...or are pregnant or trying to become pregnant. If you are breast-feeding, it is dangerous for you to be vaccinated, but those living with you can be vaccinated. If you fall into one of these groups, you should not be vaccinated unless exposed to smallpox.

For more information, go to *www.bt.cdc.gov/agent/smallpox*.

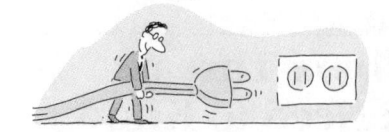

Fire Chief Reveals Most Common Causes of Household Fires

Russell E. Sanders, executive secretary, Metropolitan Fire Chiefs Section, National Fire Protection Association, Quincy, MA, *www.nfpa.org*. Mr. Sanders, a firefighter for 30 years, retired as chief of the Louisville, KY, Fire Department in 1995.

During my 30-year fire fighting career, I frequently responded to home fires that caused less than $500 in property damage—but the occupants still died from smoke inhalation.

When I was chief of the Louisville, KY, fire department, we passed an ordinance requiring all homes to have smoke detectors. Over the next three years, fire deaths dropped by 30%.

The most common causes of household fires and how to prevent them...

COOKING

Cooking is the number one cause of home fires. People often worry about grease fires. These can be very dangerous—but if you do not panic, you can extinguish one easily by sliding a lid over the flaming pan and then turning off the heat.

Caution: Do not use baking soda, flour or salt to try to smother the flames. It can cause the fire to flare and burn you. Don't use a fire extinguisher. It may send the burning grease out of the pan onto towels, curtains, cabinets, etc.

Another big danger is unattended cooking. Someone may turn on the stove to simmer a pot of stew or soup, then take a nap or run errands. The contents start to burn, and the flames ignite nearby combustibles.

Example: Bean soup seemed to be popular when I was a novice firefighter in the 1960s. We could smell it blocks away when it burned and caused a house fire.

Stay safe: Never leave the house when something is cooking. You could be delayed—and your house could burn to the ground before you get home.

When preparing slow-cooking foods, set a timer for 15- or 30-minute intervals. This will remind you to check the stove.

SMOKING

Fires caused by cigarettes, pipes and cigars are among the deadliest. Smokers fall asleep and drop them—and don't wake up when the fire starts. People also dump their ashtrays in the trash without making sure that the butts are completely extinguished.

Stay safe: Never smoke in bed, especially if you have been drinking alcohol. Always extinguish smoking materials completely—don't just give them a quick stub in the ashtray. Run water over ashtray contents before throwing them away.

Better still, quit the habit—or at least don't smoke in the house.

CLOTHES DRYERS

There are more than 14,000 clothes-dryer fires each year. The number one cause is lack of maintenance—lint collects and catches fire.

Another cause is stacking laundry or other combustibles near the dryer, especially around gas dryers that have open flames.

Stay safe: Clean the dryer filter after every use. Once a year, detach the hosing from the back of the machine and clean it. Keep combustibles three feet or more from any heat-generating equipment, including clothes dryers ...electric, gas and kerosene heaters...furnaces ...and water heaters.

CANDLES

Candles cause more than 12,000 home fires annually. About half of those fires start in a bedroom. A burning candle can fall over and set fire to furniture, curtains, carpets or other combustible materials.

Stay safe: Put candles in sturdy holders that won't tip over. Don't assume that a candle in a glass holder is safe. The glass might break. Clear the surrounding area of all flammable objects. Blow out candles before leaving the room or going to sleep.

ELECTRICAL WIRES

People often assume that most electrical fires start inside the walls. While it can happen when wiring is old or improperly installed, *visible* wires usually cause the trouble.

Example: When inspecting homes after fires, I often saw an unbelievable arrangement of tangled extension cords—sometimes eight lamps or appliances were plugged into a single outlet. The overheated wires sparked the fire.

Stay safe: Don't use more than one extension cord per outlet. And only use cords with a testing laboratory label attached—this means that safety professionals have determined that the cord is safe for its intended use.

When using power tools or appliances, be sure to check the manuals for the proper extension cord size to use.

Never run extension cords under carpets or rugs. Pressure from walking can fray the wires and cause them to spark.

COMBUSTIBLE FUMES

Gasoline fumes are more combustible than the gasoline itself. Unvented vapors can be ignited by a source that is a long distance from the actual fuel.

One of the worst fires I ever saw occurred when a man brought his motorcycle into the house and was cleaning it with gasoline. The water heater ignited the vapors—and both of his small children died in the flames. That happened on Mother's Day in the 1970s, and I will never forget it.

Stay safe: Gasoline and other flammable products, such as paint thinner, should never be kept inside the house. Only use these products for their intended purposes.

Example: Never use gasoline as a cleaning agent. Store all rags that have been used

■ *Your Life* ■ ■ ■ ■

with a flammable product in a metal container that has a tight-fitting lid.

If you have a kerosene heater, don't store extra kerosene in the house. And don't refill the heaters when they are hot or in use. Spilled kerosene can spread a fire almost instantly.

Open doors and windows before using any flammable substance, including paint, polyurethane and chemical cleaning agents.

MORE ADVICE

•**Install smoke and carbon monoxide detectors all over the house,** certainly on every floor and especially in or near bedrooms. People might believe that they will wake up if they smell smoke—but the carbon monoxide in smoke *deepens* sleep.

•**Keep fire extinguishers in the kitchen and garage.** Purchase extinguishers that are labeled "ABC." These put out common household fires, including those involving wood, paper, gas and electricity. Make sure that everyone in your family knows how to use them.

•**Identify two exits from each room in the house whenever possible.** The whole family should practice exiting. Quiz your children periodically to help them remember.

Helpful: Keep chain ladders in bedrooms on the second and third floors. But be aware that these are too heavy for young children to put in place.

•**Establish a meeting place**—in the yard or other safe location outside the house—where everyone should meet if there is a fire.

I responded to one fire in which a mother got out of the house through the front door. When she couldn't find her children outside, she ran back in the house to find them. She died in the fire, while her children were safe in the backyard.

Protect Your Children

To increase the odds of finding a lost child quickly, take these measures...

•**Dress him/her in bright clothes.**

•**Keep a recent color photo of him** in your wallet or purse.

•**Carry a description**—height, weight, hair and eye color, birthmarks—and update it every six months.

•**Sew small tags with his name,** address and phone number inside the tongues of his shoes or inside clothing.

•**Make sure your child knows where you are staying when on vacation**—and give him the address in writing.

Jean O'Neil, research director, National Crime Prevention Council, Washington, DC, *www.ncpc.org*.

Choosing a Home-Security System

Clark Howard, self-made millionaire and author of *Get Clark Smart: The Ultimate Guide to Getting Rich from America's Money-Saving Expert* (Hyperion). He also hosts *The Clark Howard Show,* a nationally syndicated radio program on consumer advice.

Before purchasing a home-security system, be sure you take a look at these helpful tips...

•**Select a company that doesn't require you to sign a contract.** But if you must sign one, never agree to more than one year. And be sure the contract doesn't have a "rollover" clause that renews automatically.

•**Monitoring should not cost more than $15 to $20 a month.**

•**When shopping for a new company,** start with those at the end of the *Yellow Pages* ads. These are usually less expensive and less likely to require a contract.

•**Get smoke and fire monitoring as part of the system.** It's relatively cheap and fire is usually a bigger danger than burglary.

•**Never lease an alarm system.** If it's a good one, you'll want it for the long term.

Is Someone Watching You?

Assume you are being videotaped anytime you go outside your home. The average big-city resident is caught on videotape 75 times a day. Cameras are so small and well-concealed that experts usually can't spot them. They are common in the workplace and stores —but not in areas where people disrobe. By law, hotels can't use cameras to spy on guests in their rooms, but managers often hide them there to catch employees stealing. There are electronic devices that can detect hidden cameras, but they can cost upward of $2,500.

Arielle Jamil, vice president of product management, The Counter Spy Shops, New York City–based manufacturer and retailer of security, surveillance and countermeasure equipment, www.spyzone.com.

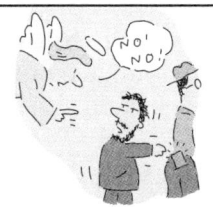

Pickpocket Protection

Be aware of this typical distraction technique used by pickpockets. Three or more people frequently are involved. One drops something in front of a victim or simply stops and blocks him/her. The second person picks the pocket or purse and hands the valuables to the third person, who very quickly gets away in the crowd.

Common distractions: Asking for directions...touching or bumping...faking an accident or fight...or forcing the victim to squeeze by while getting on or off a train, bus, subway or escalator.

Jens Jurgen, editor, TravelCompanions.com, Box 833, Amityville, NY 11701, www.travelcompanions.com.

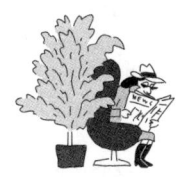

What to Do When Pulled Over by the Police

If pulled over by police, remain in your car unless you are told to get out. Be polite, but don't volunteer information. If the officer asks if you know why you were stopped, say you are not sure—if you say you were speeding or ran a stop sign, it will be used against you. If the officer says you were speeding, say, "I see" or don't respond. Don't argue. Don't hesitate to sign a ticket—doing so just acknowledges receipt but does not admit guilt.

Eric Skrum, communications director, National Motorists Association, Waunakee, WI, www.motorists.org.

How to Avoid Identity Theft...and What to Do If You've Been Victimized

Frank W. Abagnale, president, Abagnale & Associates, secure-technology consultants, 601 Pennsylvania Ave. NW, Suite 900, South Bldg., Washington, DC 20004, and author of The Art of the Steal (Broadway). Mr. Abagnale's early life was the inspiration for the film Catch Me If You Can.

Identity theft is the fastest-growing crime in the US. The Federal Trade Commission (FTC) estimates that more than one million people were victimized last year.

Each victim of identity theft spends about 175 hours and about $800 to clear his/her name.

PREVENTION STRATEGIES

Some things you can do to steer clear of identity thieves...

• **Don't disclose any personal information** until you find out how it will be used (including whether it will be shared with others).

• **Pay attention to billing cycles** so you can follow up with creditors if your bills don't arrive on time. A missing bill could mean that someone has taken over your credit card and changed the billing address to cover his tracks. If your card has expired and you haven't received your replacement, call the card issuer

■ *Your Life* ■ ■ ■ ■

immediately—someone may have obtained your new card.

• **Shred every bill** and other documents that contain personal or account information. A shredder, available at office-supply stores, costs as little as $25.

• **Install a lock on your mailbox** to prevent someone from stealing your mail to obtain your account and other personal information.

• **Remove your name, phone number and address from marketing lists** by contacting the Direct Marketing Association (*www.the-dma.org*). This does not remove your name from *all* lists, but from many of them.

• **Reduce the number of preapproved credit card offers you receive** by calling the credit reporting industry's prescreening "opt out" number at 888-567-8688.

• **Order a copy of your credit report once a year** from each of the three major reporting agencies. Make sure the information is accurate and that the report includes only legitimate transactions.

Contact: Equifax (800-685-1111 or *www.equifax.com*)...Experian (888-397-3742 or *www.experian.com*)...TransUnion (800-888-4213 or *www.transunion.com*).

• **Consider subscribing to a credit monitoring service** that alerts you within 24 hours of any changes to your credit file (for example, an application for a new credit card).

Examples: PrivacyGuard.com (877-202-8828 or *www.privacyguard.com*)...Identity Fraud, Inc. (866-4ID-FRAUD or *www.identityfraud.com*). Costs range from $69.95 to $139.95 per year.

• **Consider purchasing identity theft insurance**—a new type of policy now being offered to help identity theft victims with the high expense of restoring their good name and credit.

The insurance covers the cost of fixing credit records, lost wages for time away from work to talk with credit bureaus and investigators, long-distance phone calls, attorney fees and other costs.

Examples: Travelers Property Casualty Corp. at *www.travelers.com* and Chubb Group of Insurance Companies at *www.chubb.com*.

Premiums for $15,000 of coverage with a $100 deductible range from $15 to $30 per year. *Note:* This coverage is unavailable in some states.

• **Don't carry sensitive information,** such as your Social Security number, personal identification numbers (PINs) or passwords, in your wallet or purse.

• **Don't give out personal information** over the telephone unless you initiated the call.

• **Don't put your Social Security** or driver's license number on your checks.

• **Don't use easily available information,** such as your mother's maiden name, your birth date or the last four digits of your Social Security number, as your password for credit/debit cards, phone accounts, etc.

• **Don't have new checks sent to your residence.** Instead, pick them up at the bank or have them delivered by registered mail so that you'll have to sign for them.

• **Don't leave mail and personal information around your home** if you have outsiders there (workers, roommates, etc.).

IF YOU'VE BEEN VICTIMIZED

If you find out that someone has been getting credit using your name and personal information, do three things *immediately*...

1. Contact the fraud departments of the three major credit reporting bureaus. Report that your identity has been stolen. Have a "fraud alert" put in your file and add a "victim's statement" asking creditors to call you before opening a new account in your name.

2. Contact the security department of the creditor or financial institution of any fraudulently accessed or opened account. Close the account, and then change the password for any new account. Inform the creditor or institution that this is a case of ID theft.

3. File a report with your local police or where the identity theft took place. Request a copy of the police report in case the bank, credit card company or other creditor needs proof of the crime later on.

After these initial actions, there are things you should do to prevent additional injury as well as correct any adverse actions to date...

- **Cancel all current checking and savings accounts** and open new ones. Make sure the bank pays only the outstanding checks you've written and that it doesn't honor checks written by someone else. Contact the major check verification companies to alert them of the theft of your checks. They include Global Payments (800-766-2748), ChexSystems (800-428-9623), Cross Check (800-552-1900), Certegy (800-215-6280), SCAN (800-262-7771) and TeleCheck (800-710-9898).
- **Get new ATM cards,** and use a new PIN.
- **Contact an attorney** if credit bureaus are unresponsive or if the title to your property has been changed. Ask him to send a letter to the credit bureau or county clerk of record.
- **Report the crime to the FTC** by calling its Identity Theft Hotline at 877-438-4338 or logging on to *www.consumer.gov/idtheft*.

Important: If you are disputing fraudulent debts and accounts opened by an identity thief, the ID Thief Affidavit issued by the FTC now simplifies the procedure of cleaning up your credit history. Instead of completing multiple forms, you can use the affidavit to alert companies and the credit bureaus whenever a new account has been opened up in your name. Download the affidavit from *www.consumer.gov/idtheft*.

New Twist on Identity Theft

A skimmer—the size of a pager—can pick up the encoded data on your credit card with a single swipe. Unscrupulous waiters and store clerks swipe customers' cards through the skimmer, then turn over the devices to accomplices.

Self-defense: Keep your card in sight. Check credit card statements carefully. Report illicit charges to your credit card issuer.

Robert Finkbeiner, JD, assistant statewide prosecutor for Florida. He recently helped obtain indictments of seven people charged with running a skimming ring.

New Identity Theft Scam Uses Phony Tax Notices

In a new identity theft scam, an individual receives faked correspondence from his/her bank saying that it is updating its records to exempt the individual from paying taxes on interest or from having taxes withheld from investment accounts. Included are phony IRS forms requesting detailed personal and financial data. The forms must be faxed to a specified phone number or the individual will lose the tax exemptions, the documents say. In fact, the scammer intends to use the information to steal the victim's bank accounts, credit card numbers, etc.

This scam has been found nationwide. If you notice anything like it, call the Treasury Department's fraud hotline at 800-366-4484.

Randy Bruce Blaustein, Esq., senior tax partner, R.B. Blaustein & Co., 155 E. 31 St., New York City 10016.

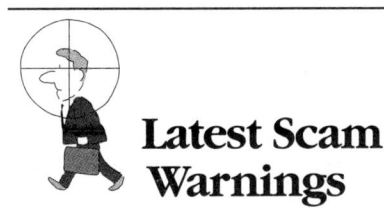

Latest Scam Warnings

Beth Givens, director, Privacy Rights Clearinghouse, nonprofit consumer education and advocacy organization, San Diego, CA 92103, *www.privacyrights.org*.

Susan Grant, director, National Fraud Information Center, Washington, DC 20006, which gives consumers advice on telemarketing, on-line offers and reporting fraud, *www.fraud.org*.

Shirley Rooker, president of Call For Action, Bethesda, MD 20816, which offers a network of hot lines that help consumers and small businesses solve disputes, *www.callforaction.org*.

Think that you're too smart to be conned? More than a half-million Americans have suffered identity theft during the past year—and many of them were tricked into divulging vital personal information.

Identity theft leads the list of scams plaguing consumers. It costs American banks and two credit card companies more than $300 million annually, the government reported in 2002. Internet scams—nondelivery of merchandise

■ *Your Life* ■ ■ ■ ■

and on-line identity theft—cost each victim an average of $427.

Three of the nation's top consumer rights advocates discuss the latest scams—and how to defend against them...

PRIVACY RIGHTS CLEARINGHOUSE
Beth Givens

APPLICATION FRAUD

How it works: You get a phone call offering a preapproved credit card at an attractive interest rate with no interest on balance transfers for one year. Interested? The caller just needs you to verify some information, including your Social Security number, date of birth and mother's maiden name.

Trap: These are the three pieces of information that allow any con artist to apply for credit in your name. The illegally obtained card is charged to the limit, and the account goes into default. Since the card wasn't sent to your address, you don't find out until you are refused for a new card or loan. Credit providers send you a notice of the default—but it goes to the address used by the scam artist.

Under federal law, you are liable for only $50 of the fraudulent charges, but restoring your credit can take years. The stolen information is often sold by the thief, causing repeated fraudulent applications in your name.

Self-defense: Place a fraud alert in your credit report with the credit-reporting agencies so issuers notify you when a credit application is made in your name. Some fail to call, so check your credit report annually.

Credit-reporting agencies...

•**Equifax** (888-766-0008 or *www.equifax.com*).

•**Experian** (888-397-3742 or *www.experian.com*).

•**TransUnion** (800-680-7289 or *www.transunion.com*).

ACCOUNT SPOOFING

How it works: You get a call or an E-mail from someone who says he/she is from your Internet service provider, bank or credit card company. The caller says that the company needs to update your security and/or billing information.

He asks for your credit card number, its expiration date and perhaps your personal identification or Social Security number. Or he might ask you to fill in the information at a Web site that looks just like the company's own Web page.

Self-defense: Ask for the caller's name and phone number, and tell him you will call back. Look up the company's customer service number, and call it to verify that the request and the Web site are legitimate.

Chances are, they aren't. Reputable companies rarely call or E-mail to verify account and security information.

NATIONAL FRAUD INFORMATION CENTER
Susan Grant

THE "NEW" NIGERIAN FEE SCAM

How it works: In the past, a letter arrived from a Nigerian "official" offering you a reward if you helped him move money out of Africa to your own bank account for safekeeping.

Now the scam also comes via an E-mail from the Middle East or Afghanistan. It targets women and religious groups, in particular.

Example: A woman says that she is the daughter of a slain rebel leader. Her father has accumulated a large fortune in gold bullion in Europe, but she can't leave the country to get it. *You are offered one-quarter of the bullion if you help by...*

•Sending thousands of dollars to her so she can arrange immigration or asylum.

•Initiating a bank transfer that requires you to deposit hundreds or thousands of dollars in a series of transfer fees, legal fees and insurance.

Self-defense: Delete these E-mails.

"NEW" SWEEPSTAKES RIP-OFF

How it works: You get a call or an E-mail saying that you have won a foreign sweepstakes. In the past, you were asked to send money to cover processing fees or taxes on the winnings.

Now, the "sweepstakes officials" send you a check first—sometimes as much as $20,000—as long as you agree to wire back the necessary taxes, bonding, customs and administrative fees when the check clears.

Trap: The sweepstakes check you deposit has a fake routing number. It appears to clear initially, but days or weeks later, the bank discovers the error. The bank then removes the money credited to your account. You are out the amount you wired to the "sweepstakes."

Self-defense: Don't believe someone who says you have won money out of the blue—especially if he requires any money from you. It doesn't matter if the ruse is a sweepstakes, lottery, etc.—you still get bilked.

CALL FOR ACTION
Shirley Rooker

MODEM DIALING FRAUD

How it works: You are offered access to an Internet site with free job postings, chat rooms, psychic readings, casino gambling, etc. All you need to do is download the required Web site viewer or dialer computer program.

The scam: The dialer program bypasses your local Internet-access phone number and instead uses an international number. You are charged as much as $350 an hour. The foreign area code functions like a 900-toll number in the US, and the foreign telephone company acts as a third-party billing service for the con artist.

Self-defense...

•**Download programs only from Web sites you know and trust.**

•**Check the "Dialing Properties" control panel on your computer** to see what number your modem is dialing.

•**Read the dialer program's user agreement.** The fine print often says the service is free, but you must pay for connection charges.

•**Monitor your children's Internet use.** Children are the frequent targets of this scam because credit cards are not necessary. Track your kids' Internet use by checking their Web browser history files.

To track all Web site visits on Internet Explorer: Click on the "History" icon in the tool bar.

In Netscape Communicator: Click on "Tools" in the drop-down menu and then click on "History."

Even if you block international calling on your phone, some modem dialers circumvent this by using a "10-10 dial-around" prefix.

Daring New Scams and How to Avoid Them

Hal Morris, veteran Las Vegas–based consumer affairs journalist who writes widely about scams, schemes and rip-offs. He is also a former bank director.

Scam artists are working harder than ever nowadays to separate you and your hard-earned money. *Among the latest rip-offs…*

DECEPTIVE LOGOS

Logos of well-known financial institutions used in communications to Internet users do not prove the sender is genuine.

Recently, a shady operator incorporated the logos of a bank, plus real estate, insurance and mortgage firms in thousands of deceptive Internet messages. The personal information the recipients were asked to give included income, mortgage balances and home values.

The Federal Trade Commission (FTC) has sued the deceptive spammer, saying it posed "as an entity it was not" simply to pry sensitive financial information from the recipients. Authorities fear others are engaged in similar shady behavior.

Self-defense: Before giving out information, verify the authenticity of the message sender by contacting the companies whose logos are used in the message. Also use a spam filter. But be cautious of any spam reduction or elimination services. The FTC recently tested such claims and found more unwanted messages rolled in *after* signing up for antispam service.

"DO NOT CALL" RIP-OFF

Fleecers are claiming to provide protection from unwanted telemarketing calls through "Do Not Call" registries. In telephone solicitations and Internet advertising, cheats falsely claim affiliation with the state attorney general's office or another government agency. They try

■ *Your Life* ■ ■ ■ ■

to secure your personal information and charge a "fee" of up to $12.

Self-defense: Sign up for the federal "Do Not Call" registry at *www.donotcall.gov*. For more details, call the FTC at 888-382-1222. Register all your phone numbers—home, cell and business.

You can also squelch unwanted phone calls through the local telephone company services such as "call intercept" or "privacy manager." When used with caller ID, the option puts a clamp on calls listed as private, unknown or out of area.

WEIGHT-LOSS SCAM

"Lose up to two pounds daily without diet or exercise!" proclaims a typical weight-loss ad. More than half of such pitches make at least one representation that "is almost certainly false," says the FTC, which has been inundated lately with complaints of unscrupulous marketers promising dramatic and effortless weight loss.

In its first law-enforcement action under a major clampdown on false weight-loss product advertising, the FTC filed suit against marketers that falsely touted substantial and permanent weight loss (20 to 40 pounds) without diet or exercise—even after consuming lots of high-calorie foods. The "secret" aid is a liquid product gulped before bedtime and at least three hours after eating or drinking.

Self-defense: There is no miracle pill for losing weight. The surest and safest route to shed pounds is by combining healthful eating and exercise. Start by cutting fatty foods and walking 30 minutes a day, five days a week.

FALSE JOB OPENINGS

Income-starved older people, lured into considering part- or full-time federal government and postal work through local newspaper classified ads placed by con artists, are being duped into paying a price (typically $39 to $160) for worthless information. Leads on job openings turn out to be merely job descriptions. Materials to improve chances of being hired and practice tests turn out to be misrepresentations. And a refund guarantee is bogus.

Self-defense: Be on guard for pitches that imply affiliation with the federal government or the Postal Service...guarantee high test scores ...offer jobs that state no experience is necessary...or provide information about "hidden" or unadvertised jobs. Toll-free numbers often connect to pay-per-call locations for more details.

Get information on postal positions from your local post office. Federal job offerings are available at the Office of Personnel Management, listed under US Government in the phone book. Web sites for postal and federal jobs—*www.usps.com, www.usajobs.opm.gov*.

FAKE CASHIER'S CHECKS

Counterfeit business and personal checks have long been the bane of the banking industry—there were more than 600,000 cases of check fraud in 2001, up 34% from 2000. But now a rash of counterfeit cashier's checks is sweeping the country, vexing bankers and hitting the wallets of unsuspecting victims.

Until now, cashier's checks have been considered as good as cash. But with sophisticated computer design and printing, scam artists are producing genuine-looking paper that purports to show checks drawn by a bank on its own funds and signed by bank officials.

Bum cashier's checks are being used primarily in auto-buying transactions. Such was the case of a Kansas woman who discovered the $21,500 "cashier's check" handed to her in exchange for her used vehicle was phony. By the time her bank told her it was worthless, her pickup truck was long gone.

The perpetrators behind this scam have been responsible for distributing other counterfeit cashier's checks in at least 17 cities in six Midwestern states.

Self-defense: Examine checks carefully for misspelled words or numbers that are unevenly spaced or misaligned. A mismatch could be a tip-off. A legitimate cashier's check usually has a watermark and the bank's logo.

How to proceed: With check in hand—and before a possible culprit makes a getaway with your vehicle or merchandise—phone the indicated financial institution. Use a number from the phone book. What appears on the check may be fake. Verify authenticity with a bank official by supplying essential details, such as check number, date, amount and authorized signature.

More from Hal Morris...

Big Cons to Watch Out For

Three rip-offs—involving health insurance, credit cards and phone bills—you should watch out for now...

•**Bogus health care plans.** Unlicensed health "insurers" are preying on individuals, small businesses and school districts nationwide. They offer unusually low premiums—$150 a month for family coverage, about $350 below normal—and generous benefits. But the plans never actually pay claims.

The insurance commissioner for the state of Texas has issued cease-and-desist orders against five such operators and is investigating 10 others.

Self-defense: Before signing anything, verify licensed firms with your state's department of insurance. Do not use an agent who claims a health insurance plan provides "benefits," not insurance...or refers to commissions as "consultant fees" and to premiums as "contributions."

Get details on this scam from the Texas department of insurance at *www.tdi.state.tx.us/consumer/unauthorized.html*.

•**Phony credit card protection.** Canada has become a hotbed for scams directed at Americans. Some Canadian telemarketing firms claiming to be affiliated with legitimate credit card issuers trick consumers into purchasing worthless credit card liability protection. The fee is typically small—say, $2.99. When the customer receives the bill, the decimal point "mysteriously" has been moved over two places, and the charge becomes $299.

Self-defense: Guard your credit card number (despite the scammer's assurance, "We already know your number but need verification"). Call your credit card issuer's customer-service number to see if the telemarketing firm is on its list of authorized marketing partners.

For more information, including names of the offenders who have been cited by the Federal Trade Commission, log onto *www.ftc.gov/opa/2002/04/consumeralliance.htm*.

•**Trick telephone charges.** A message on your voice mail, E-mail or pager requests an urgent response—to find out about a "sick" relative...claim a prize...or settle an unpaid account. You dial a phone number that you assume is for a legitimate business and are kept on hold for up to 15 minutes, listening to recorded chatter and other delaying tactics.

Worse yet, the call is to a foreign country—possibly the Dominican Republic (area code 809), the British Virgin Islands (284) or Jamaica (876). The local phone companies give the culprits a share of the international phone charges you incur.

Self-defense: If you are considering returning any such "urgent" calls, check the area code first.

If you never call outside the US, ask your long-distance provider to block outgoing international calls on your line. Report suspicious phone charges as soon as possible to the Federal Communications Commission at 888-225-5322 or *www.fcc.gov/cgb*.

Protect Yourself On-Line

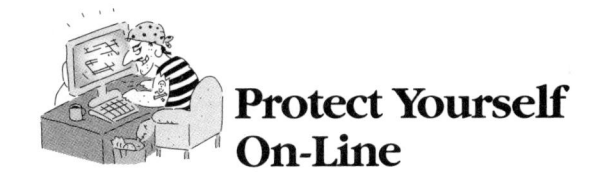

Self-defense for some common on-line scams from a director at the Federal Trade Commission (FTC)...

Internet auctions: Some buyers are sent low-quality products or nothing at all. The best self-defense is to use a credit card or an escrow service to pay for products ordered on-line.

Internet access: If you accept mailed offers that resemble checks, you may end up with long-term, noncancelable service. Read the fine print on promotional literature.

Credit card fraud: Report all suspicious charges to your card issuer's fraud department.

Travel deals: Accommodations and charges may not be as advertised. Get written details of the trip *and* cancellation policies.

■ *Your Life* ■ ■ ■ ■

If you have been defrauded, contact the FTC at 877-382-4357 or *www.ftc.gov.*

Nat Wood, assistant director, consumer business education, Federal Trade Commission, Washington, DC 20580.

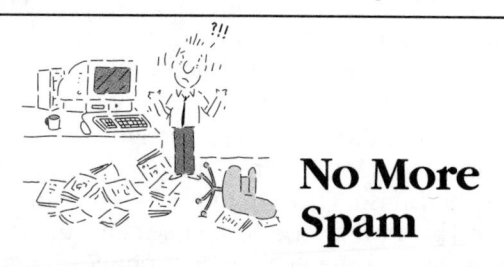

No More Spam

Jonathan Zittrain, JD, founder and faculty director, Harvard Law School's Berkman Center for Internet and Society, Cambridge, MA.

To reduce the spam (junk E-mail) you receive, but at the same time still get all the E-mail you do want...

•**Read a company's privacy policy carefully** before divulging any data about yourself. The policy is usually found at a link at the bottom of the home page. Don't do business with companies that fail to provide such a link.

•**Don't post your E-mail address on Web pages,** electronic bulletin boards or public chat rooms—spammers use software that can readily scan it and add it to a database.

•**Consider signing up for a separate, free E-mail account** from Yahoo! Mail or Hotmail, and give that address to merchants.

•**Report spammers to** *www.spamcop.net.* SpamCop will report the spammer to its service provider, which will then deny it Internet access by closing its account. Or report the spammer to the Federal Trade Commission at *www.ftc.gov/spam.*

Better Cell Phone Protection

To protect your cell phone from hackers or viruses, have your service provider deactivate features you don't need.

Examples: Internet and E-mail access... stock market alerts.

Many cell phones in Europe and Asia—more advanced than US phones—have suffered from hacker and virus attacks. Such attacks have been rare in the US. Personal firewalls for cell phones are now being developed. They will be similar to those used on desktop computers with full-time Internet access through a digital subscriber line (DSL) or cable modem.

John Featherman, personal privacy consultant and president of Featherman.com in Dayton.

More from John Featherman...

A Good Reason to Balance Your Checkbook

A thief who obtains just one of your checks may use it to create many counterfeits and loot your bank account.

Warning example: A nationally known TV host lost two checks to thieves. They made at least 26 copies of them, stealing $25,000 from his account over nine months. Because the individual thefts were relatively small and he did not balance his checkbook each month, he didn't discover the false checks until it was too late to report most of them—and the bank repaid only $3,000 to him.

Lessons: Don't throw checks in the trash or put them where anyone else can get them. And balance your checkbook on a monthly basis.

Index

A

AARP, discounts and, 225
Abdominal pain, getting right diagnosis for, 24
Accelerated death benefits as tax-free income, 125
Acetaminophen
 alcohol and, 21
 overuse of, 86
Achilles tendon strain, 51
Acupressure for hiccups, 39
Acute pain, herbs versus drugs for, 69
Acute sinusitis, relief for, 19
Adoption
 assistance for employees, 299
 credit, 137
 expenses as tax-free income, 125
Adult-education programs, 232
Adult students, financial aid for, 318
Adventure vacations, safer, 231
Aging
 human growth hormone and, 14
 money management and, 107-109
 sex and, 89
Air-conditioning costs, cutting, 187
Air travel. *See also* Travel; Vacations
 buying frequent-flier miles, 223
 conversion of hotel points to frequent-flier miles, 223
 faster check-in, 221
 fees for, 173, 221, 223-224
 food on, 222
 getting bumped on purpose, 221
 last-minute deals, 220-221
 loss of luggage and, 224-225
 recirculated air and, 222
 refunds on nonrefundable tickets, 223
 security on, 222
Alcohol
 acetaminophen and, 21
 as fat trigger, 44
 getting help for addiction to, 96
 sexual appetite and, 86

Allergies. *See also* Asthma; Hay fever
 folk remedies for, 40
 preventing food, 83
Alternative minimum tax, 131
Alternative treatments, tax deduction for, 130
Alzheimer's disease
 natural treatment for, 73
 new test for, 13
 statins and, 8
Amenorrhea, 93
Anemia, traveling and, 229
Annuities, 196-197
 passing on, to heirs, 211-212
 in paying less tax on Social Security benefits, 201
Antibiotics, oregano oil as alternative to, 70
Antidepressants, bananas and, 21
Antihistamines for children, 20
Antioxidants, aging and, 72
Aphrodisiacs, natural, 87-88
Appetite suppressants, 48
Appliances
 repairs on, 190
 saving on, 186, 188
Art, decorating tips with, 260
Arthritis, knee surgery for, 13
Artificial sweeteners as fat trigger, 44
Aspirin
 colon health and, 14
 heart attack risk and, 9
Assets, listing on balance sheet, 205
Asthma. *See also* Allergies; Hay fever
 exercising with, 54
 triggers of, 83
Atkins diet, 49
ATMs, overseas, 220
Attic insulation, maintenance of, 254-255
Auctions, on-line, 178-179
Audits. *See also* Tax audits
 home energy, 186
Autographs, collecting, 244
Automobile(s). *See also* Rental cars
 buying on-line, 248-249
 buying used, 174, 175

 checklist for new, 250
 company, for employees, 299
 driving with spouse, 250
 reporting accidents with, 117
 safety of children in backseats, 250
 tax deductions for hybrid, 136
 whiplash protection and, 250
Automobile care
 getting better repairs, 248
 mistakes owners made in, 245-246
 oil changes in, 245
 oil filters in, 245-246
 saving money on, 177
 tinted glass as gas saver, 247
Automobile donation programs, tax audits and, 142
Automobile insurance
 buying on-line, 249
 for college students, 320
 saving on, 117-118
Automobile loans, refinancing, 105

B

Baccarat, winning strategies for, 236-237
Bad debts, identifying, 303
Baggage
 fees for air travel, 223-224
 keeping airlines from losing, 224-225
Balancing exercises, 51
Bank(s)
 choosing Internet, 103
 fees at, 173
 safety of money in, 109
Bankruptcies, travel-company, 228
Bargaining for the best price, 171-173
Baseball cards, collecting, 242-243
Bathroom, redoing, 263
Bed & Breakfasts, 232
Bequests
 life insurance in funding, 205
 reviewing, 206
Berries, aging and, 72
Beta carotene in preventing breast cancer, 90

337

Bills
  cutting medical, 180-182
  getting government help in paying medical, 130-131
  tax deductions on medical, 130-131
  tips for paying, 176-177
Black cohosh for inhibited sexual desire, 88
Blackjack, winning strategies for, 234-236
Blood pressure, dizziness and, 11
Boat interest deduction, 126
Body image, enjoying better, 56-58
Bone-building exercises, 52-53
Bone loss, signs of, 93
Bones
  benefits from tea in building strong, 68
  emergency care for broken, 61
  painkillers for broken, 17
  ultrasound in healing broken, 16
Borrowed funds, as tax-free income, 125
Bottled water. *See also* Water
  avoiding fancy, 175
  food safety and, 22
Brain function, diet and, 75
Brainstorming, better, 273
Breakage in retail stores, 177
Breakfast, weight loss and, 50
Breast cancer. *See also* Cancer
  detection of, 90
  grape juice as preventive, 90
  HRT and risk of, 91-92
Broccoli, dietary benefits from, 76
Broken bones, emergency care for, 61
Brokerages, safety of money in, 109
Business
  creating Web site to boost, 297
  employing children in family, 303-305
  protecting, in estate planning, 206
  selling your, 305
  succeeding in, without working so hard, 287-289
  tax deductions for, 299-301
Business cards, tips for, 294
Business tax return, getting refund on, 301-303
Business trips
  tax break for, 132
  tax deductions for spouse's expenses on, 148
B vitamins
  benefits of, 73-74
  in lowering cholesterol, 78

C

Caffeine
  benefits of, 3-5
  as fat trigger, 44
  in increasing fat burning, 50
Calcium
  dietary benefits of, 63
  blood testing for, 32
Cancer. *See also* Breast cancer; Colon cancer; Ovarian cancer; Prostate cancer; Skin cancer
  green tea in reducing risks of, 68
  mistletoe extract in fighting, 76
  turmeric in fighting, 76
Capital gain property as tax-free income, 125

Carbohydrates, food cravings and, 46
Cardiac medications, time of day for taking, 8
Cardiovascular disease. *See also* Heart disease
Carpal tunnel syndrome, treating, 39
Carpet cleaners, avoiding scams with, 185-186
Carrots in combating ovarian cancer, 90
Casinos. *See also* Gambling
  money management and, 102
  safety and, 237
  winning strategies for, 234-237
Cataract removal, alternatives to, 59-60
Cats. *See also* Pets
  dangers with, 253
Cell phone company, selecting, 175
Central air-conditioning, maintenance of, 254
Certified public accountants as tax professionals, 145
Charitable contributions, rules of proof for, 213
Charity
  giving collectibles to, 140
  tax break for travel, 132
Checkwriting, dangers in, 103
Cherries as sleep aid, 84
Chest pain, getting right diagnosis for, 24
Child-care facilities, tax credit for, 300
Children
  antihistamines for, 20
  dangers from drinking water, 255-256
  discussing money with, 112
  keeping track of, in crowds, 286
  loaning money to, 204
  managing college savings for, 203-204
  predicting height of, 268
  talking to, 266-267
Chimney care, 256-257
Chives in reducing prostate cancer risk, 95
Chocolate
  benefits of, for heart, 80
  food cravings and, 46
Cholesterol. *See also* LDL cholesterol
  exercise in lowering, 80
  home test for, 5
  lowering, without medication, 78-79
  normal results on, 32
Chronic sinusitis, relief for, 20
Cleaning products, low-cost alternatives to, 185
Clothes dryers, energy-efficient, 188-189
Clutter, minimizing, 260-261
COBRA, 306
Co-enzyme Q10 in improving mental abilities, 286
Cognitive decline, olive oil in preventing, 73
Cognitive dissonance, 290
Collaborative law for divorce, 110
Collectibles
  autographs as, 244
  baseball cards as, 242-243
  giving, to charity, 140
  hottest, 240-242
College(s). *See also* Education
  financial aid for, 312, 317, 318, 320

insurance for students in, 319-320
investing for, 318
resources on, 312-313
saving on textbooks, 320
tax breaks in paying for, 315-317
Web sites that help children in choosing, 313
College essays, writing winning, 311-312
College savings plans. *See also* Coverdell Education Savings Account; Section 529 plan for college
  evaluating, 313-315
  protecting, 318
Colon, aspirin and health of, 14
Colon cancer. *See also* Cancer
  aspirin and, 14
  home test for, 5
  statins and, 8
  in women, 2-3
Common cold
  consumption of wine in preventing, 83
  effect of vitamin E on, 19
  exercise in reducing, 38
  feeding, 38
  recirculated air on planes and, 222
Company car for employees, 299
Company owners, fringe benefits for, 297-298
Compassionate use programs for medications, 25
Computer, keeping old monitor, 179
Condominiums, buying, 263
Confrontation, defusing angry, 278-279
Constipation, natural way of treating, 38-39
Contact lenses, getting cheaper, 182
Contests, winning, 233-234
Contractors, finding good, 189-190
Contracts, negotiating, 310
Conversations, handling difficult, 274-276
Coronary-bypass surgery, alternatives to, 60
Cosigning loans, 104
Cosmetic surgery, saving on, 180
Coupons
  free, 181
  saving with, 176
Coverdell Education Savings Account, 136, 203, 315, 320
  as tax-free income, 125
Cranberries for protection against disease, 67
C-reactive test, in predicting heart attack, 10
Creativity, rekindling, 283-284
Credit, checking, before job search, 309
Credit cards
  dangers involving, 104
  getting better deal, 104
  parental-control, 320
  paying off balance faster, 174
  paying taxes with, 140
Creditors, protecting Keogh retirement plans from, 200
Credit report, improving, 104
Crowds, keeping track of children in, 286

Cruises. *See also* Travel; Vacations
  better cabins on, 228
  for first-timers, 228
  healthier food on, 227
  security on, 227
  self-defense against viral illness on, 227
CT scan, full-body, 7
Cushing's syndrome, weight gain and, 47
Customer service via E-mail, 295
Cuts, emergency care for, 61

D

Debt(s)
  bad, as business deduction, 300-301
  easing burden of, 104-105
  getting out of, 97
Debt consolidator, choosing, 105
Decongestant, natural, 38
Decorating, tips for home, 259-260
Deeds, swapping good, 179
Deer, keeping, out of garden, 258
Deferred compensation, job loss and, 307
Dental care
  DentiPatch in, 18
  heart problems and, 18
  relaxation during, 33
  removal of fillings, 17
Depreciated deductions for business, 301
Depression, herbs versus drugs for, 69
Detergent, saving on, 185
Diabetes, dangers of drugs for, 13
Diamond jewelry, buying, 173, 184
Diarrhea, natural treatment for traveler's, 231
Diet(s). *See also* Food(s)
  brain function and, 75
  cataract removal and, 59
  coronary bypass and, 60
  disease-fighting, 62-64
  eggs in heart-healthy, 79-80
  high-carbohydrate, 48
  hip replacement and, 60
  sources of potassium in, 84
  thyroid disease and, 15-16
  wrinkle-cure, 71-72
Digestion, avoiding problems with, 81-82
Disability insurance
  for business owners, 298
  need for, 100
Discount health care clubs, 180-181
Disease, protection against, with cranberries, 67
Disease-fighting diet, 62-64
Dishwashers, energy-efficient, 189
Dividend-paying stocks, new tax law and, 122-123
Divorce
  collaborative law for, 110
  estate planning after, 207
  protecting legacy from child's, 212
  tax deductions for costs of, 134
Dizziness, blood pressure and, 11
Doctors
  in emergency room, 23-24
  house calls by, 33
  responsibilities for medical history, 30
  surviving medical emergency without, 61-62
  talking about medical research with, 31

Dogs. *See also* Pets
  dangers with, 253
Dong quai for inhibited sexual desire, 88
Drug addiction, getting help for, 96
Drug companies, influence of, on medication choice, 28
Drug use, home test for, 5-6
Durable power of attorney, 205, 216

E

Early retirement withdrawals without penalty, 199
Education. *See also* College(s)
  credits on income taxes for, 317
  tax deductions for expenses, 131, 136, 317
Educational assistance program, 298
Education Resources Institute, 318
Elasticity test in determining functional age, 70
Elderly, protecting, from financial abuse, 112
Electrical system, maintenance of, 256
Electric hedge clippers, handling, 251-252
Electricity, saving money on, 177
Electronics, discounts on, 185
E-mail. *See also* Internet
  controlling overload, 294-295
  customer service via, 295
  spam strategy for, 295, 336
Emergency, getting money for, 100-101
Emergency child medical-care form, 205
Emergency room. *See also* Hospitals
  guarantees from, 24
  surviving trip to, 23-24
  Triage Cardiac System in, 10
Employees
  fringe benefits for, 298-299
  rewarding, 293
Employer aid for college, 315-316
Employer-paid parking as tax-free income, 125
Employer-provided insurance as tax-free income, 125
End-of-life decisions, Web sites for, 216
Endorphins, food cravings and, 46
Energy expenses, saving on, 186
Enrolled agents as tax professionals, 145
Entertainment, saving money on, 177
Erectile dysfunction (impotence), treating, 87-88
Escrow account, checking, 106
Essays, winning college, 311-312
Estate planning
  after divorce, 207
  providing documents in, 211
  revisions in, 211
  in tricky times, 203-205
Estate taxes, changes in, 206
Estimated taxes
  getting overpaid back, 301-302
  reviewing, 122
Europe, getting money back when traveling in, 220
Evening primrose oil in avoiding hip replacement, 60
Executors, liability of, for unpaid estate taxes, 210

Exercise
  with asthma, 54
  avoiding injury in, 51-52
  balancing, 51
  best time for, 53
  bone-building, 52-53
  guidelines for, 54
  heartburn from, 53
  in improving sex life, 89
  in lowering cholesterol, 80
  in managing digestive problems, 82
  in protecting against impotency, 89
  relaxation, 57
  sexual fitness and, 86
Expense reimbursements as tax-free income, 124
Exposure therapy in handling common phobias, 277-278

F

Fainting, treating, 39
Family
  need for medical history in, 29-31
  securing future of, 205-206
Family business, employment of children in, 303-305
Fasting, presurgery, 34
Fat-blockers, 48
Fat burning, increasing, 50
Fatigue, thyroid disease and, 14-16
Fat triggers, weight loss and, 43-45
Fecal occult blood tests, 5
Fellowships, 318
  as tax-free income, 125
Fever, treatment of, 18
Feverfew for migraines, 70
Fiber, too little, as fat trigger, 44
Financial abuse, protecting elderly from, 112
Financial mistakes, impact of, on retirement, 195-196
Financial planner, need to see, 122-123
Financial security, hidden threats to, 99-100
First aid
  for poison ivy, 252
  for splinters, 252
First impression, improving, 282-283
Fishing, strategies for, 238-239
Fishing collectibles, collecting, 241
Fitness. *See also* Exercise
  benefits of, 56
Fitness walking, 54
Flavonoids
  bone density and, 68
  dietary benefits of, 63
Flea markets, 218
Flexible spending accounts as tax-free income, 124
Flextime, 299
Flu
  effect of vitamin E on, 19
  medications for, 18
Flu vaccine in cutting stroke risk, 12
Flying debris, dangers with, 252
Folate
  in lowering stroke risk, 81
  in protecting heart, 73-74

339

Food(s). *See also* Diet(s)
  airline, 222
  healthier, on cruises, 227
  reduced-fat, and weight gain, 46-47
  saving money on, 177
  weight loss and cravings for, 45-46
Food allergy, preventing attacks, 83
Food Pyramid, 48, 49
Food safety
  food storage and, 21-22
  undercooked meat and, 252
Fractures. *See also* Bones
Frequent-flier miles
  buying, 223
  conversion of hotel points to, 223
  for employees, 298
  as tax-free income, 125
Friends, evaluating, 280-282
Fringe benefits, making most of, 297-299
Fruits, dietary benefits of, 63
Full-body CT scan, 7
Funerals, being overcharged for, 184
Furnace, maintenance of, 254
Furniture
  arranging, 259-260
  taking advantage of bargains in, 175-176

G

Gambling. *See also* Casinos
  tax planning and, 133-134
  winning strategies for blackjack, 234-236
Garden, keeping deer out of, 258
Garlic in reducing prostate cancer risk, 95
Gasoline, avoiding premium, 174-175
Gas station collectibles, collecting, 241
Gastroenterologist, recommendations from, for staying healthy, 65
Gastroesophageal reflux disease, management of, 82
Generic products, buying, 176
Genetic oncologist, recommendations from, for staying healthy, 66
Gifts as tax-free income, 124
Gift taxes for business, 304
Ginger
  in easing knee pain, 81
  for motion sickness, 40, 70
Ginkgo biloba
  for erectile dysfunction, 88
  in improving mental function, 286
Ginseng
  for inhibited sexual desire, 88
  prior to surgery, 34
Gleason score in diagnosing prostate cancer, 94
Glucosamine sulfate in avoiding hip replacement, 60
Golden oak furniture, collecting, 241
Golf, mistakes by pros, 239
Government bonds as tax-free income, 125
Government education loans, 318
Grandchildren
  loaning money to, 204
  spoiling, 267-268
  teaching, about money, 112
Grandparents, free hotel rooms for, 226

Grants, 318
Grape juice as breast cancer preventive, 90
Green tea, benefits from, 67-68
Group term life insurance for business owners, 297
Group travel, 232
Guaranteed replacement coverage in home insurance, 116
Gym, choosing, 58

H

Hay fever. *See also* Allergies; Asthma
  drug-free relief for, 38
  triggers of, 83
Headaches. *See also* Migraines
  bacteria in triggering, 20-21
  caffeine in relieving, 4
Health
  job loss and, 308
  protecting, while traveling, 229-230
  recommendations from doctors on staying in good, 65-67
Health care proxy, 205
Health club, joining, 58
Health insurance
  for business owners, 297-298
  checking payments from, 118
  for college students, 319
  co-pays and, 119
  job loss and, 306
  minimizing costs, 119
  premiums for, as tax deduction, 130
  problem resolution and, 119
Hearing, reversing loss of, 83-84
Heart
  benefits of chocolate for, 80
  drinking water to protect, 79
  folate in protecting, 73-74
Heart attacks. *See also* Heart disease
  aspirin and risk for, 9
  C-reactive test in predicting, 10
  emergency care for, 62
  during sex, 86
Heartburn
  from exercise, 53
  management of, 82
Heart-bypass surgery
  dangers for women, 10
  side effects of, 11
Heart disease. *See also* Heart attacks
  green tea in reducing risks of, 68
  honey in protecting against, 80
  impotence and, 90
  medications for, 7-8
  traveling and, 229-230
  waist measurement and, 10
  in women, 2
Heart problems, dental care and, 18
Heart surgery, vitamins after, 80
Heat for injuries, 40
Heating costs, cutting, 186-187
Heatstroke, emergency care for, 61
Herbal tea, benefits of, 68-69
Herbs
  in avoiding cataract removal, 60
  in avoiding hip replacement, 60
  for insomnia, 36
  for phobias, 278

safety of, 69-70
stopping, before surgery, 34
Hiccups, acupressure for, 39
High blood pressure, ibuprofen and, 9
High-carbohydrate diet, 48
Hip replacement, alternatives to, 60-61
Hiring, improved, 289
HIV, home test for, 6
Home(s)
  avoiding dangers at, 251-253
  chimney care and, 256-257
  clutter control in, 260-261
  decorating hints for, 259-260
  do-it-yourself tips for, 259
  gain on the sale of, as tax-free income, 124
  getting maximum tax benefit from, 126-127
  increasing the value of, 261-263
  maintenance for, 254-256
  pricing, for sale, 264
  strategies for moving, 261
  weatherproofing, 257-258
Home energy audit, 186
Home equity loans
  in easing debt, 104
  as source of emergency money, 101
Home-health-care costs, paying for, 120
Home improvements as tax deduction, 131
Home insurance
  increased premiums for, 116-117
  lowering costs, by paying on time, 116
Home medical tests, 5-6
Home-office expenses, tax deduction for, 127, 299, 301
Homeowners' association, joining, 262
Home rental as tax-free income, 124
Home sale, tax-free gain on, 129
Home-security company, avoiding multiyear contracts with, 174
Honey in protecting against heart disease, 80
Hormone therapy
  alternatives to, 92
  for prostate cancer, 95
Hospital bills, checking, 182
Hospitals. *See also* Emergency room
  visiting patients in, 24
Hotels
  cheaper rates at, 226
  conversion of points to frequent-flier miles, 223
  fees at, 173
  free rooms at, for grandparents, 226
  getting discounts for the over age 50, 225-226
  lowest rates at, 228
  safety at, 226-227
Hot tubs, health risks for, 11
Housecleaning products, making your own, 176
Household care, as tax deduction, 130
Household chemicals, dangers of, 252-253
HRT, breast cancer risk and, 91-92
Human growth hormone, aging and, 14
Hunger, turning off, 45
Hypertension, link to rosacea, 10
Hyperthyroidism, signs of, in menstrual cycle, 93

340

Hypothermia, emergency care for, 61
Hypothyroidism, 14-15
  weight gain and, 47

I

Ibuprofen
  broken bones and, 17
  link to high blood pressure, 9
Ice for injuries, 40
Illness
  handling, after trip, 231
  during vacation, 230
Immune system, strengthening, 64-65
Immunoglobulin A, 53
Impotence
  exercise in protecting against, 89
  link between cardiovascular disease and, 90
Incentive stock options, job loss and, 306-307
Incentive trusts, 212
Income
  guaranteeing, for life, 196-197
  sources of tax-free, 124-125
Income taxes. *See also* Internal Revenue Service (IRS); Tax audits; Tax deductions
  avoiding underpayment penalties, 138-139
  avoiding underreporting penalties, 140
  deduction of education expenses, 317
  education credits on, 317
  electronic refund for, 141
  filing, 129
  on inheritance, 213
  paying, on installment plan, 140-141
  paying, with credit card, 140
  paying less, on social security benefits, 200-201
  reasons to file an amended return, 146-147
  rules of proof for charitable contributions, 213
  setting up foundation and, 208-210
  state interception of refund check, 141
  for unmarried couples, 134-136
Indigestion
  getting right diagnosis for, 24
  management of, 82
Indoor mold, 254
Infection, roundworm, 253
Infectious diseases, avoiding, 37-38
Inheritance
  income tax on, 213
  of IRA, 199
Injury
  avoiding, when working out, 51-52
  ice versus heat on, 40
Insomnia
  causes of, 35-36
  herbs versus drugs for, 70
  treatments for, 36
Insurance. *See also* Automobile insurance; Health insurance; Home insurance; Life insurance; Long-term-care insurance
  for college students, 319-320
  college-withdrawal, 319

  increasing deductibles on policies, 174
  vacation, 219
Interest-free loans, as tax-free income, 125
Internal Revenue Service (IRS). *See also* Income taxes; Tax audits
  handling accusations by, 141-142
  knowledge needed about tax audits, 143-144
  taking, to court, 148
Internet. *See also* E-mail; Web sites
  buying car insurance on, 249
  buying car on, 248-249
  choosing bank on, 103
  comparing available homes on, 264
  financing car on, 249
  getting best prices on, 179
  pharmacies on, 183
Internet service, selecting discount provider, 175
Interviews, improved hiring and, 289
Intuition, ignoring, in money management, 101-102
Inventory, tax credit for excess, 301
Inventory write-downs, 301-302
Investment loans as source of emergency money, 101
Investments for college, 318
IRA. *See also* Roth IRA
  converting regular to Roth, 198
  inheritance of, 199
  naming of beneficiaries through will, 212
  rolling 401(k) over to, 199
  withdrawals from versus 401(k) withdrawals, 199
Irritable bowel syndrome, management of, 82
Isoflavones for prostate cancer, 95

J

Jet lag, caffeine in fighting, 4-5
Job loss
  health and, 308
  making the most of, 306-307
Jobs and Growth Tax Relief Reconciliation Act of 2003, 121
Job search
  on-line résumés in, 310
  secrets for getting pass the receptionist, 310
Job sharing, 299
Joint ownership, property in, 213
Jukeboxes, collecting old, 241-242

K

Keogh plan, protecting against creditors, 200
Kidney stones, soy foods and, 83
Kitchen, redoing, 262-263
Kites, tips in flying, 239-240
Knee pain, ginger in easing, 81
Knee surgery for arthritis, 13

L

Las Vegas, VIP treatment in, 232
Lawn mowing, 258
Lawsuits, umbrella policies to protect against, 115

Layoff candidates, identifying, 293
LDL cholesterol. *See also* Cholesterol
  level of, 7-8
  trans fatty acids and, 9
Leaders, tips for being successful, 291-293
Leg cramps
  folk remedies for, 40
  nighttime relief from, 37
Life annuities, 211
Life insurance
  in funding bequests, 205
  group term, 297
  job loss and, 306
  maintaining adequate, 99-100
  missing policy, 115
  proceeds as tax-free income, 124-125
  reviewing, 113-115
Lifestyle changes in avoiding cataract removal, 59-60
Lifetime learning credit, 317
Lightbulbs, saving with, 187-188
Lighting
  decorating tips with, 260
  saving on, 186, 187-188
Light therapy for insomnia, 36
Like-kind exchanges as tax-free income, 125
Living trusts in providing for pets, 212
Living will, 205
Loans. *See also* Mortgage
  cosigning, 104
  debt-consolidation, 105
  government education, 318
  home equity, 101, 104
  interest-free, 125
  refinancing automobile, 105
Long-term-care insurance, 98, 195
  checking coverage, 120
  cutting costs in, 120
  tax breaks on, 143
  as tax-free income, 125
Low-glycemic foods, aging and, 72
L-tryptophan in promoting sleep, 36
Lycopene in tomatoes, 84
Lyme disease, test for, 16

M

Magnesium, benefits of, 50-51
Mail, receipt of bills by, 103
Mammography, 90
  improving accuracy in, 90-91
  in predicting stroke risk, 91
Marriage
  hope for unhappy, 266
  money fights and, 110-112
  retirement and, 198
Mattresses
  discounts on nonallergenic, 181
  time to buy new, 184
Meals, skipping, 44
Meat, dangers of undercooked, 252
Medical aids, as tax deduction, 130
Medical benefits, retirement and, 198
Medical bills
  cutting, 180-182
  getting government help in paying, 130-131
Medical costs, reducing, 182

341

Medical emergency, surviving, without doctor, 61-62
Medical history, need for family, 29-31
Medical insurance. *See also* Health insurance
Medical research, doing your own, 31-32
Medical tests, home, 5-6
Medical travel as tax deduction, 131
Medications. *See also* Pills; Prescriptions
 avoiding mistakes with, 25-26
 compassionate use programs for, 25
 cutting costs on, 183-184
 generic, 27, 28
 getting free, 181
 for heart disease, 7-8
 for insomnia, 36-37
 lowering cholesterol without, 78-79
 overdosing on, 26-27
 for phobias, 278
 for psoriasis, 16
 stocking up on, for vacation, 230-231
 switching, 27
 weight-loss, 48
Meetings, need for less, 288
Melanoma. *See also* Skin cancer
 common sites for, 16
Melatonin as sleep aid, 36, 84
Memoirs, writing your, 244
Memories, letting go of painful, 276-277
Men
 osteoporosis in, 2
 skin cancer in, 1-2
Menopause
 home test for, 6
 insomnia and, 35
Menstrual cycle, signs of hyperthyroidism in, 93
Mental abilities, improving, 285-286
Merchandise, easier returns, 179-180
Microwave, disinfecting sponges in, 259
Midlife, improving marriage and, 264-266
Migraines. *See also* Headaches
 bacteria and, 20-21
 herbs versus drugs for, 70
 medications for, 21
Misplacement of things, 286
Mistletoe extract (Iscar) in fighting cancer, 76
Molds
 in cars, 247-248
 indoor, 254
Money
 converting, to foreign currency, 219-220
 discussing, with children, 112
 fights over, in couples, 110-112
 getting, for emergencies, 100-101
 guide to saving, 173-175
 safety of, 109-110
 teaching grandchildren about, 112
 tips for saving, 176-177
Money management
 aging and, 107-109
 ignoring intuition in, 101-102
 in a volatile economy, 97-99
Mortgage
 checking escrow account and, 106
 handling buyout, 106-107
 money management and, 102

paying off, 109
prepaying, 126
refinancing, 105, 107
size of, 99
Mortgage broker, reasons for using, 105-106
Mosquito bites, folk remedies for, 40-41
Motion sickness
 folk remedies for, 40
 herbs versus drugs for, 70
Moving
 strategies for, 261
 tax deductions for expenses, 123
Moving company, hiring, 190
Municipal bonds, new tax law and, 122
Mutual funds, safety of money in, 109-110

N
Napkin rings, collecting silverplated figural, 241
Naturopathic physician, recommendations from, for staying healthy, 67
Negotiations
 on contracts, 310
 with integrity, 270
Networking, 306
 in job search, 308
 making time for, 294
Niacin in lowering cholesterol, 79
Nicotine as fat trigger, 44
911, calling in life-threatening emergencies, 23
Nonqualified stock options, job loss and, 307
Norwalk virus on cruises, 227
Nose filters for hay fever, 38
NSAIDs, broken bones and, 17
Numbness, getting right diagnosis for, 24
Nursing home
 expenses as tax deduction, 131
 paying for, 120

O
Oat bran in lowering cholesterol, 78
Olive oil
 aging and, 72
 in preventing cognitive decline, 73
Omega-3 foods, dietary benefits of, 63-64
On-line auctions, 178-179
On-line résumés, 310
Open house, holding, 263-264
Ophthalmologist, recommendations from, for staying healthy, 65
Orange juice as source of vitamin C, 84
Oregano oil as alternative to antibiotics, 70
Organic produce, pesticides and, 22
Osteoporosis
 in men, 2
 screening for, 17
Outplacement services, job loss and, 307
Ovarian cancer, carrots in combating, 90
Overseas ATMs, 220
Ovulation, home test for, 6

P
Pain
 getting right diagnosis for abdominal, 24
 getting right diagnosis for chest, 24

 herbs versus drugs for acute, 69
 knee, 81
 self-hypnosis in stopping, 76-78
 in women, 1
Panic attack, coping with, 278
Paralysis, getting right diagnosis for, 24
Parental-control credit cards, 320
Parties, feeling more comfortable at, 283
Pass-through entity, effect of new tax law on, 122
Peanut butter, healthier, 47
Pedometer, 53, 55
Pensions. *See also* Retirement
 lump-sum payout, 197
 mistakes with, 197-198
Perfectionist tendencies, controlling, 272
Personal gifts as source of emergency money, 100
Personality conflicts, resolving, at work, 289-290
Personal loans as source of emergency money, 100-101
Pesticides, organic produce and, 22
Pets. *See also* Cats; Dogs
 providing for, with living trusts, 212
 saving, via the Internet, 244
 toxocariasis in, 253
Pharmacoepidemiology and Drug Safety, 26-27
Phobias, cures for common, 277-278
Phone companies, fees at, 173
Physical exam, need for annual, 29
Physically active, staying, 285-286
Phytosterol in lowering cholesterol, 78
Pickup tax, 206
Pills. *See also* Medications; Prescriptions
 exercise in, 54
 hints for swallowing, 42
 splitting, 21
Plastic packaging, cutting, 251
Plumbing, maintenance of, 255
Poison ivy
 emergency care for, 61
 first aid for, 252
 preventing, 41
Postmenopausal women, breathing difficulties in, 93
Postnuptial agreement, 110
Potassium, food sources of, 84
Poultry, food safety and, 22
Power of attorney versus durable power of attorney, 216
Prepaid college tuition plans, 315
Prescriptions. *See also* Medications; Pills
 avoiding mistakes in, 26
 savings on, 182-183
 as tax deduction, 130
Prices, bargaining for best, 171-173
Priceline, learning how to bid at, 219
Problem solving, stress-free, 274
Produce, canned or fresh, 84
Prostate cancer. *See also* Cancer
 detecting, 96
 garlic in reducing risk, 95
 isoflavones for, 95
 surgery for, 94, 96
 therapies for, 93-95
Protein, aging and, 71
Provisional income, calculating, 200

342

Psoriasis, new medications for, 16
Psychiatrist, recommendations from, for staying healthy, 66

Q

Qualified personal residence trusts (QPRT), 135-136
Qualified terminable interest property (QTIP) trusts, 207-208
Qualified tuition programs, 136

R

Radiation therapy for prostate cancer, 94-95
Radios, collecting vintage, 240-241
Ramada Inns, senior discounts for, 226
Recreational vehicle interest deduction, 126
Reduced-fat foods, weight gain and, 46-47
Refrigerators, energy-efficient, 188
Relaxation exercises, 57
Rental cars
  avoiding rip-offs, 229
  fees at, 173
Renter's insurance for college students, 319
Restless legs syndrome, 36
Résumés, on-line, 310
Retail store, breaking items in, 177
Retirement. *See also* Pensions
  early withdrawals without penalty, 199
  financial needs in, 191-194
  getting married and, 198
  impact of financial mistakes on, 195-196
  location for, 191-192, 202
  lump-sum payout versus pension for life, 197
  medical benefits and, 198
  money strategies in, 109
  projecting income, 193
  working during, 192-193
Retirement plan
  contributions to, 137
  job loss and, 307
Retirement planning, tax-free, 298
Retirement savings
  catch-up provisions for, 108
  effect of new tax law on, 122
Reverse mortgage as tax-free income, 125
Road trips, preparing for, 229
Roof, maintenance of, 256
Roof gutters, buying right, 258
Rosacea, link to hypertension, 10
Rotator cuff strain, 52
Roth IRA. *See also* IRA
  converting regular IRA to, 198
  as tax-free income, 124
Rugs, decorating tips with, 260

S

Safety. *See also* Food safety; Security
  adventure travel and, 231
  at casinos, 237
  children in backseats of cars, 250
  of children in crowds, 286
  hotel, 226-227
  of money, 109-110
  whiplash protection and, 250
Safety recalls, 177
Salmon, aging and, 71-72

Salt, food cravings and, 46
Satellite dish, TV from, 176
Savings bonds for college, 316
Scholarships, 316, 318
  as tax-free income, 125
Screening for osteoporosis, 17
Seasonal tax return preparers, 145
Secondhand smoke, 12, 67
Second-home mortgage deduction, 126
Second opinions, HMO and, 119
Section 529 plan for college, 123, 203, 313, 315, 319, 320
  as tax-free income, 125
Security. *See also* Safety
  airport, 222
  company for home, 174
Selenium in boosting health, 64
Self-employed, effect of new tax law on, 122
Self-esteem, boosting, 282
Self-hypnosis in stopping pain, 76-78
Senior discounts, 192
  for hotels, 225-226
Septic system, maintenance of, 255
Serotonin
  food cravings and, 45
  mood and, 3
Severance pay, 306
Sewer, maintenance of, 255
Sex, aging and, 89
Sexual fitness, boosting, 85-87
Shin splints, 52
Shopping bargains, 177
  getting the best, 217-219
Sinus
  relief for, 19-20
  surgery for, 20
Sinusitis
  acute, 19
  chronic, 20
Skill-development workshops, 232
Skin cancer. *See also* Cancer; Melanoma
  in men, 1-2
Sleep, tips for getting and staying, 35-37
Sleep aid, cherries as, 84
Sleep apnea, 35
Slot machines
  collecting old, 241
  myths of, 236
Small-employer retirement plan start-up tax credit, 300
Smoking
  secondhand, 12, 67
  warning for women, 12
  weight gain and, 13
Snoring, injection snoreplasty for, 14
Social Security, retaining W-2s in confirming earnings, 202
Social Security benefits
  paying less tax on, 200-201
  as tax-free income, 124
Social Security integration, 198
Solo traveling, 231-232
Soy foods
  kidney stones and, 83
  in lowering cholesterol, 78-79
Spanish fly, for inhibited sexual desire, 88
Splinters, first aid for, 252
Spousal bypass trusts, 204

Sprains, emergency care for, 61
Sprinkle trusts, 205
Stafford Loan Program, 318
Stair climbing, 52-53
Static balance test in determining functional age, 70-71
Statins, uses of, 7-8
St. John's wort for depression, 69
Stock, limiting ownership in company, 108
Stock market, money management and, 102
Stock mutual funds, new tax law and, 122-123
Stock options, job loss and, 306-307
Stop-smoking programs as tax deduction, 130
Stress
  as cause of disability, 289
  getting more done with less, 272-274
  problem solving with less, 274
Stress management, tips for, 41-42
Strokes
  cutting risk of, 80-81
  flu vaccine in cutting risk, 12
  folate in lowering risk of, 81
  mammography in predicting risk, 91
  prevention of, 12
Student load interest, 316
Sunburn, folk remedies for, 40
Sunglasses, buying, 184-185
Surgery
  bloodless, 34
  bypass, 60
  fasting before, 34
  heart, 80
  heart bypass, 10, 11
  knee, for arthritis, 13
  for prostate cancer, 94, 96
  saving on cosmetic, 180
  sinus, 20
  stopping herbs before, 34
  tests prior to, 33
  for weight loss, 48
Sweepstakes, winning, 233-234
Swimmer's ear, folk remedies for, 40

T

Tax attorneys, 145
Tax audits. *See also* Internal Revenue Service (IRS)
  auto donation programs and, 142
  knowledge needed about, 143-144
Tax avoidance, secrets of, 143
Tax credits for business, 300
Tax deductions. *See also* Income taxes
  for alternative treatments, 130
  for business, 299-301
  for divorce costs, 134
  for education, 136, 317
  for health insurance premiums, 130
  for home-office expenses, 127, 299, 301
  for household care, 130
  for hybrid cars, 136
  for medical aids, 130
  for mortgage refinances, 107
  for moving expenses, 123
  for nursing home expenses, 131
  for prescriptions, 130
  for recreational vehicle interest, 126

343

for second-home mortgage, 126
for sweepstakes and contest
  winnings, 234
for weight-loss programs, 130, 132, 137
Taxes. *See also* Income taxes
  estate, 206
  pickup, 206
  state death, 206
  value-added, 218, 220
Tax-free gifts, exclusions for, 213-214
Tax-free income, sources of, 124-125
Tax-free retirement planning, 298
Tax-friendly states, 123
Tax law, profiting from new, 121-123
Tax planning for gamblers, 133-134
Tax professionals
  evaluating, 144-146
  penalties and, 147-148
Tax returns
  filing amended, 303
  Social Security number on, 138
Tea, benefits of herbal, 68-69
Teaching hospitals, saving at, 180
Telecommuting, 299
Telephone, paying less for long
  distance, 174
Term life insurance, 113
Theobromine, food cravings and, 46
Thyroid disease, 14-16
Tipping, guide to, 220
Tires
  blowouts, 246-247
  winter, 247
Tomatoes, lycopene in, 84
Trans fatty acids, problems with, 9
Travel. *See also* Air travel; Cruises;
  Vacations
    carrying whistle and, 225
    protecting health and, 229-230
    saving money on, 177
    saving on last-minute, 219
    tips for, 225
    warning and help for overseas,
      221-222
Travel agents, benefits of, 221
Travel-company bankruptcies, 228
Traveler's diarrhea, natural treatment
  for, 231
Trees, checking for problems, 254
Triage Cardiac System in predicting
  heart attacks, 10
Trusts
  funding foundation with, 210
  incentive, 212
  living, in providing for pets, 212
  Qualified terminable interest property
    (QTIP), 207-208
  spousal bypass, 204
  sprinkle, 205
  tax audits and, 142
Tuition payments, gifts of, 317
Tuition reimbursement as tax-free
  income, 125
Turmeric in fighting cancer, 76

Television
  extras in shows on, 243-244
  getting from satellite dish, 176
  minimizing time watching, 285

U

Ultrasound in healing broken bones, 16
Umbrella insurance, need for, to protect
  against lawsuits, 115
Unemployment compensation, 307
Uniform Transfers to Minors Act, 208
  in saving for college, 203
Unincorporated businesses, tax refunds
  for, 301
Universal life insurance, 114
Unmarried couples, income taxes for,
  134-136
Urinary tract infections, home test for, 6
Used automobiles, buying, 174, 175

V

Vacation homes, tax break for, 132-133
Vacation insurance, 219
Vacations. *See also* Air travel; Cruises;
  Travel
    getting sick on, 230
    safer adventure, 231
    saving money on, 174, 175
    solo, 231-232
    tax breaks for, 131-132
Vaccines
  booster shots for adults, 18
  flu, 12
Valerian for insomnia, 36
Variable universal life insurance, 114
Vegetables
  aging and, 72
  dietary benefits of, 63
VIP treatment in Las Vegas, 232
Viral illness, self-defense against on
  cruises, 227
Vitamin A, warning on, 17
Vitamin C
  in improving mental abilities, 286
  orange juice as source of, 84
Vitamin E
  effect on colds and flu, 19
  in improving mental abilities, 286
Vitamins, after heart surgery, 80
Vitamin supplements, in lowering
  stroke risk, 80-81

W

Waist, right measurement of, 10
Walking, fitness, 54
Washing machines, energy-efficient, 188
Water. *See also* Bottled water
  dangers from chemicals added to,
    255-256
  dietary benefits of, 64
  in protecting the heart, 79
Watermelon, dietary benefit from, 76
Wealth planning for blended families,
  207-208

Weatherproofing home, 257-258
Web sites. *See also* Internet
  creating, to boost business, 297
  health, 6-7
  in helping children choose college,
    313
  for making end-of-life
    decisions, 216
Weight gain
  hidden causes of, 47
  reduced-fat foods and, 46-47
  smoking and, 13
Weight loss
  breakfast and, 50
  caffeine in, 4
  drugs for, 48
  fat triggers and, 43-45
  food cravings and, 45-46
  secrets of, 47-48
Weight-loss programs, 47-48
  tax deductions for, 130, 132, 137
Whole-grain foods, dietary benefits
  of, 63
Whole life insurance, 113-114
  with secondary guarantees, 115
Wills, naming of IRA beneficiaries
  through, 212
Windows, decorating tips with, 260
Wine, consumption of, in preventing
  common cold, 83
Women
  colon cancer in, 2-3
  dangers of heart-bypass surgery
    for, 10
  heart disease in, 2
  pain in, 1
  screening for osteoporosis, 17
  warning for smoking, 12
Work
  controlling E-mail overload
    at, 294-295
  during retirement, 192-193
  rekindling creativity at, 283-284
  resolving personality conflicts at,
    289-290
Workouts
  caffeine in maximizing, 4
  no-exercise, 53
Wrinkle-cure diet, 71-72
Writing, college essays, 311-312
W-2s, retaining, in confirming earnings,
  202

Y

Yard sale, making money at, 261
Yeast infections, self-diagnosis of, 93
Yoga in avoiding hip
  replacement, 60

Z

Zoning rules, checking before buying
  house, 264